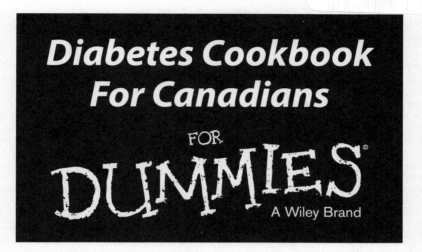

Diabetes Cookbook For Canadians

FOR DUMMIES®

A Wiley Brand

by Ian Blumer, MD, FRCPC
Cynthia Payne, RD, CDE

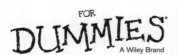

FOR DUMMIES®
A Wiley Brand

Diabetes Cookbook For Canadians For Dummies®

Published by
John Wiley & Sons, Inc.
111 River Street
Hoboken, NJ 07030

www.wiley.com

For general information on John Wiley & Sons, Inc., including all books published by John Wiley & Sons, Inc., please call our distribution centre at 1-800-567-4797. For reseller information, including discounts and premium sales, please call our sales department at 416-646-7992. For press review copies, author interviews, or other publicity information, please contact our publicity department, Tel. 416-646-4582, Fax 416-236-4448.

For technical support, please visit www.wiley.com/techsupport.

Wiley also publishes its books in a variety of electronic formats. Some content that appears in print may not be available in electronic books.

Library and Archives Canada Cataloguing in Publication Data

Blumer, Ian
        Diabetes cookbook for Canadians for dummies / Ian Blumer, Cynthia Payne.
Also available in electronic formats.
ISBN 978-1-119-01396-9 (pbk.)
ISBN 978-1-119-04552-6 (ebk); ISBN 978-1-119-04566-3 (ebk)
        1. Diabetes—Diet therapy—Recipes.
I. Payne, Cynthia II. Title.
RC662.B59 2010   616.4'620654   C2010-903847-9

Printed in the United States

2 3 4 5 15 14 13 12 11 10

Contents at a Glance

Recipes at a Glance

Appetizers

Potatoes, Rice, Pastas, Beans

Vegetable Side Dishes

Fish and Seafood Entrées

Chicken Entrées

Meat Entrées

Vegetarian Entrées

Table of Contents

Introduction

•••

*I*f you're living with diabetes (either because you have diabetes or you have a loved one with diabetes), you likely already know that one of the most important tools to help you keep your diabetes under control is to eat healthfully. Hopefully, you also know that healthy eating with diabetes doesn't mean you have to sacrifice taste, variety, or the simple, sheer pleasure of eating well.

We believe passionately that there is no such thing as a "diabetic diet." A so-called diabetic diet is simply a nutritious, healthy eating program that balances the appropriate amounts of the key nutrients and supplies the right amount of calories for your needs.

The recipes in *Diabetes Cookbook For Canadians For Dummies* are suitable for anyone who wants to eat healthfully, whether or not you have diabetes. The recipes are also suitable for low-fat diets and lower sodium diets as well.

On these pages you will discover a huge variety of recipes that will not only satisfy your hunger, but will do so in a nourishing way. Breakfasts, lunches, dinners, snacks, party foods, treats for kids, and treats for adults — it's all here.

And because staying healthy with diabetes is so very dependent on being empowered — the more you know, the more you can master your diabetes — we devote the first few chapters of this book to looking at key aspects of diabetes care, including the roles that nutrition, exercise, and medications can play.

About This Book

This book was written with a single overriding purpose: to help people living with diabetes prepare foods that are as tasty and enjoyable to eat as they are nutritious. We're also hoping that as you create the recipes in this book you'll find the time to read some (or even all) of Part I, where we examine all sorts of ways that you can use nutrition (and other strategies) to stay healthy with your diabetes.

The recipes in this book were chosen based on several guiding principles.

- Feature ingredients that are easy to find. (Cynthia lives in a small community and was able to readily find all the ingredients in stores in her town.)

- Emphasize healthy eating for a person living with diabetes — therefore, low sugar, lower fat, and lower sodium content were priorities — but they are appealing for *everyone*. If you don't have diabetes, no worries: You don't have to miss out on these recipes; you're going to love them, too!

  (We do use sugar in a number of this book's recipes. Sugar is not a "bad word" when it comes to diabetes, although, of course, you need to limit quantities.)

- Have met with glowing approval (yeah, we were tough on ourselves; *good* simply wasn't going to be good enough) by our diverse — and painfully honest — taste-testing panel of friends, neighbours, relatives, kids, and others.

- Reflect the wonderfully diverse nature of the Canadian population and the increasing desire of Canadians to try non-traditional foods.

- Are not only enjoyable to eat, but also enjoyable to prepare.

- ☺ Recipes are designated as vegetarian by using a little tomato icon.

We list the amount of carbohydrate in each recipe; this will help you as you balance out the nutrients in your diet and will be especially helpful if you're carbohydrate counting. (The recipes refer to "Carbohydrate Choices." Each Carbohydrate Choice consists of 15 grams of carbohydrate.) We also list the amount of sodium (avoiding excess sodium is important for everyone and especially important if you have high blood pressure), phosphorous, and potassium (avoiding excess phosphorous and potassium is important if you have kidney failure).

We'd love to hear from you. Whether it's to tell us you especially liked one of our recipes (please!) or, perish the thought, found some cooking instruction insufficiently clear, please do share your comments with us by sending an e-mail to diabetes@ianblumer.com. (We apologize in advance, however, for our being unable to provide medical advice.)

Foolish Assumptions

We have written this book based on the assumption that you are living with diabetes (either because you have diabetes yourself or because you have a loved one with diabetes) and that, whatever your knowledge of cooking, you want to learn more. Period.

If you know nothing about cooking, you'll find this book enables you to readily discover the basics, and if you're already a wizard in the kitchen, you'll discover additional recipes and food preparation ideas to meet your needs.

Icons Used in This Book

Icons act as little flags or identifiers — bookmarks, if you will — that let you know what information you're going to find in the paragraph that follows.

This icon signifies that we're sharing a story about a patient. These stories have been specifically selected because they contain elements that you may well relate to. (The names and other identifiers have been changed to maintain confidentiality.)

This icon lets you know we're recommending that you speak to a member of your health care team (be it your family physician, registered dietitian, diabetes specialist, and so forth), in order to get help.

This icon lets you know that we're about to drop some medical jargon on you. Don't be alarmed; we then define or explain the term before we move on.

When you see this icon, it means the information is essential and you would be well served to pay special attention.

This icon indicates that we're sharing a practical piece of information that will arm you with a time-saving or grief-avoiding measure.

This book is all about creating healthy, appealing recipes. It's also about living healthfully with diabetes. This icon means we're discussing a critical health issue that you shouldn't ignore.

Beyond the Book

In addition to the material in the print or e-book you're reading right now, this product also comes with some access-anywhere goodies on the web. Check out the free Cheat Sheet at www.dummies.com/cheatsheet/ diabetescookbookforcanadians for tips on how to eat healthy at home, or when you're out and about. You can also find links to several web-pages to help you with everything from calculating your BMI, to understanding how to read nutrition labels.

Where to Go from Here

We wrote *Diabetes Cookbook For Canadians For Dummies* in a format that allows you to open the book to any chapter and jump right in without feeling lost. So, if as you read this paragraph you realize it's 6:00 at night and you have to get dinner ready pronto, feel free to flip to Part III to find a recipe that suits your fancy. Same goes if you're looking for breakfast, lunch, or snack ideas. If, however, you're new to diabetes, and if you don't need to rush into the kitchen, sit back and spend some time familiarizing yourself with diabetes by reading some (or all) of Part I.

Whichever section of this book you first turn to, rest assured — there's no "wrong" place to start your reading.

Part I

Getting Started with Diabetes & Cooking

In this part . . .

Diabetes is far more than "just a sugar problem." Having diabetes means that you need to look after all of you, from your head down to your toes. In this part we explore how diabetes can affect you and what you can do to master diabetes and stay healthy.

Chapter 1

Diabetes 101: Discovering the Basics

*T*his is a cookbook with a twist.

This book begins not with recipes or a discussion on food handling or food shopping or the like, but rather starts right here, in Chapter 1, with a discussion on diabetes.

Beginning this book by talking about the basics of diabetes — Diabetes 101, if you will — is in keeping with the very special nature of diabetes. Diabetes is special in many ways, but none more so than this: If you're living with diabetes, the more you know about your diabetes and the more actively you are involved in your own health care, the more you can do to ensure you stay healthy.

Your diabetes therapy begins anew every day when you first get up and decide what you're going to eat. And your therapy continues all day with every morsel you put in your mouth. If you have diabetes it's not your doctor or nurse or dietitian or any other person who ultimately makes your nutrition choices; it is *you*.

Healthy eating affects diabetes in many different and crucial ways: The food choices you make will influence your blood glucose ("blood sugar"), your weight, your blood pressure, your cholesterol, your bowel habits, your sense of well-being, and much more. Indeed, we are routinely, absolutely, *blown away* by the dramatic improvement in the health of our patients with diabetes who carefully practise healthy eating.

In this chapter, we look at the different types of diabetes and we explore how to manage them. Because diabetes is (as we look at in a moment) a condition characterized by high blood glucose, we look in detail at blood glucose, how high (and low) levels can make you feel, and how you can control your blood glucose through nutrition, exercise, and medication. For most people with diabetes, a combination of these therapies works best in achieving and maintaining both good blood glucose control and good health in general.

This chapter is an overview of key elements of diabetes. For detailed information on the material we cover here, we unabashedly refer you to another book that Ian co-wrote: *Diabetes For Canadians For Dummies* (Wiley).

Examining the Types of Diabetes

Diabetes is a condition in which you have elevated *blood glucose* (blood sugar) either because you don't make enough insulin, or you make enough insulin but it doesn't work well, or, in some cases, both. *Glucose* is the type of sugar that the body uses as fuel to provide energy for metabolism, muscle action, and brain function. *Insulin,* a hormone made by the pancreas, works by acting on muscle and fat cells to allow them to extract glucose from the blood, and by acting on the liver to suppress its production of glucose. You could think of it as insulin grabbing onto the glucose and opening the door to take the glucose into the cells to be used for energy.

There are three main types of diabetes:

- ✔ Type 1 diabetes
- ✔ Type 2 diabetes
- ✔ Gestational diabetes

All three types of diabetes are, by definition, characterized by a tendency for having high blood glucose levels. With proper therapy, however, you can (and indeed, must) bring high blood glucose levels under control.

Type 1 diabetes used to go by two other names that, although outdated, you still may come across: *juvenile diabetes* and *insulin-dependent diabetes mellitus* (IDDM). Type 2 diabetes also used to go by two other names: *adult onset diabetes* and *non-insulin dependent diabetes mellitus* (NIDDM). These older names were abandoned because they led to confusion. For example,

---

Diabetes *insipidus:* The "other" form of diabetes

Although most people (including us in this book) talk about diabetes as if there were only one form, in fact there are actually two. Diabetes *mellitus* refers to the form of diabetes we discuss in this book: that is, the form of diabetes characterized by elevated blood glucose.

The other form, called diabetes *insipidus,* is an entirely different condition: an uncommon disease in which a problem with *antidiuretic hormone* puts you at risk of excess urine production and, as a result, dehydration.

---

type 1 diabetes frequently begins in adults (so it's not actually a "juvenile" condition) and people with non-insulin dependent diabetes frequently depend on insulin treatment. No wonder these old terms were abandoned!

Type 1 diabetes

Type 1 diabetes is an *autoimmune disease,* meaning that the body's immune system malfunctions and creates antibodies that target its own tissues. In the case of type 1 diabetes, the body makes antibodies that attack and destroy the insulin-producing *islet cells* in the pancreas. (More specifically, they attack one type of islet cell called a *beta cell.*)

These are some important things to know about type 1 diabetes:

- ✔ It most commonly develops in adolescents, but also often occurs in young children and young adults. (Increasing scientific evidence suggests that, in fact, in most cases the first onset is in adults.)

- ✔ Symptoms typically appear soon after the condition first develops. (We discuss these symptoms later in this chapter.)

- ✔ It is far less common than type 2 diabetes. Type 1 diabetes accounts for between 5 and 10 percent of all cases of diabetes.

- ✔ Urgent treatment with insulin is required as soon as this condition is discovered; delaying therapy can be life-threatening.

Type 2 diabetes

Type 2 diabetes is caused by a combination of the body's insulin not working as effectively as it should (a condition called *insulin resistance*) and the pancreas making insufficient quantities of insulin.

These are some important things to know about type 2 diabetes:

✔ It most commonly occurs in middle-aged or older individuals, most of whom are overweight and sedentary. (However, many people with type 2 diabetes don't fit this mould.)

✔ It is often preceded by years of *prediabetes,* a condition in which blood glucose levels are higher than normal but not high enough to make a diagnosis of diabetes.

✔ It is far more common than type 1 diabetes. Type 2 diabetes accounts for between 90 and 95 percent of all cases of diabetes.

✔ The most important component of therapy is lifestyle, including healthy eating, exercise, and weight control.

Gestational diabetes

Gestational diabetes (GDM) is a temporary form of diabetes that, by definition, occurs only during pregnancy. It develops in anywhere from 4 to 18 percent of pregnancies depending on what criteria are used to make the diagnosis (there are two different sets of criteria in use, each with its pros and cons), and is routinely tested for at about the midway point of a pregnancy. As in the other types of diabetes, women with gestational diabetes have a tendency toward elevated blood glucose levels that, with proper therapy, can be kept under control.

Gestational diabetes does not harm or risk harming the affected woman, per se. Its importance lies in its potential impact on the developing fetus. If the diabetes is insufficiently treated, the fetus can become overly large, which can make delivery difficult. Also, after delivery, the newborn often has low blood glucose. (Medical staff routinely test for this in a baby born to a woman with gestational diabetes.) Low blood glucose in the newborn is not serious and is easy to treat by giving the baby sugar water to drink. Other complications from gestational diabetes seldom occur.

Gestational diabetes is treated by following a special nutrition program (as we discuss in Chapter 4). Regular exercise also helps. If despite these measures the woman's blood glucose levels remain elevated, insulin therapy is typically used. Because of limited scientific evidence regarding their use in pregnancy, oral hypoglycemic agents (see "Taking Oral Medications to Help Control Your Blood Glucose" later in this chapter) are seldom used. This may change in the future.

If you've had gestational diabetes, it means you're at high risk of later developing type 2 diabetes so it's essential that you follow a very healthy lifestyle after the delivery and that your doctor test your blood glucose levels from time to time thereafter. This testing includes both a glucose tolerance test within a few months of your delivery and a measurement of your fasting blood glucose from time to time.

If you've had gestational diabetes, get your blood glucose level checked before trying to conceive again; that way, if you've developed type 2 diabetes it can be brought under control before you get pregnant. Uncontrolled diabetes present at the time of conception and during early pregnancy is very dangerous as it can damage the fetus's developing organs.

Investigating How Diabetes Is Diagnosed

Diabetes — in any form — is a serious disease and, befitting this, is diagnosed according to strict criteria. According to the Canadian Diabetes Association's criteria, you have diabetes if you have any one of the following:

- A **random** blood glucose level equal to or greater than 11.1 millimoles per litre (mmol/L). *Random* is defined as any time of day or night, without regard to how long it's been since the last time you ingested anything containing calories.

- A **fasting** blood glucose level equal to or greater than 7.0 mmol/L. Fasting is defined as eight or more hours without calorie intake.

- A blood glucose level equal to or greater than 11.1 mmol/L, when tested two hours after ingesting 75 grams of glucose as part of what is called a **glucose tolerance test.**

- An **A1C** level equal to or greater than 6.5 percent. The **A1C** is measured on a blood test and allows for an estimate of one's average blood glucose level for the preceding three months. The **A1C** should not be used as a diagnostic test for diabetes if you are a child, an adolescent, are pregnant, if type 1 diabetes is suspected, or if you have a condition which can affect its accuracy.

Testing positive for one of the preceding criteria on a single occasion is not enough to make a diagnosis of diabetes (although important exceptions exist, which we discuss next). Any one of the tests must be also be positive on another day to establish the diagnosis. Also, the diagnosis of diabetes should be based on a blood sample taken *from a vein* and *analyzed at a laboratory;* the diagnosis should *not* be made based on a blood glucose level measured with a blood glucose meter.

Waiting for another day to have a second test performed after having an initial high blood glucose discovered is *not* required — and indeed, can be dangerous in two circumstances:

✔ If your initial blood glucose level is 11.1 mmol/L or higher *and* you have symptoms of high blood glucose (frequent urination, increased thirst, loss of weight)

✔ If your doctor thinks you may have type 1 diabetes (especially if you are a child)

In either of these circumstances, the diagnosis of diabetes is made without a second test, and you need to start treatment *immediately*.

Looking at Target Blood Glucose Levels

You can drastically reduce your risk of developing many types of diabetes complications by keeping your blood glucose levels in check. The Canadian Diabetes Association (CDA) has established these target blood glucose levels for most adults living with diabetes:

✔ Blood glucose before meals: 4.0 to 7.0 mmol/L

✔ Blood glucose two hours after meals: 5.0 to 10.0 mmol/L (5.0 to 8.0 if your **A1C** is above 7.0)

The **A1C** is an important test to determine whether your blood glucose control is where it should be. The **A1C**, which is performed on a blood sample taken from a vein in your arm at the lab, and should be done about every three months or so, reflects your overall blood glucose levels over the preceding several months. It uses a different scale from the usual blood glucose test, and the target value is 7 percent or less for most adults with diabetes.

Although the preceding blood glucose targets are appropriate for the great majority of adults, targets differ for elderly infirm or frail individuals, and for people with a limited life expectancy. In these circumstances targets are:

✔ Blood glucose before meals: 5.0 to 12.0 mmol/L.

✔ **A1C** up to 8.5 percent.

You can learn more about the **A1C** on Ian's website (www.ourdiabetes. com/key-definitions.htm).

Although you should strive to achieve CDA target blood glucose (and **A1C**) levels, it is important to be aware that *nobody* with diabetes has every single blood glucose reading within target; that is virtually impossible. It's also unnecessary. If you can keep the majority of your blood glucose readings within target, you'll be at low risk of developing most complications.

Understanding How High and Low Blood Glucose Can Make You Feel

Having diabetes means that you will be prone to higher than normal blood glucose levels. Popular wisdom to the contrary, diabetes does not, in fact, cause *low* blood glucose; rather, it is certain drugs used *to treat* diabetes that sometimes leads to this. In this section, we look at how high or low blood glucose levels can make you feel.

High blood glucose

High blood glucose is not an "all or none," yes or no kind of thing. Rather, elevated blood glucose levels run a continuum ranging from only slightly higher than normal to up into the stratosphere. A person without diabetes seldom has blood glucose levels higher than 8 mmol/L or so, and symptoms of high blood glucose develop only if blood glucose is higher than 10 mmol/L or so.

Looking at the symptoms of high blood glucose

These are the most common symptoms of high blood glucose:

- Frequent urination
- Increased thirst
- Blurred vision
- Fatigue
- Hunger
- Weight loss
- Persistent vaginal infections

Not everyone with high blood glucose experiences all these symptoms. Indeed, many people have only one or two of these symptoms and some people have none at all. Also, the severity of the symptoms can vary widely.

Some people have profound thirst, are running to the bathroom 24/7, and lose many pounds, whereas other people feel slightly tired and that's it.

The fact that symptoms can be minimal or nonexistent partly explains why so many people with diabetes don't know they have it. After all, if you feel perfectly fine it only makes sense you won't suspect you've got a problem and thus won't be knocking on your doctor's door to get checked out.

Because people can have diabetes yet feel perfectly well and therefore not know they have the condition, the Canadian Diabetes Association recommends all people 40 years of age or over be tested periodically for diabetes. You should have the test sooner if you have an increased risk of diabetes (for example, if you have a parent with type 2 diabetes).

Considering the complications of high blood glucose

Having high blood glucose can do two main things: It can cause symptoms like those we discuss in the previous section, and, if severe or if longstanding, it can damage the body.

If you have very high blood glucose levels (more than 15 to 20 mmol/L or so) and you are feeling very unwell, then this may be an emergency and you should seek immediate medical attention.

If your blood glucose levels exceed target year after year, you will be at risk of a number of different types of complications. But if you keep most of your blood glucose levels within target you can dramatically reduce your risk of running into problems. In other words, diabetes complications are not inevitable!

Chronically elevated blood glucose levels can lead to complications like these:

- Eye damage *(retinopathy),* which, if severe, can lead to blindness
- Kidney damage *(nephropathy),* which, if severe, can lead to kidney failure and the need for dialysis
- Nerve damage *(neuropathy),* including abnormal or loss of sensation in the feet, which can be a factor leading to amputation

The role of high blood glucose in causing heart attacks and strokes is more complicated, but it likely plays an important role. Your risk of a heart attack or stroke is much higher if you are overweight, sedentary, smoke, have inadequately controlled high blood pressure, or if you have elevated LDL cholesterol. See a common denominator? We do. These are all things that, working with your diabetes team, you can control! In Chapter 4, we look at the ways healthy eating can help you control your blood pressure and your cholesterol.

Low blood glucose

Low blood glucose *(hypoglycemia)* is defined as a blood glucose level below 4.0 mmol/L. As we mention earlier in this chapter, diabetes, per se, does not cause low blood glucose; rather, it is certain drugs — such as insulin or glyburide — used to treat diabetes that can lead to this condition.

Looking at the symptoms of low blood glucose

These are the common symptoms of low blood glucose:

- ✔ Anxiety
- ✔ Hunger
- ✔ Sweating
- ✔ Palpitations (noticing a rapid or excessively forceful heartbeat)
- ✔ Trembling of the hands

If hypoglycemia is severe, it can lead to other symptoms, including confusion, difficulty concentrating, difficulty speaking, and even loss of consciousness. Fortunately, the great majority of the time when people with diabetes experience hypoglycemia they will quickly recognize its symptoms and ingest some sugar-containing food, which will quickly bring their blood glucose level back to normal.

Treating low blood glucose

If ever you have low blood glucose, you need to treat it quickly in order to return your blood glucose to a safe level.

As recommended by the Canadian Diabetes Association, these are the steps you should take if you have low blood glucose:

1. **Eat or drink 15 grams of a fast-acting carbohydrate** such as

    - Four 4-gram glucose tablets (for example, Dex4 tablets; this totals 16 grams)

    - ¾ cup (175 ml) of juice or regular (not diet or sugar-free) pop (but see the warning following this list)

    - 3 tsp (15 ml) honey or maple syrup; or 3 tsp (15 ml) of table sugar dissolved in water

    - Seven jelly beans

2. **Wait 15 minutes, and then retest your blood.**

    If your blood glucose level is still less than 4 mmol/L, ingest another 15 grams of fast-acting carbohydrate (as listed in the previous step).

3. **If your next meal is more than one hour away, or you are going to be physically active, eat a snack, such as half a sandwich or cheese and crackers.**

   The snack should contain 15 grams of carbohydrate and a source of protein.

If you have low blood glucose and you're about to eat a meal, you must *instead* first treat your hypoglycemia with the measures we just described. Only when your blood glucose is back to normal (above 4 mmol/L) should you then eat your meal.

Controlling Your Blood Glucose through Nutrition

Not a day goes by when we aren't totally blown away by the tremendous power that healthy eating has on helping improve blood glucose control. Indeed, nutrition therapy can reduce your **A1C** up to 2 percent (which is far greater than most drugs ever achieve). Nutrition is so vital in the management of diabetes that we felt it deserved an entire cookbook devoted to the topic. That would be this book.

When coupled with regular exercise and weight control, the impact of healthy eating is all the greater.

Achieving better health — and needing fewer pills — through the magic of lifestyle therapy

Martha was a very overweight, sedentary 55-year-old woman who had been living with type 2 diabetes for five years. She was taking three different types of medicine per day — totalling more than ten pills — to control her blood glucose. One day, after witnessing her grandson's look of alarm as he saw her swallowing a fistful of pills, she decided there had to be a better way of managing her health. Working with a dietitian and her local YMCA,

she adopted healthy eating strategies, began regularly exercising, and progressively shed weight. With each passing day her health improved, and within a year she was able, under Ian's guidance, to reduce the number of her pills from ten down to two.

"I'm going to soon not need these last two," she said as she left her doctor's appointment. "I bet you're right," Ian said to her as she left.

As we discuss in detail in Chapter 2, there are three basic types of nutrients: carbohydrates ("sugars"), proteins, and fats. Each of these has important roles in healthy eating, but when it comes to blood glucose control it is carbohydrates that have the key role. We look at carbohydrates next.

Watching your carbohydrate intake

Carbohydrates are found primarily in those foods that are grown in the ground (such as rice, potatoes, grains, and fruits), and in dairy products. They provide energy for your body; when consumed in excess of your needs, this extra energy is stored as fat. Also, the carbohydrates you eat are responsible for raising your blood glucose levels. For these reasons, you need to make sure you're eating the appropriate amount of carbohydrate; consuming too much or too little is unhealthy.

The Canadian Diabetes Association recommends that between 45 to 60 percent of the calories you consume come from carbohydrates, the remainder being divided up between protein (15 to 20 percent) and fat (20 to 35 percent).

Not all carbohydrates have the same impact on blood glucose. Carbohydrates that are especially likely to raise blood glucose are said to have a high *glycemic index* and, as you might expect, those that that don't raise blood glucose levels as much are said to have a low glycemic index. We discuss the glycemic index in detail in Chapter 4. Also, fibre, which is a form of carbohydrate, doesn't raise blood glucose at all.

When discussing meal plans, we often refer to "Carbohydrate Choices." One Carbohydrate Choice is equivalent to 15 grams of carbohydrate (excluding fibre). Knowing about Carbohydrate Choices will allow you to map out a meal plan that contains the appropriate amount of carbohydrates. Your dietitian is the best person to teach you about Carbohydrate Choices and how to incorporate them into your nutrition program. (Each recipe in *Diabetes Cookbook For Canadians For Dummies* — wow, that's a mouthful of a title! — has the number of Carbohydrate Choices in a serving.)

Timing when you eat

Having diabetes, you should eat three square meals a day rather than engaging in that popular and ill-advised Canadian pastime of eating almost nothing all day, getting home ravenous after a long day's work and chowing down on a big supper, and then grazing at the fridge and pantry the rest of the night.

The goal is to not go longer than six hours between meals during waking hours. If your next meal is going to be longer than six hours from your last one, have a snack to hold you over until meal-time comes around.

Consuming a small mid-morning and mid-afternoon carbohydrate-containing snack may, depending on your specific situation, also be helpful in maintaining good blood glucose control. See the next section for more information on scheduling your meals.

Getting nutritional assistance: How a dietitian can help

If you have diabetes, you need to obtain the expert advice of a registered dietitian. The designation "registered" means that the dietitian has completed a special program of training and has achieved official certification establishing his or her credentials. Many registered dietitians, like Cynthia, have also trained as certified diabetes educators, in which case they have the initials RD, CDE after their names.

A dietitian can assist you in many ways, including helping you

- Learn the ins and outs of healthy eating in general and healthy eating when you have diabetes in particular.

- Balance the amounts of carbohydrates, proteins, and fats in your diet.

- Master carbohydrate counting. (We discuss carbohydrate counting later in this section.)

- Figure out how to read food labels.

- Know what snacks to eat, when to eat them, and how often to eat them.

- Effectively use nutrition therapy to improve your blood glucose control, your blood pressure, and your lipids, including cholesterol and triglycerides. (See Chapter 4 for information about lipids.)

- Determine how to get the appropriate amounts of vitamins and minerals in your diet and, when necessary, what supplements of these nutrients you should take.

- Develop a meal plan that takes into account your particular food preferences as well as any food needs (or restrictions) related to religious, cultural, ethnic, or other factors.

- Calculate how many calories you need to consume to lose weight, maintain a steady weight, or, when necessary, gain weight; and how best to adjust your diet in order to achieve whatever weight change you require (if any).

✔ Adjust your diet to accommodate your exercise program, travel schedule, sleeping in, shift work, and other factors.

✔ Find great recipes; indeed some dietitians are so expert at cooking they even co-write entire books on this subject . . . like this book!

A good dietitian will not ask you to follow a regimented, unrealistic, unpleasant diet. A good dietitian will help you find a culturally appropriate, tasty, interesting, nutritious, and varied eating program. Not happy with the diet you've been asked to follow? Let your dietitian know; he or she'll be glad to have the opportunity to modify your diet to better suit your needs.

Finding a registered dietitian

These are a few ways you can find a registered dietitian to assist you:

✔ **Call your local diabetes education centre (DEC).** Most diabetes education centres allow self-referral, but if the one local to you doesn't, then ask your doctor to refer you. The cost of the services provided by dietitians working out of a DEC are typically covered by the hospital or other health care facility where they are located, so you will not have to pay.

✔ **Contact a private registered dietitian.** You can find the name of a registered dietitian local to you in your phone book or online at http://dietitians.ca. Also your doctor can likely recommend one to you. Remember, it is a *registered* dietitian you want to see. Expect to pay a charge for the services provided by a private dietitian; however, if you have private insurance, your insurer may cover some or all of these costs.

✔ **If your family physician works in a clinic setting, ask whether the clinic has a registered dietitian on staff.** If so, you can book an appointment to see that clinic's dietitian.

Exercise and Blood Glucose

Exercise has a powerful effect in controlling blood glucose. Indeed, if you've been sedentary and your blood glucose control hasn't been very good, you'll likely find yourself very impressed by how much your newfound exercise program helps bring your blood glucose down. This effect is made all the greater when coupled with nutrition therapy and weight loss. (Exercise also helps control blood pressure and cholesterol, lowers the risk of heart disease, and makes one feel generally better. Not too shabby, eh?)

Cardiovascular (cardio) exercise causes your muscles to use oxygen and your heart to speed up and beat more forcefully. As the name suggests, cardiovascular exercise works — and benefits — the heart (hence the term *cardio*) and circulation *(vascular)*. Examples of cardiovascular exercise are walking, running, and skating.

The Canadian Diabetes Association recommends you perform cardiovascular exercise for *at least* 150 minutes per week, spreading it out over a minimum of three days of the week. Also, you should avoid going more than two days in a row without performing cardiovascular exercise.

Resistance exercise uses muscular strength to move a weight or to work against a resistance. If you lift weights or exercise with weight machines, you're performing resistance exercise. This type of exercise improves muscle strength and, as shown by pioneering Canadian research undertaken by Dr. Ron Sigal, also helps control blood glucose levels.

The Canadian Diabetes Association recommends that you perform resistance training at least two times per week (and preferably three times per week), starting with one set of 10 to 15 repetitions using a moderate weight, and gradually progressing toward a goal of three sets of eight repetitions three times per week using a heavier weight.

Before you take up a new exercise program, be sure to first speak to your physician. He or she will need to ensure you are sufficiently healthy to perform the activity. Also, exercise can affect your blood glucose levels both while you're performing the activity *and afterward,* so you'll need to keep a close eye on them to see how they respond to your activities. Be sure to keep a fast-acting carbohydrate (as we discuss earlier) with you in case you develop hypoglycemia during or after your exercise.

Taking Oral Medications to Help Control Your Blood Glucose

If you have type 2 diabetes, taking oral medication or insulin to control your blood glucose should always be considered complementary to lifestyle therapy (including healthy eating, regular exercise, and weight control).

These are the classes of oral medications (and the generic names of the drugs within the classes) used to control blood glucose in people living with type 2 diabetes:

- *Alpha-glucosidase inhibitors* (acarbose) work by slowing down the rate of absorption of glucose into the body from the intestine.
- *Biguanides* (metformin) lower blood glucose primarily by reducing how much glucose the liver makes.
- *DPP-4 inhibitors* (linagliptin, sitagliptin, saxagliptin) work by reducing how much glucose the liver makes and by stimulating the pancreas to make more insulin.
- *Meglitinides* (repaglinide, nateglinide) work by stimulating the pancreas to make more insulin.
- *Sulfonylureas* (gliclazide, glimepiride, glyburide) work by stimulating the pancreas to make more insulin.
- *SGLT-2 inhibitors* (canaglifozin) work by allowing greater amounts of glucose to pass through the kidneys and be excreted from the body in the urine.
- *Thiazolidinediones* (pioglitazone, rosiglitazone) work primarily by helping glucose move from the blood into fat and muscle cells.

Of the various oral medications available, metformin is the preferred initial drug for most people.

GLP-1 analogues (exenatide, liraglutide) have similar properties to DPP-4 inhibitors, but have the additional benefit of facilitating weight loss. GLP-1 analogues, however, are given by injection; they are not taken orally.

Using Insulin to Help Control Your Blood Glucose

As many Canadians know — and proudly declare — insulin was discovered in Canada. (Want to learn more about the amazing story behind the discovery of insulin? We highly recommend reading the superb book *The Discovery of Insulin,* by Michael Bliss, University of Chicago Press.)

All people with type 1 diabetes require insulin therapy from the time of diagnosis. Many people with type 2 diabetes, given a sufficiently long time living with the condition, will also require insulin therapy because the pancreas in a person with type 2 diabetes gradually loses its ability to make insulin.

Insulin is given by a painless injection with a tiny needle into the abdominal wall, arms, legs, or buttocks. It is most easily administered using a pen device. Pens are small, convenient, portable, and available for free from pharmacies and diabetes education centres.

Looking at the types of insulin

A variety of different types of insulin therapy are available, each with its own specific properties. Combinations of different types of insulin are also available.

The various insulins can be grouped into three main categories:

- *Rapid-acting* and *short-acting* insulins are given before meals and prevent the carbohydrates you ingest from making your blood glucose levels rise excessively. The trade names for the available rapid-acting insulins are Apidra, Humalog, and NovoRapid.

- *Intermediate* and *long-acting* insulins are given to prevent your blood glucose level from rising too high between meals and, especially, overnight. The only intermediate-acting insulin used in Canada is called NPH. The trade names for the available long-acting insulins are Lantus and Levemir. Lantus and Levemir have a main advantage over NPH insulin in that they are far less likely to cause hypoglycemia.

- *Premixed* insulins are mixtures of both rapid-acting (or short-acting) insulin with intermediate-acting insulin and, as such, act to control both between-meal and after-meal blood glucose levels. Premixed insulins are typically given before breakfast and before dinner.

Using insulin and nutrition together: A recipe for success

Used individually, insulin and nutrition therapies are very helpful in keeping blood glucose levels in control. Used together they provide a simply awesome one-two punch.

The key element to achieving success with insulin therapy is to give the right amount of insulin to match your body's needs. Your body's needs will depend on many factors including, importantly, the types and amounts of food you eat, and the types and amounts of exercise you do.

Of the various types of foods you eat (and liquids you drink), the *carbohydrates* influence your blood glucose levels and insulin requirements the most. In general, the more carbohydrates you ingest, the more your blood glucose level will potentially go up and thus the more insulin you need to take to prevent this from happening. (The main exception to this is if you're eating carbohydrates in the form of fibre; fibre does not make blood glucose levels go up.)

If everything else in your life is stable (exercise, stress, general health, and so forth), and if you ingest a very similar amount of carbohydrate day-to-day, then you will likely find the amount of insulin you need to take to keep your blood glucose levels in check will be quite consistent. If, however, the amount of carbohydrate you eat (both in terms of types and quantities) varies quite a bit, then you will need to regularly adjust your insulin dose to match your intake. The best way to do this is to use a technique called *carbohydrate counting*. We look at this topic next.

Carbohydrate counting

Carbohydrate counting involves calculating how many grams of carbohydrate ("carbs") — excluding fibre — you are about to eat and giving an amount of rapid-acting insulin proportionate to this. For most people, the formula works out to about one unit of insulin for every 10 grams of carbohydrate. For example, if you are about to eat a meal that contains 50 grams of carbohydrate (again, fibre isn't included in the calculation), you would need to give yourself five units of insulin.

The other key factor in determining how much rapid-acting insulin you require before a meal is your blood glucose level before the meal. If your blood glucose level is high before your meal, you'll need to take extra insulin to bring it down. This extra insulin is called a *correction factor* or *sensitivity factor* and is usually about one unit of insulin for every 3 mmol/L your blood glucose level is above 7 or so.

Carbohydrate counting isn't rocket science, but it isn't easy either. To master carbohydrate counting requires quite a bit of guidance from a skilled dietitian. And even when you've learned the ropes, periodic visits to the dietitian to reinforce the skills you've learned are a good idea.

Using carb counting and a correction factor

Here's an example of how to use carb counting and a correction factor.

Let's say you're about to eat a dinner that has 70 grams of carbohydrate (including 10 grams of fibre) and your before-meal blood glucose level is 13 mmol/L. You are, say, using a carbohydrate counting ratio of 1 unit of insulin per 10 grams of carbohydrate and a correction factor of 1 unit of insulin per 3 mmol/L your blood glucose level is above 7.

You will be eating 70 grams of carbohydrate but you exclude the 10 grams of fibre you'll be eating from your calculations because the fibre doesn't raise blood glucose. (The amount of fibre in a product is listed on the Nutrition Facts table.) Therefore, 70 grams of carbohydrate minus 10 grams of fibre leaves you with 60 grams of carbohydrate to use for your remaining calculations.

Because you're now dealing with 60 grams of carbohydrate and you take one unit of insulin per 10 grams, that would mean you need six units of insulin to "cover" the food you're about to eat.

Because your blood glucose is 13 mmol/L and you need to take an extra one unit for each 3 mmol/L above 7, you need to take an extra two units of insulin to "correct" the elevated blood glucose level.

You add the six units (from your carb counting) and the two units (from your correction factor), and thus you'd take a total of eight units of insulin.

In the accompanying sidebar ("Using carb counting and a correction factor"), we give an example of how to effectively use carbohydrate counting and a correction factor.

Even if you aren't taking insulin, being familiar with the number of grams of carbohydrates in the foods you eat is helpful. This will help you stay on track with making sure you get the proper quantities of carbohydrates in your diet and that you maintain balance between the amount of carbohydrates, proteins, and fats you consume.

Fibre is a carbohydrate that doesn't influence blood glucose. In the recipes in this book, we note the *available carbohydrate*, which is the total carbohydrate minus the fibre. This is the carbohydrate amount you need to keep track of.

Chapter 2

You Are What You Eat

Doctors seem to have an obsession with analogies to food. When describing certain diseases, doctors talk about nutmeg liver, strawberry tongue, and cauliflower ear; and when it comes to the risk of diabetes, whether you are pear-shaped (meaning your body is fuller around your buttocks, hips, and thighs) or apple-shaped (meaning being round around the middle). Being apple-shaped increases your risk of acquiring type 2 diabetes.

Eating healthfully is, pardon the pun, an essential ingredient to maintaining good health in general, and controlling diabetes in particular. Indeed, we can think of no better example of the phrase "You are what you eat." How important is it to fuel your body with healthy nutrients if you have diabetes? Oh, no more important than having oxygen in the air that you breathe.

In this chapter, we look at how your food choices can help you manage your diabetes and keep you healthy. In particular we consider how your nutrition plan can help you

✔ Keep your blood glucose levels under control

✔ Lower your blood pressure

✔ Improve your cholesterol and triglyceride levels (that is, your *lipids*)

✔ Achieve and maintain a healthy weight

The recipes in this book were created with the preceding factors in mind; that is, the recipes provide healthy food choices that are geared toward assisting you in your quest to control not just your blood glucose levels but your blood pressure, your lipids, and your weight also.

What Is a "Diabetic Diet"?

This could be the shortest section in this entire book because, truth be told, we don't believe a "diabetic diet" exists, and certainly not in a restrictive or limiting sense. Indeed, virtually *any* food can be accommodated if you have diabetes. A "diabetic diet" really means a well-balanced, nutritious, healthy eating program.

Because the word "diet" often conjures up so many negative connotations — crash diets, fad diets, failed diets, and so on — all replete with frustration and aggravation, we're hesitant to even use the word. (Perhaps it's no coincidence that *diet* is a four-letter word!) Our preferred term for a "diet" is "meal planning" or simply "healthy eating." When we refer to a "diet" in this book it is this healthy eating strategy we're referring to.

The Canadian Diabetes Association (CDA) recommends — as do we — that people with diabetes follow *Eating Well with Canada's Food Guide* (which you can find online at www.healthcanada.gc.ca/foodguide, or in an abbreviated form in the colour insert of this book). Health Canada created this guide (typically referred to in its short form: Canada's Food Guide) to help Canadians plan meals based on choosing appropriate amounts of food from the various food groups.

Canada's Food Guide offers these sensible eating tips:

- Enjoy a variety of foods from the four food groups (vegetables and fruit, grain products, milk and alternatives, and meat and alternatives).
- Emphasize vegetables, fruits, and cereals, breads, and other whole-grain products.
- Choose lower-fat dairy products, leaner meats, and food prepared with little or no fat.
- Achieve and maintain a healthy body weight by enjoying regular physical activity and healthy eating.
- Limit salt, alcohol, and caffeine.

We look more closely at the recommendations in Canada's Food Guide later in this chapter (see "Eating Well with Canada's Food Guide").

In addition to general healthy eating principles as discussed in this chapter, you can undertake several other CDA-approved strategies to enhance your health.

✔ **The Mediterranean diet** can improve blood glucose control and lower the risk for cardiovascular disease. The Mediterranean diet emphasizes consuming olive oil, legumes, unrefined cereals, fruits, vegetables, nuts, seeds, dairy products, and fish. Meat is consumed in only small amounts.

✔ **A vegan or vegetarian diet** can improve blood glucose control and lipid levels. (Though definitions vary, generally speaking a vegan diet excludes all animal products, including dairy products, and a vegetarian diet excludes meat, fish and poultry, but includes dairy products such as cheese, eggs, yogurt, or milk.)

✔ **A DASH ("Dietary Approaches to Stop Hypertension") diet** can lower blood pressure, improve blood glucose control, and lower the risk for cardiovascular disease. The DASH diet emphasizes fruits, vegetables, fat-free or low-fat dairy products, whole grains, fish, poultry, fibre, and nuts, and avoids saturated fats, cholesterol, and red meats.

The CDA also notes that diets high in "dietary pulses" (examples of dietary pulses are beans, peas, chickpeas, and lentils) can be consumed to improve blood glucose and lipid levels.

In order for you to succeed with your diabetes nutrition plans, you must know what to eat. This chapter provides helpful information, but nothing replaces the guidance that a registered dietitian provides. If you haven't seen one, you're missing out and we would strongly encourage you to arrange an appointment. In Chapter 1, we look at how you can find a dietitian.

A prescription for a healthy eating program

Doug hadn't seen a doctor for years but, having turned 40, he figured it was time to get "checked out." Although he was quite a bit overweight, he felt reasonably well and was very surprised when his family physician told him that not only did he have diabetes but he also had high blood pressure and high cholesterol.

"Gee doc, I guess this means you're going to recommend I take a whole bunch of pills, eh?" he said dejectedly.

To Doug's surprise, his doctor responded by saying, "Well, we *could* use a whole bunch of pills, but your blood glucose levels aren't *all that high* and your blood pressure and cholesterol aren't *all that bad,* so it's up to you."

"Up to me?" Doug said with surprise.

"Yes, it's up to you," the doctor continued. "If you think you can change your eating habits, cut down on your calories, and reduce your salt and fat intake, you may be able to avoid medication."

Doug was all for that, so the doctor arranged an appointment with Cynthia, who got Doug set up with a healthy eating program, and it didn't take long before his blood glucose, blood pressure, and cholesterol were on the way down. Was Doug on a "diabetic diet"? As Shakespeare said, a rose would smell as sweet by any other name . . .

Exploring the Key Ingredients

Most of what people eat is made up of carbohydrates, proteins, and fats. Other necessary ingredients in a person's diet are vitamins, minerals, and, in abundant quantities, water.

Although everybody needs to pay attention to how much of each of these things he or she eats, in order to stay healthy, people with diabetes need to be especially careful to ensure they get the right amounts of the right nutrients.

The Canadian Diabetes Association (CDA) recommends that you divide your diet (based on energy, or calories) as follows:

- Carbohydrate: 45–60 percent
- Protein: 15–20 percent
- Fat: 20–35 percent

Carbohydrates, proteins, and fats each provide different amounts of energy (measured in calories). The number of calories contained in 1 gram is

- Carbohydrate: 4 calories
- Protein: 4 calories
- Fat: 9 calories

Vitamins and minerals do not provide calories.

In the following sections, we look at each of the key ingredients of a healthy diabetes nutrition program.

Carbohydrates

Carbohydrates — often simply called *carbs* — are found in dairy foods and in foods that start their journey as seeds in the ground. Here are some examples of carbohydrates:

- Fruit
- Potatoes
- Rice, pasta, and corn
- Grains, breads, and cereals
- Dairy products

Glucose: The critical carb

Although many types of carbohydrates exist, the carbohydrate most closely connected to diabetes is glucose. Indeed, diabetes is defined by how much glucose is present in your blood. (We discuss blood glucose levels in more detail in Chapter 1.)

Although you can eat or drink foods or liquids that contain glucose, most of the glucose in the body comes from two sources:

- The breakdown, during digestion, of other carbohydrates
- The liver, which manufactures glucose

What carbohydrates do

Carbohydrates play a number of very important roles in the body, including the following:

- Providing energy for muscles.
- Supplying the brain with fuel. (Hmm, how apt that one talks about "food for thought.")
- Stimulating the pancreas to make insulin.
- In the case of fibre, helping prevent constipation.

"Sugar" (in the form of *sucrose* as present in sweet items such as candy) is a form of carbohydrate. Popular wisdom to the contrary, eating sugar does not cause diabetes and is not directly harmful (except, perhaps to your teeth) as long as the total number of calories you ingest is not excessive.

Because sweets lack health value and contain significant calories, you need to limit the amount of sweets in your diet. The CDA recommends that sweets make up no more than 10 percent of your daily calorie intake.

The glycemic index

Different types of carbohydrates raise blood glucose levels to different degrees. The *glycemic index* (GI) of a food is a measure of this tendency. The higher the glycemic index of a food, the higher it tends to raise blood glucose. In theory, therefore, because a key goal of treating diabetes is to prevent high blood glucose levels, it would make sense to emphasize low GI foods in one's diet. In practice, however, things get a lot more complicated. For example, the GI of *the same* food can vary depending on whether you eat it alone or as a part of a mixed meal, and is also affected by, among other things, how the food is prepared. Also, following a low glycemic index diet can be difficult. We discuss the glycemic index in more detail in Chapter 4.

Carbohydrate counting

Carbohydrate counting is a system in which people calculate how many grams of carbohydrate they are eating; it is of special importance if you are taking rapid-acting (meal-time) insulin because it allows you to determine the appropriate insulin dose based on how many grams of carbohydrate you are about to eat. The more the amount of carbohydrate, the higher the required insulin dose. We discuss carbohydrate counting in detail in Chapter 1. (Nutritional breakdowns of the recipes in this book include the number of grams of carbohydrate present per serving.)

Fibre

Fibre is a carbohydrate that is not absorbed into the body and thus does not add calories.

Because fibre isn't absorbed into the body and therefore provides no calories, it isn't included when performing carbohydrate counting (see the preceding section and Chapter 1).

Fibre is found in most fruits, grains, and vegetables, and can be categorized into two distinct types:

- **Soluble fibre** can dissolve in water. Ingesting soluble fibre can help to lower your blood glucose and cholesterol. An example of soluble fibre is oatmeal.

- **Insoluble fibre** cannot dissolve in water; it absorbs water in the intestine and helps prevent constipation by providing bulk to the stool. Because insoluble fibre swells in the intestine, it helps to make you feel full and may aid in weight loss. An example of insoluble fibre is the skin of an apple.

It is recommended you ingest 25 to 38 grams of fibre daily. Because too much fibre can lead to diarrhea and flatulence, you need to increase the fibre content in your diet fairly slowly. Also, make sure you drink plenty of water.

Protein

For most people, the main source of dietary protein is meat products — specifically, muscle — from animals such as chicken, turkey, beef, and lamb. Fish, eggs, and cheese are also sources of protein. Certain meat alternatives, such as soybeans, legumes, nuts, and seeds, contain protein, but for most people these alternatives make up a much smaller proportion of their daily protein intake.

The most important function of the protein you eat is to provide the nutrients to maintain the health of tissues such as muscle. This is sometimes mistakenly interpreted to mean that in order to build up muscle bulk — such as bigger biceps — you need to consume large amounts of protein. The reality, however, is that the only way to develop bigger muscles is by exercising them regularly, and the normal quantities of protein found in a healthy diet are sufficient to allow for increased muscle bulk if that's your desire.

The protein you eat does not affect your blood glucose levels significantly.

Protein sources also contain variable amounts of fat, so you need to give careful thought to the protein sources you eat. For example, 30 grams (1 oz.) of very lean meat, fish, or meat alternative (such as skinless white-meat chicken or turkey, or tuna canned in water) has 7 grams of protein and 1 gram of fat and a total of 37 calories, whereas, on the other side of the spectrum, 30 grams (1 oz.) of high-fat meat (such as pork sausage, bacon, or processed sandwich meats) contains the same amount of protein (7 grams) but 8 grams of fat and 100 calories.

Fat

Pretty well anyone who has ever purchased meat at the butcher or grocery store or ever thrown some meat on the barbecue has at least some familiarity with what fat looks like.

Not all fat is created equal. Consuming some types of fat, particularly in excess quantities, can be harmful, but ingesting other types of fat has potential health benefits.

Cholesterol

Cholesterol is a fat like substance that, when present in elevated levels in the blood, contributes to the development of atherosclerosis ("hardening of the arteries"), which, in turn, can lead to heart attacks and strokes. For this reason, you are typically best off minimizing the amount of cholesterol you ingest. The Canadian Diabetes Association recommends that, if you have diabetes, you limit your cholesterol intake to no more than 300 milligrams a day. (To put this in perspective, one large egg has about 215 mg of cholesterol.) Other sources of cholesterol include liver, kidney, whole milk, and hard cheeses such as Monterey Jack and cheddar.

When we tell patients that they have high cholesterol, we are often met with a puzzled look and a comment along the lines of, "But that doesn't make sense; I don't eat much cholesterol." This conundrum is explained by the fact that most cholesterol in the body comes not from what you *eat,* but from what your liver *makes.*

People with diabetes are more prone to high cholesterol levels and, although limiting your cholesterol consumption is important in reducing your cholesterol level, medication is often required to effectively slow down how much cholesterol the liver is making.

Many types of lipids exist. Far and away the most important one for you to be aware of — and to have within target — is your LDL cholesterol; however, there are other lipid levels that are also measured. These are lipid tests for you to be aware of:

- **LDL:** This stands for *low density lipoprotein*. LDL is thought of as the *bad* cholesterol because elevated levels of LDL cholesterol increase the risk of developing atherosclerosis ("hardening of the arteries"). You want your LDL to be low. To remember this, think "**L**DL is **l**ousy and should be **l**ow." For most adults with diabetes the target LDL is 2.0 mmol/L or less.

- **HDL:** This stands for *high density lipoprotein*. HDL is thought of as the *good* cholesterol. You want your HDL to be high because it helps protect your blood vessels (by removing cholesterol from the walls of your arteries). You can remember this by the phrase "A **h**igh **H**DL keeps you **h**ealthy."

- **Total cholesterol:** This is the total level of all the different types of cholesterol in your blood.

- **Non-HDL cholesterol:** This is your total cholesterol minus your HDL cholesterol. The lower the number, the better. Your target non-HDL cholesterol level is less than or equal to 2.6 mmol/L.

- **Total cholesterol/HDL ratio:** Just as it sounds, this is a ratio of total cholesterol to HDL cholesterol and is used by your doctor to help decide if you require treatment. The lower the ratio, the better. A ratio less than 4.0 is considered good.

- **Apolipoprotein B ("apo B"):** This is a component of LDL cholesterol. The target apo B level is less than or equal to 0.8 grams per litre.

- **Triglycerides:** These are the main fats in the blood. Their role in the development of atherosclerosis is not quite as proven as LDL and HDL; however, keeping your triglycerides in the normal range is wise (see later explanation). Although the Canadian Diabetes Association guidelines do not have a specific treatment target for triglycerides, a level less than 1.5 mmol/L is considered optimal.

The CDA recommends that you have your lipid levels checked at the time your diabetes is diagnosed and then yearly (more frequently if treatment has been initiated or changed).

Traditionally, people are asked to fast when their blood is taken to measure their lipids because the results are more precise, but even on a non-fasting blood sample a very good idea of a person's lipid levels can be determined. (Apo B and non-HDL testing does not require fasting.) Also not to be ignored are the logistical difficulties in going for fasting blood work: getting up even earlier than usual in order to get to the lab, long lineups at the lab as you stand there beside dozens of other people who were also sent for fasting blood work, potentially being late for work, and, importantly, risking hypoglycemia if you are on certain blood glucose-lowering medications. Not surprisingly, many people end up not going for the blood test at all! And that serves nobody well. Therefore, feel free to ask your doctor, if he or she asks that you have a fasting blood test, if you may instead go for a nonfasting test.

Saturated fat

Saturated fat comes from animal food sources. Examples of saturated fat are the fatty streaks found in meat such as steak or bacon, butter, cream, and cream cheese.

Because consuming saturated fat can make your LDL cholesterol go up, minimizing your consumption of it is a good idea. The Canadian Diabetes Association recommends that less than 7 percent of your total daily calories come from saturated fat.

Trans fatty acids

Over the past few years trans fatty acids have garnered all sorts of attention, and for good reason. Trans fatty acids raise LDL cholesterol levels and promote the development of atherosclerosis.

Trans fatty acids have traditionally been used in many commercially baked goods such as cookies, cakes, potato chips, doughnuts, pastries, French fries, and breaded foods. The commercial food industry, in response to public pressure (and, in some cases, legislation), has been working quickly at reducing or eliminating the amount of trans fatty acids present in its products.

You should minimize how much trans fatty acid–containing food you eat. To do this, avoid commercially fried foods and high-fat bakery products. The Nutrition Facts table on a food label will also tell you how much trans fat a product contains. (We talk more about the Nutrition Facts table in Chapter 6.)

Unsaturated fat

Unsaturated fat comes from vegetable food sources.

Consuming *monounsaturated* fat (as is found in avocados, olive oil, canola oil, almonds, and peanuts) helps raise your HDL cholesterol and does not affect your LDL cholesterol.

Consuming *polyunsaturated* fat (as is found in corn oil, mayonnaise, and soft margarine) helps lower your LDL, but may also lower your HDL. Polyunsaturated fats should be less than 10 percent of your total daily calorie intake.

Omega-3 fatty acids

Omega-3 fatty acids are a healthy form of fat that helps protect against the development of atherosclerosis. Some evidence links a diet rich in omega-3 fatty acids with a reduced risk of other health problems, including cancer, arthritis, depression, lupus, and asthma.

In your Internet (and other) travels you may come across terms regarding three specific types of omega-3 fatty acids, each with its own sources (and its own incredibly complicated name!):

- ✔ *Docosahexaenoic acid* (DHA) is found in fatty fish and some commercially grown algae.
- ✔ *Eicosapentaenoic acid* (EPA) is found in fatty fish.
- ✔ *Alpha-linolenic acid* (ALA) is found in walnuts, flax, canola, and soy.

Omega-3 fatty acids are found in certain fish such as salmon, herring, mackerel, and trout. Eat fish rich in omega-3 fatty acids at least twice per week. If you don't fancy fish, try crushed flaxseed, omega-3 eggs, or canola oil.

Whether or not the same benefits of ingesting omega-3 fatty acids in food sources can be achieved by taking them in supplement form remains to be determined.

Getting Enough Vitamins, Minerals, and Water

In your healthy eating program, you need to include a sufficient quantity of vitamins, minerals, and water. Most people can meet their daily needs of these nutrients by eating a balanced diet. In this section, we look at the important vitamins and minerals required to maintain good health.

Munching on minerals

The minerals you require to maintain good health are readily available in the foods you eat as part of a healthy eating program.

Calcium

Ingesting sufficient calcium is important for good bone health and, especially, to avoid osteoporosis.

Good sources of calcium include milk and other dairy products, calcium-fortified tofu, canned salmon and sardines (if containing bones), calcium-fortified orange juice and soy milk, almonds, and beans.

Be sure to ingest, depending on your age, at least 800 to 1,200 milligrams of elemental calcium per day. Depending on your dietary calcium intake, you may require calcium supplements to obtain all the calcium you need. Because of the increased calcium needs of pregnancy, pregnant women often require calcium supplements. Many other people also need them, so checking with your dietitian to see if you would benefit from taking extra calcium is a good idea. When buying calcium supplements, be sure to take note on the label of the *elemental* calcium content, not the total calcium content; it is the elemental calcium content that you need to factor into your nutrition program.

For more on calcium, see Chapter 21.

Chromium

Chromium is required for certain internal chemical reactions to take place normally. Principal sources of chromium are brewer's yeast, meat, and cheese. The North American diet is sufficiently rich in chromium that deficiency of this nutrient is highly unlikely and chromium supplements are neither necessary nor helpful.

Iodine

Iodine is necessary for normal thyroid gland function. Iodine is found in iodized salt, dairy products, and seafood. Again, a North American diet is sufficiently rich in iodine that deficiency doesn't occur and supplements are unnecessary.

Iron

Iron is used to make red blood cells. Being deficient in iron leads to *iron deficiency anemia.* Iron deficiency (and iron deficiency anemia) is very common in women who menstruate because of menstrual blood losses (blood is rich in iron). Men almost never have iron deficiency on the basis of insufficient iron ingestion unless they are strict vegetarians. Women who are strict vegetarians are also at increased risk of iron deficiency.

Good sources of iron include red meat, turkey, chicken, clams, eggs, and whole grain cereals. Women who menstruate often require iron supplements.

Several different types of iron supplements are available; your doctor can advise you as to which one is best for your particular situation.

Magnesium

Magnesium is required for a number of different chemical reactions to occur. Sources of magnesium are soybeans, wheat germ, almonds, and dairy products. Magnesium deficiency is seldom a problem, and routine supplements are unnecessary.

Phosphorus

Phosphorus is required for healthy, strong bones. Sources of phosphorus include milk products, meat, fish, legumes, and nuts. As Canadian diets contain sufficient phosphorus, routine supplements are not required.

Sodium

Getting enough sodium (salt) in one's diet is never a problem in Canada; quite the opposite in fact! Excess salt consumption may be a factor leading to high blood pressure or, if you already have high blood pressure, making it worse. Avoid adding salt to your food, and if you have high blood pressure, make a point of buying foods that are low in salt to begin with. In Chapter 4, we look at how healthy eating can help control blood pressure.

Zinc

Zinc is required for certain normal chemical reactions to take place in the body. Zinc is found in beef, lamb, chicken, pumpkins seeds, dried beans, and lentils. Zinc is present in sufficient quantities in a Canadian diet and supplements are not required.

Vitality through vitamins

Whether or not you have diabetes, you should take vitamins with the same due diligence and caution that applies to taking prescription drugs or over-the-counter medications. Consider these three important factors about taking vitamin supplements:

✔ **Do you actually need a vitamin supplement?** With a few specific exceptions (which we discuss in a moment), if you are eating a healthy, well-balanced diet, you're unlikely to benefit from taking a vitamin supplement.

✔ **If you do need a vitamin supplement, take the specific one you need.** Most vitamin preparations are a grab bag of different vitamins. If you need a vitamin supplement, take only the specific vitamin supplement you actually require.

✔ **Don't take too much.** Taking too high a dose of a vitamin supplement can damage your body.

Most people, whether or not living with diabetes, can obtain all the vitamins that are needed from consuming a well-balanced, healthy diet following Canada's Food Guide. These are the most important exceptions to this rule:

✔ If you are pregnant or breastfeeding, elderly, a strict vegetarian, on a very low calorie diet, or for some other reason consume a diet insufficient in vitamins, you should take a daily multivitamin.

✔ If you are a woman with diabetes who is looking to become pregnant, you should take 5 mg of folic acid daily starting three months before stopping contraception. You should then continue to take 5 mg of folic acid daily until you are 12 weeks pregnant, at which time you can reduce the dose to 0.4 to 1 mg per day. You should then stay on this lower dose until you have completed breastfeeding.

✔ If you are over the age of 50, you should take vitamin D supplements totalling 400 units per day. This is a general rule of thumb. Depending on your particular situation you may need more than this amount or you may need to take a vitamin D supplement at a younger age or, possibly, only seasonally. We discuss vitamin D in more detail later in this chapter.

In the remainder of this section, we look at the roles that certain vitamins have in maintaining good health.

Vitamin A

Vitamin A is found in a variety of food sources, including certain meats (liver, beef, chicken), dairy products (eggs, cheese, milk, butter), vegetables (carrots, sweet potatoes, spinach, and other green vegetables), and fruits (mangoes and oranges).

If you are deficient in vitamin A, you will be at risk of developing impaired vision, reduced immune function, dry hair and dry skin, miscarriages, and, in children, poor bone development.

In and of itself, diabetes does not put you at risk of vitamin A deficiency.

Vitamin B_9 (folate or folic acid)

Vitamin B_9, more commonly known as *folate* or *folic acid,* is found in dried beans, green, leafy vegetables (such as spinach, Swiss chard, cabbage, kale, broccoli, and Brussels sprouts) and citrus fruits.

If you are deficient in folic acid you may develop anemia and/or a sore, inflamed tongue. If you are pregnant, folate deficiency puts your fetus at increased risk of spinal cord damage; for this reason, pregnant women are advised to take folic acid supplements routinely. (We discuss the recommended folic acid supplement dose earlier in this section.)

Vitamin B_{12}

Vitamin B_{12} is found in animal (meat and dairy) products.

Deficiency of vitamin B_{12} can lead to anemia, nerve damage (leading to difficulty walking), impaired thinking, and soreness and inflammation of the tongue.

If you have diabetes you will be at increased risk of vitamin B_{12} deficiency:

- ✔ Having type 1 diabetes increases your risk of having *pernicious anemia,* which, like type 1 diabetes, is an autoimmune disorder (that is, a condition in which antibodies attack one's own body). Pernicious anemia commonly causes impaired absorption of vitamin B_{12} from the intestine into the body.

- ✔ Taking *metformin* to treat type 2 diabetes increases the risk of vitamin B_{12} deficiency because metformin, for reasons that aren't yet fully sorted out, can interfere with the ability to absorb vitamin B_{12} into the body.

Also, because vitamin B_{12} is found only in animal products, if you don't consume animal products you will be high risk of deficiency of this vitamin.

If you have type 1 diabetes, type 2 diabetes treated with metformin, or if you do not consume animal products, discuss with your doctor about checking your vitamin B_{12} level with a blood test from time to time.

Vitamin D

Vitamin D is found naturally in eggs and fatty fish and is added to many other foods (such as milk). Sun exposure allows your own skin to make vitamin D (which is pretty darn cool we think). Because of limited dietary intake of vitamin D, and because of limited sun exposure, many Canadians are deficient in this vitamin.

Deficiency of vitamin D can lead to osteoporosis (in adults) and rickets (in children). These are conditions in which bone mass and strength are reduced, which, in turn, increases the risk of fractures. Low vitamin D levels also can lead to low calcium levels and decreased immune function. In recent years, rapidly accumulating evidence has linked vitamin D deficiency to other health problems, including an increased risk of some types of cancer and atherosclerosis ("hardening of the arteries").

As we mention earlier in this section, Canada's Food Guide recommends that people over the age of 50 should take 400 international units of vitamin D supplements daily. Osteoporosis Canada recommends 400-1,000 IU (international units) of vitamin D_3 a day.

Speak to your doctor or dietitian to find out what your specific vitamin D needs are.

Vitamin E

Vitamin E is found in almonds, sunflower seeds and oil, safflower oil, hazelnuts, wheat germ, green, leafy vegetables (such as spinach, Swiss chard, cabbage, kale, broccoli, and Brussels sprouts), cauliflower, asparagus, and avocado.

Deficiency of vitamin E can lead to anemia, nerve damage, and muscle injury.

Having diabetes does not put you at increased risk of having vitamin E deficiency.

Vitamin K

Vitamin K is found in green, leafy vegetables (such as kale, spinach, Swiss chard, cabbage, broccoli, and Brussels sprouts), avocado, and kiwi fruit. The human gut also has the ability to make vitamin K from other nutrients that are eaten. (We never fail to be amazed at what the human body can do. Making its own vitamins . . . Wow.)

Deficiency of vitamin K can lead to impaired ability of the blood to clot, which, in turn, can lead to bleeding (ranging from the minor, such as a nose bleed, to the life-threatening, such as internal hemorrhaging).

Having diabetes does not increase your risk of having vitamin K deficiency.

What about water?

The single most important reason to ensure you drink enough water is to help your body maintain hydration. If your body doesn't have enough water (that is, you are dehydrated), you are at risk of becoming very ill; indeed, if dehydration is severe enough, you are at risk of profoundly low blood pressure, kidney failure, and even death.

In addition to maintaining hydration, drinking water can help you control your weight as it may help reduce your appetite by giving you a feeling of fullness.

Hydration is maintained not only by drinking water (and other fluids), but also from eating food. Vegetables and fruits are almost entirely made up of water and, perhaps surprising to you, uncooked meat is 70 percent water. (Gee, next time we're at the butcher shop maybe we'll ask for 70 percent off the price!) Another source of water is a by-product of normal metabolism, as water is created when the body breaks down proteins, fats, and carbohydrates.

Everyone is aware that a fair bit of water is lost from the body through urine, but water is also lost in sometimes less obvious ways (and amounts). Here are some estimates of daily water losses from the body:

- Urine: 0.5 L to 1.5 L
- Breathing: 0.4 L (water is present in your exhaled breath)
- Skin (through sweating, perspiring, and simple evaporation): 0.5 L
- Bowel movements: 0.1 to 0.2 L

In order to maintain hydration, you need to ingest sufficient fluids to make up for these losses from your body. In general, you should drink a minimum of 1.5 L (6 cups) per day.

Some situations result in far greater than normal losses of water from the body and, hence, the need to drink similarly far greater quantities of water to maintain hydration. For example, vigorous exercise — especially in hot, dry climates — can result in fluid losses in the form of sweat as great as *1.5 litres per hour!* Another example is diarrhea, which, if severe enough, can lead to fluid losses of several litres per day.

Poor blood glucose control, with values up into the high teens or greater, can lead to greater urine production, which, in turn, puts you at risk of dehydration. Therefore, if your blood glucose levels are high, in addition to taking measures such as adjusting your medications (under the guidance of your doctor), make sure you drink enough water to maintain your hydration.

Internet (and other) rumours to the contrary, tap water is just as healthy as — and a lot less expensive than — bottled water, spring water, mineral water, or any other packaged water.

Eating Well with Canada's Food Guide

Whether or not you have diabetes, eating healthfully is essential. To help Canadians succeed with healthy eating, Health Canada developed *Eating Well with Canada's Food Guide.* (This title is typically abbreviated as Canada's

Food Guide.) The guide is chock-a-block full of information to help people make good food choices.

Canada's Food Guide is available online (www.hc-sc.gc.ca/fn-an/food-guide-aliment/index-eng.php), in a shortened form in this book's colour insert, and in hard copy from your dietitian.

Following Canada's Food Guide brings these important benefits:

✔ Getting the appropriate amounts of vitamins.

✔ Consuming the right amount of minerals.

✔ Ingesting a healthy number of calories (thereby helping with weight control).

✔ Reducing your risk of developing heart disease, cancer, osteoporosis, and certain other health problems.

The guide uses the colours of a rainbow to illustrate the recommended amounts of nutrients that should be consumed from each of the four food groups:

✔ **Green: Vegetables and Fruits.** This is the biggest arc of the rainbow. More of your daily food choices should come from this food group than any other group.

✔ **Yellow: Grain Products.** This is the second biggest arc of the rainbow and thus grains should be the second greatest type of food you should eat daily.

✔ **Blue: Milk and Alternatives.** This is the third biggest arc of the rainbow. "Alternatives" here refers to foods such as cheese, yogurt, and soy-based beverages.

✔ **Red: Meat and Alternatives**. This is the smallest arc of the rainbow and fewest of your food choices should come from this food group. "Alternatives" here refers to foods such as fish, beans, lentils, and tofu.

The guide emphasizes the importance of enjoying a variety of foods from each of the four food groups to help meet your overall nutritional needs. The guide also discusses portions in terms of "servings." It's important to know — as you will discover in the guide — what, exactly, is a serving size. (P.S. It's often a lot smaller than you might expect!)

Rather than guessing whether or not you've chosen a proper serving size, use measuring cups to help guide you. After doing this for a while you'll better be able to judge what a serving size is.

These are some important recommendations from the guide:

- Eat at least one dark green vegetable and one orange vegetable every day.
- Have vegetables and fruit more often than juice.
- Choose a minimum of half of your grain products as whole grain.
- Drink milk daily. Choose skim, 1 percent, or 2 percent milk rather than whole milk.
- Have meat alternatives like lentils, beans, and tofu regularly.
- Consume at least two servings of fish per week.
- Include unsaturated fat in small amounts daily.
- Choose foods that are low in fat, sugar, and salt.

Chapter 3

You Are How You Eat

*W*hen we discuss how to eat, we're not referring to whether your preferred utensils are forks and knives, chopsticks, or those most versatile of all implements — your own fingers; rather, we're referring to such "how-tos" as portion size, meal timing, eating out, using artificial sweeteners, and so on. (For the inside scoop on what to eat, see Chapter 2.)

Living with diabetes presents many eating challenges. What many of our patients tell us is that discovering which foods are healthy and which foods are unhealthy is the easiest part of the diabetes nutrition education process. Far trickier for most people to master are the more nuanced, less black-and-white essentials like figuring out how much is a serving or portion size, how to divide up the different types of nutrients, and how to eat healthfully when you're away from home at a restaurant, at a party, on the road, and so forth. In this chapter, we look at these challenges and provide tips to help you meet them.

Keeping Portions under Control

Making healthy food choices is tremendously important, but also important is eating *the right amount* of these healthy choices — that is, keeping portion sizes under control.

Ian recalls years ago seeing an industrious, enthusiastic, older woman who, newly diagnosed with type 2 diabetes, was committed to "turning her eating habits around" so that she could "stick around" until her grandchildren were married. She gave up her predilection for cakes, chips, and the like and took up eating vegetables, fruits, and other healthy choices. Nonetheless, try as she might, the extra pounds she carried wouldn't fade away. Upon reviewing her eating habits, Ian discovered that his keen patient was indeed eating very healthy foods, including nutritious, scrumptious, Granny Smith apples . . . over a dozen a day! Ian advised her to reduce her apple consumption to one to two a day and, lo and behold, the excess pounds gradually started to fall. Moral of the story: Healthy foods still contain calories, and like most things in life, you can have too much of a good thing.

A helpful way to determine what, for most people, is a healthy portion size is to compare an amount of a food to something else:

- One deck of playing cards equals 3 ounces (90 grams) of cooked fish, poultry, or meat.
- A chequebook represents 3 ounces (90 grams) of cooked roast beef or fish fillet.
- Half a tennis ball equals ½ cup (125 ml) of mashed potato, pasta, or fruit salad.
- A golf ball is the equivalent of ½ cup (125 ml) of nuts.
- A fist is the size of a medium-sized piece of fruit or potato.
- Four dice are the size of 1 ounce (30 grams) of cheese.
- The end of your thumb (from the tip to the first joint) is the size of 1 teaspoon (5 ml) of soft margarine.

Here are some excellent aids to help you learn more about portion sizes:

- *Health Canada's Eating Well with Canada's Food Guide* (www.healthcanada.gc.ca/foodguide or in this book's insert)
- The Canadian Diabetes Association's (CDA's) *Just the Basics* (www.diabetes.ca)
- The CDA's *Beyond the Basics* (www.diabetes.ca)

How much is half a cup?

Here's a tip that Cynthia shares with her patients to help them estimate how much is ½ cup (125 ml) without needing to get out a measuring cup each time:

Pour water into a measuring cup until you've measured out ½ cup.

Pour the water into one of your frequently used glasses.

Take a mental snapshot of where the level came to.

Now whenever you use that glass you'll readily know how much is ½ cup (125 ml) of your favourite drink.

Do the same thing with a bowl to be able to estimate how much is 1 cup (250 ml) of soup. You can also use a dry measuring cup to measure out ½ cup (125 ml) of cereal or vegetables (or pasta, and so forth) and then pour this into a favourite bowl.

This technique will help you to be more aware of portion sizes and what you're consuming at a meal.

Don't be misled by the term "serving size" on the Nutrition Facts tables on the foods you buy. Despite what you may think, a serving size isn't based on hard scientific evidence. In other words, just because a label says a certain amount of a product constitutes a serving size, that doesn't mean it's the best size *for you*.

In this book's recipes, serving sizes are based on the principles of healthy, balanced eating as set out by the Canadian Diabetes Association and Canada's Food Guide.

Timing Is Everything

If you have diabetes you should aim to eat three meals per day with your meals spaced no longer than six hours apart. This schedule will help you keep your blood glucose levels in check and will also help you avoid falling into that all too common trap of starving yourself all day then, once you get home in the evening, raiding the fridge or pantry and grazing until you go to bed.

If your meals will be more than six hours apart, eating a snack midway between your meals is often a good idea. This is particularly important if you are on medication (such as insulin or a sulfonylurea medication such as glyburide; see Chapter 1) that may cause hypoglycemia.

Eating a bedtime snack may be necessary if you are taking medicine — especially NPH insulin given in the evening — that can cause your blood glucose levels to go too low overnight. Bedtime snacks should contain both carbohydrate and protein. We talk more about snacking to prevent hypoglycemia later in this chapter.

Balancing Out a Meal's Ingredients

Cynthia reminds her patients to always think of balance at mealtimes. A meal shouldn't consist solely of carbohydrates nor should it be made up exclusively of proteins. (And most definitely it should not be comprised purely of fat! Oh my, even the thought of that is too much to handle.)

Meals should have at least one serving each of a carbohydrate and a protein. (In Chapter 2, we discuss the roles that these nutrients play in maintaining good health.)

Jeff was a 35-year-old patient of Cynthia's. He was evenly balanced when it came to his temperament, his exercise, his work, and pretty well everything else in his life, except, that is, for his eating habits. He came to see Cynthia because he was having recurring problems with hypoglycemia (low blood glucose) occurring an hour or two after his lunch. As Cynthia discovered, for lunch Jeff always had a tossed salad with lettuce, tomato, cucumber, and celery topped with diet dressing and washed down with a glass of water. Although these were healthy food choices, Jeff was not eating any carbohydrate or protein. Because Jeff took long-acting insulin every morning, the insulin was pulling his blood glucose level down and, with no carbohydrate in his lunch to keep it up, he was developing hypoglycemia. Cynthia advised Jeff to have some milk, cheese, and crackers with his salad; after that he seldom ran into problems with after-lunch hypoglycemia. (Also he wasn't quite so hungry come suppertime and, as a result, ate a more modestly sized supper.)

Eating Vegetarian

Vegetarian diets are generally low in cholesterol and fat (especially saturated and trans fats), high in fibre, and, compared to non-vegetarian diets, often lower in calories and less expensive to boot.

Vegetarian diets have many health advantages, including an association with lower blood pressure and cholesterol, less obesity, and a decreased risk for stroke, heart disease, and cancer.

In order to ensure you get all the nutrients you require, following a vegetarian diet requires careful planning. This is especially true for children, teens, and pregnant and lactating women. Be sure to speak to your dietitian to receive his or her expert advice.

In Chapter 16, we present a delectable assortment of healthy vegetarian recipes.

Sorting Out Snacks

If you have had diabetes for a while, you likely recall being told at some time that you should eat three snacks per day. This longstanding recommendation has recently been changed. The Canadian Diabetes Association now advises that the need to snack and the number of daily snacks to eat should be determined on a case-by-case basis taking into account your personal preferences, medications you take that might cause hypoglycemia, the type of work and exercise you do, and so on. Your dietitian can work with you to help you sort out your personal snacking needs and how best to fulfill them.

The exception to the preceding recommendation is if you have diabetes and you are pregnant, in which case you should, indeed, make a point of eating three snacks per day, one of which should be at bedtime.

The term "snacking" often carries negative connotations. And sure, if snacking automatically meant pulling out a tub of ice cream from the freezer or a box of cookies from the pantry then snacking's bad reputation would be justified. Snacking, however, can be done perfectly healthfully and can help complement your daily nutrient needs.

A snack for someone with diabetes should generally contain a carbohydrate, or a carbohydrate with a protein from the Milk and Alternatives group or the Meat and Alternatives group. (We discuss the food groups in Chapter 2.)

Here are some examples of healthy snacks:

- 1 medium apple
- 1 medium pear
- 15 cherries
- 1 small banana
- ½ cup (125 ml) fruit salad
- 1 cup (250 ml) low-fat milk

- ¾ cup (175 ml) unsweetened flavoured yogurt
- 1 slice multigrain bread with soft margarine and diet jam
- 1 slice pumpernickel toast with 1 tbsp (15 ml) peanut butter
- ½ sandwich

- ½ small bagel with 1 oz. (30 g) melted low-fat cheddar
- 1 small bran muffin
- ⅓ cup (75 ml) dal with 1 small chapati
- 3 cups (750 ml) plain popcorn
- 1 low-fat granola bar
- 1 low-fat pudding cup
- 3 arrowroot cookies
- ⅓ cup (75 ml) trail mix
- ½ cup (125 ml) chocolate milk with ¼ cup (50 ml) almonds
- 1 oz. (30 g) cheese with 4 whole-grain crackers
- ¼ cup (50 ml) low-fat cottage cheese with ½ cup (125 ml) fruit

- ¼ cup (50 ml) hummus with ½ pita
- 1 egg and 1 slice rye toast
- Tossed salad with ½ cup (125 ml) chickpeas and 1 tbsp (15 ml) light dressing
- ¼ cup (50 ml) hummus with raw veggies
- Spinach salad with ½ cup (125 ml) mandarin oranges and ¼ cup (50 ml) walnuts
- 15 grapes and 1 oz. (30 g) cheese
- ½ cup (125 ml) cereal and 1 cup (250 ml) low-fat milk
- 1 small slice of pizza

As you can see, there is certainly no shortage of variety in the types of snacks available. For other healthy snack suggestions have a look at our Month of Menus (see Appendix B).

Take nutritious snacks from home to eat at school, work, sports events, or on the run. Having these snacks on hand will help reduce the temptation to purchase less nutritious snacks.

If you don't want to snack but you need to in order to avoid hypoglycemia, speak to your doctor about having your medications adjusted. With so many different drugs to treat diabetes now available, your doctor will almost certainly be able to find medications and doses that will be less likely to cause hypoglycemia and, therefore, won't force you to snack (and consume unwanted calories with the potential for weight gain) when you don't want to. If changing the types or doses of your medications doesn't help or is not an option, then speak to your dietitian; adjusting your diet could improve the situation.

Ian recalls meeting Mary, a 42-year-old woman who had been living with type 2 diabetes for five years. Mary was being treated with NPH insulin at bedtime. Her problem was that even though she had no desire to take a bedtime snack, if she didn't she would invariably awaken in the middle of the night with hypoglycemia. Things had gotten so bad she was afraid to go to sleep.

Ian changed Mary's NPH insulin to Levemir insulin (see Chapter 1), which, like Lantus insulin, tends to cause less overnight hypoglycemia than NPH insulin. Mary had no further overnight hypoglycemia and she was thrilled to be able to abandon her unwanted bedtime snacks.

Despite what many people believe, sugar (in the form of *sucrose* or table sugar) isn't forbidden from your diet if you have diabetes. Indeed, the Canadian Diabetes Association *Clinical Practice Guidelines* (www.diabetes.ca) note that up to 10 percent of calories can come from sugar. These guidelines don't advocate for you to make a point of consuming sucrose; just that it's okay to have sugar so long as you limit the quantities. We use sugar in the dessert recipes in this book (see Chapters 17 and 18) — in keeping with the principle that sugar isn't a "dirty word." Also — and in keeping with the need to be careful with the amount of sugar you consume — some of the dessert recipes provide a choice of using less sugar or a sugar substitute.

If you have diabetes, consuming excess sugar will make it harder to control your blood glucose levels. Also, whether or not you have diabetes, the surplus calories in sugar will promote weight gain.

Artificial sweeteners

Although limiting sugar intake is important, humans naturally enjoy sweet things. Many food manufacturers have addressed this conundrum by replacing (or reducing) the sugar in certain foods with artificial sweeteners or sugar alcohols. These are the artificial sweeteners in use in Canada:

- **Acesulfame potassium:** Trade names for acesulfame include Sunette and Sweet One.

- **Aspartame:** Trade names for aspartame include NutraSweet and Equal. Do not use aspartame if you have PKU, which is a rare genetic disorder.

- **Cyclamate:** Cyclamate is found in Sucaryl, Sugar Twin, and Sweet'N Low. Do not consume cyclamate if you are pregnant.

- **Neotame:** A new sweetener that is very similar to Aspartame, but more stable.

- **Saccharin:** Saccharin is contained in Hermesetas. It is available in Canada only in pharmacies. Do not consume saccharin if you are pregnant.

- **Stevia:** Steviol Glycoside has been approved for use in foods and beverages. Stevia is a natural sweetener.

> ✔ **Sucralose:** The trade name for sucralose is Splenda.

> ✔ **Tagatose:** A new sweetener made from lactose (milk sugar), but is poorly absorbed causing abdominal problems.

> ✔ **Thaumatin:** A new sweetener and flavour modifier.

Some artificial sweeteners, despite having the same name in different countries, may contain different ingredients. For example, in Canada Sweet'N Low contains cyclamate whereas in the U.S.A. it does not.

Many of the dessert recipes we describe in this book have the option of substituting sugar with artificial sweeteners.

Sugar alcohols

Sugar alcohols (erythritol, isomalt, lactitol, maltitol, mannitol, sorbitol, and xylitol) are another type of sweetener. Though the term "sugar alcohol" is scientifically correct, these sweeteners contain neither table sugar nor ethanol (that is, the alcohol found in alcohol-containing drinks).

Sugar alcohols vary in the degree to which our bodies absorb them. Sugar alcohols convert slowly to glucose, but this is variable and often minimal, which leads to no significant effect on blood glucose. The Canadian Diabetes Association recommends that rapid insulin not be matched to sugar alcohols. Therefore, don't include sugar alcohols in carbohydrate counting!

Many brands of chewing gum contain sugar alcohols. Sugar alcohols are also found in some types of hard candies, ice cream and other frozen desserts, jams, and syrups.

Consumption of more than 10 grams per day of sugar alcohols can cause abdominal cramping and diarrhea.

Cynthia recalls speaking to a group of people living with diabetes. When she mentioned that excess consumption of sugar alcohol–containing products can lead to diarrhea, a middle-aged man leaped to his feet and excitedly announced, "So that's what the problem is!" Turned out he was working as a long-distance truck driver and had recently taken to consuming bags full of "diet" chewy treats made with sugar alcohols. He had then started having bothersome diarrhea but hadn't made the connection with his new dietary habits. Cynthia recommended he cut down on his treats and in short order his rig was up and running, and his bowels weren't.

Alcohol

Most people enjoy drinking alcohol from time to time. If you have diabetes and you would like to consume alcohol, you can continue to do so safely (unless you're pregnant, in which case you must consume no alcohol at all), but you should follow certain precautions:

✔ **Limit your quantity.** You should limit the quantity of alcohol you drink to no more than two drinks per day if you're a man and one drink per day if you're a woman.

Note that this is not the same as "saving up" your drinks and having a dozen on a Saturday night while watching *Hockey Night in Canada!* In the same way you can't save up your week's calories for one big night of food debauchery, you can't save up your alcohol consumption either; both need to be spread out over time.

✔ **Know that a drink is a drink is a drink.** Because alcohol has calories, you must account for the alcohol you drink in your diet. Depending on the strength of the individual product, 12 oz. (350 ml) of beer, 5 oz. (150 ml) of wine, and 1½ oz. (45 ml) of hard liquor all count as one drink and all have similar quantities of alcohol.

Despite what many people think, drinking beer or wine is not "better for you" than drinking hard liquor. To your liver they all taste the same.

✔ **Watch out for hypoglycemia.** Consuming alcohol increases your risk of developing hypoglycemia — even many hours after the alcohol is consumed — if your diabetes is being treated with medications, such as insulin, that reduce blood glucose. You can reduce this risk by making sure you eat some carbohydrate-containing food when you drink alcohol.

✔ **Help your friends keep an eye on you.** Tell your companions that if you're "acting drunk" or, especially, if you have passed out, it may not be from the alcohol — similar symptoms can be due to low blood glucose. Also, make sure you educate them in advance on what to do if you are hypoglycemic (see Chapter 1). If nothing else, at the very least tell them to call 911 if you are unconscious.

Healthy Eating at Home

Eating at home has certain advantages, many of which apply whether or not you have diabetes. For instance, you have more control over the type of food served, the way it is prepared, the serving size, and meal timing. If you have diabetes and you are carbohydrate counting (see Chapter 1), you have likely already discovered how much easier it is to determine how many grams of carbohydrates are present in food you've prepared yourself or bought pre-packaged for cooking at home rather than ordered in a restaurant.

Here are some healthy eating tips you can use at home:

- ✔ Eat breakfast every day.
- ✔ Limit your use of margarine or butter.
  - • Use light mayonnaise instead of margarine or butter on your bread. Just one teaspoon of margarine or butter has 35 calories and a teaspoon of light mayonnaise has 15 calories.
  - • If you're going to be adding peanut butter to your toast, don't also use margarine or butter. Stick, ahem, to the peanut butter alone.
  - • Use salsa or light sour cream on top of a baked potato instead of butter or margarine.
- ✔ Bake, broil, roast, microwave, or stir fry more often; avoid deep frying.
- ✔ Remember that with easier access to food in the home (compared to a restaurant) you need to keep an eye on how much food you're eating.

One of Cynthia's patients knew that eating breakfast is important and that eating fruit is a healthy thing to do, too, so she routinely ate three cups (750 ml) of fruit salad and one banana as part of her breakfast. When Cynthia pointed out to her that these fruits contained a total of almost 450 calories and 100 grams of carbohydrate, the patient was flabbergasted. She reduced the amount to one cup (250 ml) of fruit salad, saving herself hundreds of calories and many grams of carbohydrate per day, and over the next few weeks lost several pounds and lowered her blood glucose!

For more calorie-saving tips, see our discussion in Chapter 4 on behaviour modification strategies.

Healthy Eating When You're Away from Home

For some people, eating away from home is a special treat; for others it's a way of life. Whether you are at a restaurant, deli counter, cafeteria, vending machine, or corner store, making healthy choices is almost always possible. This is quite a contrast from even a few short years ago when healthy eating was a near impossibility once you left the confines of your own kitchen.

Healthy eating in restaurants

Canadians are eating more and more of their meals in restaurants. This is not necessarily a bad thing, but it does pose some additional challenges if you have diabetes. For instance, when dining out in a restaurant you may not know how a dish was prepared, portions are often overly large (and so very hard to turn down!), and, if you are carbohydrate counting, determining how many grams of carbohydrate are in a dish can be very hard. Also, restaurant foods often contain more fat and salt than homemade recipes.

Here are some general strategies you can follow to make eating out a healthful, not harmful, experience:

✔ Choose foods in the appropriate amounts from the different food groups (see Chapter 2).

✔ Resist the temptation to be "super-sized."

✔ Ask the waitstaff how big the portions are. If the portions are large, try one of the following:

- Share the serving with your dinner-mate.
- Eat half and take the other half home for your next day's lunch.
- Order the "lunch" sized portion for your dinner.
- Order a kid's sized serving.

✔ Avoid "all you can eat" buffets. We wouldn't want to speak for you, but if you're like us you've likely seldom (if ever) left such a restaurant without saying to yourself, "Oh my, I ate too much."

✔ When ordering a salad, ask for low-calorie dressings like oil and vinegar rather than creamy dressing. Ask for your dressing to be on the side so you can choose how much to put on. Also, rather than pouring the dressing on the salad, instead pick up pieces of salad with your fork and dip a small portion of the piece in the dressing. You'll end up with much less dressing and save calories and fat.

✔ Ask to see the nutritional information for the food and look at the content of the various food choices you're considering so that you can be sure to select appropriate items. Also, increasingly often restaurant menus have symbols to let you know what are healthier food choices.

✔ Make sure the waitstaff are paying attention when you order a "diet" soft drink. Waitstaff sometimes bring a non-diet soft drink to the table even when a diet drink has been ordered.

These are good food choices when ordering in a restaurant:

- Baked, steamed, or broiled foods
- Tomato-based dishes
- Grilled chicken
- Fish (non-battered)
- Sandwiches made with chicken, turkey, pastrami, or Black Forest ham. When ordering a sandwich ask for extra lettuce, tomatoes, or other vegetables to be added. If mayonnaise is being used, ask for it be "light" and have them apply it to only one piece of bread, not both. Add mustard on the other piece of bread. Instead of two pieces of bread, choose a whole grain bun, pita, or wrap.

- For dessert, order a piece of fruit or a fruit salad.

These are food choices usually best avoided:

- Deep-fried, heavily battered, or breaded foods
- Foods that are served with rich, creamy, cheesy, or other heavy sauces
- Sandwiches made with salami, mock chicken, or bologna
- Bacon cheeseburgers (If you want a cheeseburger, get it without the added bacon.)
- Cakes and pies

Diabetes is a long-term condition and requires a long-term commitment to healthy eating. This is *not* the same thing as saying that you can never indulge and eat those things you normally wouldn't. Craving a double bacon cheeseburger with fries? Having this as a special, occasional treat isn't going to kill you. Enjoy it. And don't feel guilty! Then get back on track with healthy eating.

Healthy eating at vending machines

Finding healthy food choices in vending machines can be especially challenging, but even here great strides are being made with an ever-increasing variety of nutritious choices becoming available.

Here are some tips when buying food from a vending machine:

- Select sandwiches made with whole-grain breads.
- Choose vegetable juice instead of pop.
- Buy cheese and crackers, hummus and crackers, or tuna and crackers.

✔ Look for fresh or canned fruit.

✔ Avoid large muffins — they usually contain a whopping 500 calories.

✔ Stay away from canned soups unless you know they are low in sodium.

Healthy eating at the convenience store

Are we the only ones irked by those commonplace billboard ads that encourage commuters to stop in at the local convenience store to pick up needed essentials, all the while showing a picture of a shopping bag full of colas, chips, and cookies? Well, as much as we find those ads irritating, truth be told even at convenience stores you can — with some difficulty — find reasonably healthy food choices.

Here are some tips when buying foods at the convenience store:

✔ Choose milk instead of a soft drink or other sugary drink. When buying chocolate milk, choose one with reduced fat. If buying a pop, choose a diet one.

✔ Try trail mix, almonds, or whole grain pretzels for a snack.

✔ Look for healthy pre-made sandwiches.

✔ Try the slow cooker of chili or stew.

✔ Reach for the fruit, not the chocolate bars.

Healthy eating at friends' homes

If you are visiting a friend's home and you are asked what foods you can or cannot eat, often the easiest thing to say is that you are restricted only to "a healthy diet" and that "all foods can fit."

Here are some tips you can follow to help ensure you eat healthfully when you're at your friends' homes:

✔ Ask your friends at what time they will be eating. If it will be quite a bit later than your usual meal-time and if you customarily eat a snack at bedtime, eat your snack at your usual dinnertime instead. This will help you to avoid being overly hungry, which could lead to overeating when meal-time arrives. (However, if you need to eat a bedtime snack to avoid hypoglycemia overnight, then you will still need to eat your usual bed-time snack.)

✔ Offer to bring an appetizer, a vegetable dish, or a dessert. Choose one that works with your eating plan but that others will enjoy too. Check out the recipes in this book!

✔ If you will be having wine or beer with dinner, choose a non-alcohol-containing beverage before dinner.

✔ Be moderate with the number of appetizers you eat.

✔ Choose a protein-containing main dish, if available, rather than one that is high in carbohydrate (or fat).

✔ Be moderate in the portions of your side dishes such as potato or rice.

✔ Heap on the vegetables.

✔ If you elect to eat a sugar-rich dessert, ask for a small serving. (As we discuss in Chapter 2, sweets are not forbidden although you do have to limit how many sweets you eat.)

✔ If you've eaten robustly, consider going for a walk after dinner; it will likely make you feel less full and will help keep your blood glucose level in check.

Healthy eating at parties and celebrations

Christmas, Thanksgiving, Kwanza, Passover, Diwali, weddings, birthday parties, and most every other celebration involves eating. Festivities are a part of everyone's life and living with diabetes doesn't mean that you can't enjoy the event as much as everyone else. You do, however, have to follow a few precautions, which we discuss in this section.

Here are a few tips to help you enjoy your time at a party or other celebration:

✔ Try not to overindulge. (Easy to say, not easy to do.) If you think you may overindulge, eat especially modestly the rest of the day. For example, eat a low-fat breakfast and lunch and save the extra fat for later.

✔ Don't go to a party hungry; eat something healthy before you leave.

✔ Offer to bring a healthy appetizer. Then feel free to eat some of it!

✔ If you're on medicine (such as insulin) that can cause low blood glucose, eat a carbohydrate-containing snack when drinking alcohol. This will reduce your risk of developing hypoglycemia. (See earlier in this chapter for more on this topic.)

✔ Mingle *away* from the food so you're not so tempted to keep eating.

✔ Use a plate to better monitor how much you're eating.

✔ Participate in organized activities. That way it's not all about eating and drinking.

✔ If at a wedding, where the meal is typically served quite late, bring a snack to eat to tide you over until dinner is served.

✔ Dance, dance, dance. Dancing is exercise and will burn off those extra calories you just ate. Who said exercising isn't fun?

Going to a sporting event? The vendors are much more likely to be selling chips than something healthy. To help you avoid temptation, bring a piece of fruit or some nuts. Walk around during breaks in the action to stretch your legs, burn off some calories, and lower your blood glucose.

Chapter 4

Staying Healthy through Nutrition

· ·

In This Chapter

▶ Considering healthy ways to lose weight

▶ Finding out about the glycemic index

▶ Eating right with gestational diabetes

▶ Getting the lowdown on high blood pressure

▶ Controlling lipids by eating well

▶ Dealing with kidney failure through nutrition

· ·

*W*hether you've had diabetes for days or decades, healthy eating is a key component to managing both your diabetes and your general health. (Our hunch is that you know this already, but we thought it couldn't hurt to mention it anyhow.) In Chapters 2 and 3, we look at general nutrition principles, and in this chapter we look specifically at important and common dietary challenges that face many people living with diabetes.

Weight-Loss Strategies

If you have type 2 diabetes then you may be facing the very common challenge of trying to figure out how you can lose weight without feeling like you're starving or you've given up all the foods you like to eat. Indeed, for the majority of our patients with type 2 diabetes, having a satisfying diet that still facilitates weight loss is typically both their single biggest struggle and their single greatest frustration. Fortunately, you can overcome this challenge.

There are no easy ways to lose weight. There are no shortcuts, no tricks, no magic bullets, and no miracles. Losing weight is hard and persisting work. Ever wonder why there are so many bestselling diet books? It's because none of them provide the perfect answer for all people. Indeed, most of them provide the perfect answer for hardly anyone at all!

Knowing if you're overweight

The easiest and best way to determine if you're overweight is to calculate your body mass index (BMI). BMI is an indicator of whether you're the right weight for your height. (Not to be confused with the flip version, which many people jokingly say as they declare they are too short for their weight!)

A healthy (normal) BMI is 18.5 to 24.9. If your BMI is less than 18.5 you're likely underweight and if your BMI is more than 24.9 you're likely overweight. Note that the normal range for BMI does *not* apply to pregnant or breastfeeding woman, nor does it apply to infants, children, or adolescents, nor to particularly muscular individuals.

You can quickly determine your BMI by using an online calculator such as the one available at www.cdc.gov/healthyweight/assessing/bmi. Alternatively you can calculate your BMI yourself, though nobody ever does it this way: by dividing your weight in kilograms by the square of your height in metres. Uh-huh; just as we thought, we saw your eyes just glaze over.

Another way of knowing if you're overweight is based on your waist circumference. Health Canada notes that your risk of health problems goes up if your waist circumference is

- For men, 102 cm (40 inches) or more.
- For women, 88 cm (35 inches) or more.

Reviewing the benefits from weight loss if you're overweight

If you're overweight and have diabetes, these are some of the benefits you may experience from even small weight loss:

- Improved blood glucose control
- Improved blood pressure
- Improved lipids (cholesterol and triglycerides)
- Enhanced self-esteem
- Better sex life
- More energy and more incentive to exercise
- Reduced risk of some types of cancer

> ✔ Increased life expectancy
>
> ✔ Reduced need for medications (such as those for blood glucose, blood pressure, and lipid control)

Being skeptical about fad diets

When Ian's patients ask him if they would lose weight by following this or that fad diet or by adhering to the most recent celebrity-endorsed diet book's recommendations, they are typically quite surprised when Ian quickly answers in the affirmative. But Ian is then equally quick to share his self-proclaimed 95-95-95 rule: In his experience, 95 percent of people following any fad diet will lose weight for 95 days, at which point 95 percent of people will get fed up with the diet, abandon it, and will then regain all (or even more) of the weight they'd lost!

Two other points about fad diets are worth mentioning. One: Many of these diets are so restrictive they can make you feel unwell with constipation, fatigue, muscle ache, hair loss, and so on. And two: Some of these diets can be very expensive. (Hmm, a diet that doesn't provide long-term weight loss, can make you feel unwell, and often costs lots of money to boot; not exactly a recipe for success — except for the people selling the books and running the fad clinics.)

Checking out healthy weight-loss strategies

If we are skeptical of fad diets, what then do we recommend? It may not sound very sexy, but we advocate those tried and true healthy eating principles — which we describe in detail in Chapters 2 and 3 — that are espoused by bodies such as Health Canada and the Canadian Diabetes Association. And we recommend these healthy eating strategies be accompanied by behaviour modification (see the next section) and regular exercise (see Chapter 1).

A highly effective way to lose weight is to cut out 500 calories per day from your diet. Where can you find these 500 calories? A large muffin with butter, 37 potato chips, 4 chocolate chip cookies, and ½ cup (125 ml) peanuts all contain 500 calories.

By the way, it may seem like a misnomer to call a lifelong healthy eating strategy a diet, but in fact the origin of the word "diet" comes from the ancient Greek word *dieta,* meaning "way of life." Knowing this piece of trivia, we no longer consider the word *diet* to be a four-letter word!

Modifying your behaviour

Changing your behaviour is a highly effective way to lose weight. In this section, we list some tried and true behaviour modification techniques. You needn't adopt all the following tips (though you're welcome to); adopting even a few of them can have a terrific impact. If you're looking to lose weight, try some of the following:

✔ When you're eating, shut off the TV, radio, computer, or any other electronic wizardry that may cause you to lose track of how much you're eating.

✔ Slow down your eating. Slowing down is easier if you wait until you've swallowed your last bite before putting more food in your mouth, and if you put your cutlery down between mouthfuls. As you do this, think about whether or not you're still hungry. Often even a brief pause for reflection will allow you to recognize sooner when you are full.

✔ Enjoy your food. Concentrate on the taste of each mouthful before you swallow.

✔ Use a small plate and try making a point of leaving some food over.

✔ When servings have been distributed, remove the serving dishes and bread basket from the table.

✔ Keep snacks and other treats out of sight or, even better, out of the house. Like they say, out of sight, out of mind.

Considering volumetrics

Another helpful technique to help you lose weight is to add bulk to your food; something that goes by the high falutin' name of *volumetrics*.

Hunger is often satisfied by increasing the volume of food even if the number of calories is reduced. Here are a few ways you can do this:

✔ Start your meals with a glass of water followed by a broth-based vegetable soup, like Veggie Soup (see Chapter 8).

✔ Eat a tossed salad with a small amount of light dressing, or eat raw vegetables and light dip.

✔ End your meal with diet Jell-O (or some other equivalent product).

Looking at ways your attempts at losing weight can be sabotaged

A whole bunch of factors can conspire against your best attempts to lose weight. Be on the lookout for these factors and fight back against them:

- ✔ **Having unrealistic expectations.** Losing 2 to 4 pounds (about 1 to 2 kg) per month is a sufficient goal and a lofty achievement. (The CDA recommends aiming to lose 5 to 10 percent of your initial body weight over 6 to 12 months.)

- ✔ **Not preparing a food shopping list.** Bringing a list with you to the store when you buy your groceries will help you avoid making last-minute impulse purchases of unhealthy foods.

- ✔ **Keeping the wrong foods in the house.** If your pantry is chock-a-block full of chips, cookies, sweets, and other treats, you're going to face constant temptation to eat those things, which are not going to help you lose weight. Instead, stock your pantry (and fridge) with healthy, less caloric treats.

- ✔ **Following an overly restrictive diet.** As we discuss in the section "Being skeptical about fad diets," most "diet books" advocate eating strategies that are overly restrictive (both in terms of the variety of foods they advocate and the number of calories they permit) and as a result eventually get abandoned.

- ✔ **Feeling hungry all the time.** If your nutrition program leaves you feeling hungry too often, it's pretty well guaranteed you're going to abandon your nutrition program. We sure would! A registered dietitian can set you up with a healthy eating program that won't leave you feeling hungry.

- ✔ **Skipping meals.** Skipping meals tends to make you overly hungry later in the day and to then overeat, thus undoing any calorie savings you've achieved by having missed a meal.

- ✔ **Pretending that snacks have no calories.** We will be the first to admit that this is our greatest personal foible. A chip here, a cookie there, and presto, hello extra belt notch. Oops, now how'd that happen? Having a snack isn't a bad thing — indeed it is often a good thing if you have diabetes; it's just that you need to include the calories that snacks contain in your nutrition program.

- ✔ **Letting loose on weekends.** We recommend that people living with diabetes feel free to occasionally indulge and eat some favourite treat like a bowl of ice cream or a piece of cake. That's not the same, however, as eating like a saint Monday to Friday and eating indiscriminately all weekend because, well, it's the weekend. Excess calories cause the same amount of weight gain if you eat them on Saturday as if you eat them on Monday. Rats.

✔ **Feeling that an indiscriminate nibble has "wrecked the day."** If you've eaten something you know to be unhealthy, that doesn't mean the "day is shot" and you may as well go ahead and eat whatever you want the rest of the day. Each calorie counts, so if you've nibbled on something you shouldn't have, forget about it and simply get back on track. And don't feel guilty! Life happens, after all.

✔ **Ignoring the impact of exercise.** As we discuss in Chapter 1, exercise in conjunction with nutrition therapy can play a very helpful role in helping you lose weight.

✔ **Not rewarding yourself.** Losing weight is a hard-fought battle. If you win — even if it's a small, few-pounds victory — reward yourself. How about a trip to the store to buy those new shoes or that new golf club you've been eyeing?

Diabetes and the Glycemic Index

All carbohydrates aren't alike in the degree to which they raise blood glucose. This fact was recognized some years ago, and a measurement called the *glycemic index* was created to quantify the amount that each food raises blood glucose. The glycemic index (GI) uses oral glucose as the standard (or indicator) food and assigns it a value of 100. Another food containing an equal amount of carbohydrate is rated according to its capability to raise blood glucose and is assigned a value in comparison to oral glucose. A food that raises glucose one quarter as much as oral glucose has a GI of 25, while a food that raises glucose three quarters as much has a GI of 75. A glycemic index of 70 or more is considered high; 56 to 69 is medium; and 55 or less is low. The point of the index is to select carbohydrates with low GI levels to try to keep the glucose response as low as possible.

Choosing carbohydrates with a low glycemic index can help to improve blood glucose control (and lipids). You might think, therefore, that you should make a concerted effort to choose low-GI foods. Alas, the story is much more complicated:

✔ The GI of a carbohydrate-containing food may be different when it is eaten alone than when it is part of a mixed meal.

✔ The GI of a food may differ depending on how it's processed and prepared.

✔ Some low-GI foods contain a lot of fat.

✔ Figuring out the GI can be difficult and can lead to confusion.

We can think of no better illustration of the fact that a low GI food is not automatically a good food choice than this: A Snickers candy bar rates better on the GI than a bowl of cornflakes. (We are not making this up!) Does the fact that a Snickers bar has a better GI than cornflakes make it a better food choice? Of course not! The glycemic index, in and of itself, doesn't make a food choice healthy or good. The GI is just one component among many (as we discuss in this chapter) that determines if a particular food is a good choice.

Because following a low glycemic index diet can help control blood glucose and lipids, the Canadian Diabetes Association recommends following a low GI diet: however, given the challenges of following a low GI diet, the CDA wisely notes that this "should be based on the individual's interest and ability."

Healthy Eating if You Have Gestational Diabetes

Gestational diabetes is treated primarily with a nutrition program (see Chapter 1 for more information about gestational diabetes). Exercise, such as going for a daily walk, is also helpful. If you've been diagnosed with gestational diabetes, your doctor should refer you to a registered dietitian who can share with you the key dietary strategies to help you control your blood glucose, allow you to gain an appropriate amount of weight, and keep your developing fetus growing normally.

These are the key components of the nutrition program used to treat gestational diabetes:

- ✔ Three appropriately spaced meals per day.

- ✔ Two to three snacks per day (mid-morning, mid-afternoon, bedtime).

- ✔ Moderate carbohydrate restriction. Your dietitian will advise you as to the appropriate number of grams of carbohydrate that is best for you and how to divide your carbohydrates up into your various meals and snacks.

- ✔ An appropriate number of calories to provide sufficient nutrition to you and your fetus. You will likely be asked to check your urine every day to see if a substance called ketones is present. If ketones are present, you should let your dietitian or your doctor know as this may indicate that you're not eating sufficiently well or that your diet needs some other change.

If nutrition therapy and exercise aren't sufficient to keep your blood glucose levels within target, medication — most commonly insulin — is used.

The Lowdown on High Blood Pressure and Nutrition

High blood pressure *(hypertension)* is one of the most common chronic medical conditions in our society. Although medical science doesn't know for certain why most people with hypertension develop this condition, genetics (as is so often the case with chronic diseases) plays a role. Evidence also suggests that excess salt consumption is a factor.

Having well-controlled blood pressure is essential if you have diabetes. Insufficiently controlled blood pressure increases your risk of stroke, heart attack, retinopathy, kidney damage, and other complications. If you have diabetes your target blood pressure is less than 130/80.

Reducing your salt (sodium) intake is a key dietary step in controlling your blood pressure. Most of the sodium in your diet probably comes from canned and processed foods. Your daily sodium intake should be no more than 1,500 mg to 2,300 mg. One teaspoon (5 ml) of salt contains 2,300 mg of sodium.

Here are ways you can reduce your salt consumption:

✔ Buy foods that are low in sodium, are unsalted, or have no added salt. Read the food labels and avoid foods that have a sodium content of "15% Daily Value" or more. Even better, aim for 5% Daily Value or less. (We discuss food labels in detail in Chapter 6.)

✔ Avoid adding salt during cooking.

✔ Avoid adding salt to your cooked food. (Avoid temptation; don't put the salt shaker on the table.)

✔ Spice up your life with a delicious variety of herbs, spices, and other seasonings.

✔ Rinse canned legumes with water.

✔ Avoid seasonings like garlic salt, celery salt, and MSG (monosodium glutamate).

Each recipe in this book is lower in sodium and has the sodium content listed for your convenience.

Here are other measures to help you lower your blood pressure:

✔ Limit your alcohol consumption. (See Chapter 3.)

✔ Exercise regularly. (See Chapter 1.)

✔ If you are overweight, work toward shedding the extra pounds.

✔ If stress may be a contributory factor, undertake stress reduction measures.

✔ Take blood pressure ("anti-hypertensive") medications as prescribed by your physician. The preferred drugs are typically those from the *ACE inhibitor* or *ARB* families.

Helping Control Your Lipids with Nutrition

As we discuss in Chapter 2, having excellent lipids (including cholesterol and triglycerides) reduces your risk of certain types of diabetes complications, including heart attack or stroke.

Here are ways of improving your lipids:

✔ Avoid eating saturated fats, such as butter and hard margarine, and trans fatty acids such as hydrogenated oils, fried foods, and vegetable shortening.

✔ Eat soluble fibre including psyllium powder and lima beans.

✔ Consume foods rich in omega-3 fatty acids, like Atlantic or Chinook salmon and herring.

✔ Take medication as prescribed by your physician. *Statins* are the preferred class of drug. Statins' main effect is to lower LDL cholesterol.

Nutrition Strategies if You Have Kidney Failure

The kidneys perform a wide variety of functions, including helping regulate the body's salt, fluid, and mineral balance; ridding the body of certain waste products; influencing blood pressure control; and affecting the production of red blood cells (by the bone marrow).

Diabetes can lead to kidney damage or even kidney failure (which, if severe enough, requires dialysis). Having kidney failure puts you at risk of accumulating excess amounts of a number of substances in your body, including these:

- Sodium, which contributes to high blood pressure, swelling *(edema),* and, if you have heart disease, *heart failure*
- Potassium, which can lead to heart rhythm problems
- Phosphorous, which can cause a type of bone damage *(osteomalacia)*

That's the bad news. The good news is that you can drastically reduce your risk of running into kidney damage by keeping your blood glucose and blood pressure well controlled. In Chapters 1 and 2, we look in detail at the various measures you can use to keep your blood glucose and blood pressure well controlled. The recipes in this book were specifically created to assist you with achieving these goals.

If you have kidney failure, your doctor will arrange for you to meet with a dietitian who will teach you how to avoid foods that are rich in potassium, phosphorous, and sodium (and, in some situations, may also instruct you to restrict the amount of protein you consume).

To help you keep track of how much potassium, phosphorous, and sodium you are consuming, in the recipes in *Diabetes Cookbook For Canadians For Dummies* we note how much of each of these substances is present in a serving. (This will help you if, for example, you are keeping track of the amount of sodium you consume per day.)

The recipes in this book are lower in sodium because we know that so many people with diabetes, even if they do not have kidney failure, are watching their sodium intake to either avoid, or to treat, high blood pressure. The general goal for Canadians is to consume no more than 1,500 to 2,300 milligrams per day of sodium.

Part II
Cooking and Meal-Planning Essentials

Nutrition Facts
Valeur nutritive
Per 125 mL (87 g) / par 125 mL (87 g)

Amount Teneur	% Daily Value % valuer quotidienne
Calories / Calories 80	
Fat / Lipides 0.5 g	**1**%
Saturated / saturés 0 g + Trans / trans 0 g	**0**%
Cholesterol / Cholestérol 0 mg	
Sodium / Sodium 0 mg	**0**%
Carbohydrate / Glucides 18 g	**6**%
Fibre / Fibres 2 g	**8**%
Sugars / Sucres 2 g	
Protein / Protéines 3 g	
Vitamin A / Vitamine A	2%
Vitamin C / Vitamine C	10%
Calcium / Calcium	0%
Iron / Fer	2%

For Dummies can help you get started with lots of subjects, including diabetes. Visit www.dummies.com to learn more and do more with *For Dummies*.

In this part . . .

Department and specialty stores are packed with countless must-have kitchen gadgets — but what do you really need? In this part we cover the essential cooking and baking supplies you'll need for your kitchen. And to make sure you put these supplies to good use, we look at effective food-shopping strategies and how to master label-reading.

Chapter 5

Getting Equipped

• •

• •

To do a job well, having the right equipment makes all the difference in the world. Whether it's Ian relying on his favourite stethoscope, Cynthia using her teaching food models and charts, or any other person, including you, who relies on tools to assist in doing things effectively and efficiently, having trusted equipment is invaluable. So, too, with cooking equipment, as we look at in this chapter.

But it's not only about the equipment. If you're going to be able to use your cooking tools to create the tasty recipes we describe in this book, familiarizing yourself with some cooking jargon will also be helpful. In this chapter, therefore, we define some key terms to help you in your culinary journey.

Covering Basic Cooking Equipment

Before starting to follow a recipe, you need the tools of the trade. If you can afford to spend some money to buy good-quality cooking products you will save money, time, and aggravation in the long run.

You will need kitchen utensils for measuring, mixing, cutting, and cooking. You'll also need pots and pans for the oven and the stove top, and microwave-friendly products, too. And, even though you're going to be cooking up delectable foods, no doubt you're going to also require containers for storing leftovers.

Pots, pans, and plates

Nothing's worse than having gotten all the ingredients home for a meal, only to realize you don't have the proper pots or pans to cook it in. That's why, if you can, you should have a wide array, like the following:

✔ Pans. It's a good idea to have a variety of sizes and types:

- 9-x-13-inch (22 × 32 cm) baking pan
- 9-x-5-inch (22 × 12 cm) loaf pan
- 8-x-8-inch (20 × 20 cm) square pan
- 8-inch (20 cm) diameter round pan
- Cookie sheet
- Jelly roll pan
- Muffin tin
- Pie plate
- Roasting pan

✔ Casserole dishes (of various sizes) with lids

✔ Frying pans/skillets with lids

✔ Mixing bowls — various sizes

✔ Pots with lids — various sizes

✔ Wok

Handy tools

The following tools are indispensable in any kitchen, and they'll make the task of preparing a meal so much easier:

✔ Basting brush

✔ Can opener

✔ Electric mixer/egg beater

✔ Garlic press

✔ Grater with various size holes

✔ Hand juicer

✔ Knives — paring, serrated (bread knife), French (chef's) knife

✔ Lifter for eggs and pancakes

✔ Measuring cups for dry and liquid ingredients

✔ Measuring spoons

✔ Meat thermometer

✔ Pastry blender

✔ Potato masher

- ✔ Rolling pin
- ✔ Scale — if weighing foods (as is often helpful when carbohydrate counting; see Chapter 1)
- ✔ Spatulas
- ✔ Spoons — metal, slotted, soup ladle, wooden
- ✔ Strainer/colander — large and small holes
- ✔ Timer
- ✔ Tongs
- ✔ Vegetable brush
- ✔ Vegetable peeler
- ✔ Whisk

Other useful equipment

Here's a grab-bag of stuff that no cook can live without:

- ✔ Aluminum foil
- ✔ Cooling rack made of wire
- ✔ Cutting boards
- ✔ Parchment paper
- ✔ Plastic wrap
- ✔ Storage containers for leftovers

Speaking the Cooking Lingo

The world of cooking has a jargon of its own. Here are definitions for some important cooking terms:

Al dente: Pasta that is cooked firm.

Baste: Periodically spooning or brushing liquid over the food during cooking to keep it moist.

Beat: To make a mixture creamy, smooth, or filled with air by whipping in a brisk motion with a spoon, whisk, or beater.

Blend: To mix two or more ingredients until they are smooth and uniform in consistency.

Boil: To heat until bubbles rise continuously and break on the surface.

Broil: To cook food by placing it on a rack that is directly under the source of heat. This is also referred to as *grilling*.

Brown: To cook until food changes to a brown colour to help seal in natural juices.

Chop: To cut food into small pieces with a knife or other small cutting appliance.

Cream: To whip or beat with a spoon, whisk, or electric mixer until a mixture is soft and fluffy.

Cut in: To use two knives or a pastry blender to add solid fat (such as butter, shortening, or lard) to dry ingredients.

Dice: To cut food into small cubes of uniform size and shape.

Fold: To gently combine ingredients by a combination of two motions: cutting vertically through the mixture and sliding the spatula across the bottom of the bowl and up the sides turning the ingredients over.

Fry or pan fry: To cook food in a small amount of hot fat or oil. (Also see *sauté*.)

Grate: To shred food by rubbing it over the holes of a grater.

Knead: To work and press dough with the heels of your hands so the dough becomes stretched and elastic.

Mix: To stir until all ingredients are distributed evenly.

Parboil: To boil until partially cooked.

Purée: To blend a food until it is smooth and of fine texture.

Sauté: To fry lightly and briefly over high heat, turning frequently.

Simmer: To cook in liquid just below the boiling point. Bubbles form slowly and break below the surface.

Steam: To cook on a rack or strainer over a small amount of boiling water in a tightly covered container.

Stir: To mix, usually with a spoon or spatula, in a circular or figure-8 motion.

Toss: To combine two or more ingredients lightly and gently, with a slight lifting motion.

Whip: To beat rapidly to incorporate air. This increases the volume and lightens the consistency of the ingredients.

Whisk: A looped wire utensil used for whipping by hand.

Zest: To remove the "coloured" peel of a citrus fruit with a grater, peeler, or zester.

Chapter 6

Successful Food Shopping

- -

In This Chapter

▶ Stocking up on staples

▶ Shopping wisely

▶ Planning menus

▶ Filling the pantry with food

▶ Decoding labels

- -

*L*ove it or hate it, grocery shopping is a fact of life for most people. And whether you're spending an hour in an acre-sized, all-purpose grocery store or making a quick dash into the local convenience store, knowing how to shop wisely will ensure you're getting the healthy, nutritious foods you need in the most economical way you can.

In this chapter, we look at how you can save money on your groceries, how you can shop effectively, and how you can decode those invaluable but sometimes confusing food labels.

Saving Money on Staples

Getting the most for your food dollar involves time and effort. In this section, we provide a whole raft of helpful tips to help you save money when you're buying food essentials.

Healthy nutrition is always important, and it's especially important if you're living with diabetes. If you're struggling to make ends meet and as a result you're unable to purchase healthy foods, you can get help by contacting your local food bank or food pantry, or contacting your local health unit.

Buying fruits and vegetables

When it comes to fruits and vegetables:

- ✔ **Buy your fruits and vegetables at roadside stands and farmers' markets.** The food will not only be less expensive, but it will also typically be very fresh.

- ✔ **Buy fresh fruits and vegetables that are in season.** Fruits and vegetables that are in season are typically less expensive — sometimes *much* less expensive — than fruits and vegetables that are out of season. (If you want fruits and vegetables that are out of season, get the frozen variety; they'll be far less expensive than their fresh counterparts.)

- ✔ **Consider root vegetables.** Potatoes, sweet potatoes, carrots, turnips, parsnips, and onions keep well and are often good bargains.

- ✔ **When buying juice, go for frozen.** Frozen juice concentrates are usually cheaper than boxed, bottled, or chilled juices.

- ✔ **Check the "reduced stand" in the produce section for "ripe" fruits and vegetables.** (Ripe bananas are great for the Banana Bread and Banana Chocolate Chip Muffins in this book.)

Moo-ving to the dairy section

Here are a couple of ways to save money when buying your dairy products:

- ✔ **Avoid expensive yogurt.** Buy low-fat plain yogurt and then add your own fruit to it. Add a sugar substitute if needed.

- ✔ **Buy big, if you can.** Purchase the largest size of light sour cream, light cottage cheese, or low-fat yogurt you can use before the expiry date.

Picking poultry

When you're in search of protein-rich foods, consider buying eggs. Although you should eat eggs in limited quantities because of their cholesterol content, you don't need to avoid them altogether, and they're an incredibly versatile food. Omega-3-rich eggs are available but are more expensive. (Omega-3 eggs contain omega-3 fatty acids; these types of fatty acids reduce the risk of heart disease.)

Because buying a whole chicken is typically cheaper than buying a similar amount of chicken in parts, consider buying a whole chicken and cutting it into parts yourself or roast the whole chicken and use leftovers. (We have a whole bunch of chicken dishes in this book. Spread your wings!)

Seeking alternate sources of protein

Beans are a good source of protein and carbohydrate, are low in fat, and have no cholesterol, and they're cheap to boot. In addition to buying fresh beans, buy some canned beans as well to keep on hand as backup for unexpected company. (Check out our helpful-in-a-pinch Mixed Bean Salad in the recipes section.) Baked beans are always handy to have on hand, too and they have a long shelf life. You can save money by purchasing dry beans, soaking and cooking them, then storing them in your freezer in small serving sizes.

When it comes to peanut butter . . . ah, sigh; peanut butter — Ian's all-time favourite food. Yes, well, when it comes to peanut butter, it's a good source of protein and is not overly expensive. Remember to check the ingredient list of the peanut butter you're buying as you want to avoid those many brands that have sugar and salt added.

When looking for an economical source of protein, consider buying tofu (also known as soybean curd; we think "tofu" sounds much more appetizing). You can use tofu to quickly prepare the Vegetarian Curry Tofu with Noodles recipe in this book.

Going fishing

Fish are healthy to eat. Heck, even other fish know that. Alaskan pollock and Boston bluefish are cheaper alternatives to haddock and cod. Don't forget to stock up on water-packed canned tuna and salmon when they're on sale.

Smart Shopping

Everyone has his or her own particular preferences when it comes to shopping, but we all want to be smart shoppers. In this section, we offer some shopping techniques that will help you be an efficient and thrifty shopper.

Here's Cynthia's shopping strategy: When possible, she buys her fresh fruits and vegetables at the local farmers' market and roadside stands. She buys spices at the bulk food store. Cynthia purchases her non-perishable foods and toiletries at big box stores. And she does the rest of her food shopping at one of a variety of local grocery stores (depending on who has the best prices on whatever goods she needs).

Plan your week's menu ahead of time

Planning your week's menus *before* you shop will save you time *when* you shop because you will know specifically what you're looking for rather than trying to think through a whole raft of meals while you're shopping.

Another advantage to planning your meals in advance is that it may help you save money because you're buying food for many meals at a time so you'll be buying some of your food in bulk, which, as we discuss earlier in this chapter, typically offers cost savings.

Another way planning your week's menus ahead of time can save you money is that, with more food on hand from your grocery store trip, you will be less in need of last-minute trips to more expensive convenience stores.

Make a list

Making a list of the foods you need will help you avoid the temptation of impulse purchases. A list will also help save you time when you're at the grocery store as it will make you a more efficient shopper.

Make your list of needed foods after you've planned out your week's menus (see the preceding section). If you're going to be preparing one or more of the recipes in this book — and we sure hope you will! — be sure to write down the types and amounts of the different ingredients you'll require so that you can be sure to pick up what you need at the grocery store. Keep your grocery list on your fridge door or another convenient spot in the kitchen and update it every time you run out of an item.

Consider organizing your grocery list according to one of the following:

- **Food groups:** Cynthia uses this strategy as it helps her ensure she won't forget any important foods and it's a quick way to add foods to the grocery list through the week. Also, she doesn't always shop at the same grocery store.

- **Grocery store layout:** This will help you stay organized when you're in the store.

Bring a pencil to cross off the items on your grocery list as you add them to your cart. Stick to your grocery list, but be flexible to take advantage of in-store bargains.

Estimate your food needs

Try to estimate how much food you'll need because large or "bonus sized" products or bulk products end up being no bargain if you have to throw away half of what you bought because it's spoiled. Buy the size that is most economical and convenient for you.

Be a grocery-store guru

Navigating through a grocery store is sometimes like playing chess, trying to figure out what moves will help you succeed in your food shopping quest and what moves will end up costing you (literally). Here are some helpful tips to help you keep more of your hard-earned money in your pocket:

- **Eat before you shop.** Having hunger pains as you walk the aisles makes you more likely to make non-essential impulse purchases. Trust us on this one; we know from personal experience!

- **Look for specials.** Grocery stores often have specials or promotions. Keep an eye out for these in your newspaper and in flyers.

- **Shop around.** Check out the stores in your community and compare their prices. Certain stores or chains often feature better prices than other stores. You may, however, find that some stores offer lower prices than a competitor for some types of products and higher prices for others. If so, you'll need to decide if it's worth your while to make trips to multiple stores.

- **Use coupons.** Many companies offer coupons that will allow you to get a reduced price on the item you're buying. Check your newspaper, store flyers, or magazines. (Cynthia recently saved $17 by using coupons during a trip to the grocery store. The man behind her in the line was getting a little impatient, but when she told him how much she saved, his mouth dropped and he asked her for advice about where to get the coupons!)

- **Leave the kids at home (if and when you can).** Kids are kids. And that means as they walk (or ride) the grocery store with you they will want you to buy many of the treats they see advertised on TV. (And sometimes, unbeknownst to you, they will take even greater initiative and put things in the cart themselves, as Ian's wife discovered years ago when she was checking out of the grocery store and found the cashier ringing up four boxes of condoms that their 3-year-old daughter had added to the cart!)

✔ **Bring reusable grocery bags with you.** In some areas of Canada, stores are now obliged by governments (as part of environmental initiatives) to charge you for the plastic grocery bags they provide you. Avoid this cost by bringing your own reusable bags.

✔ **Plan your path.** Grocery stores are designed with essential items such as milk and bread in the back of the store, which obliges you to walk past all sorts of tempting but non-essential items that call out "choose me, choose me," in order for you to get to these staples.

One way of dealing with this situation is, in advance of your trip to the grocery store, to think through where the location is of each of the different items you need to buy. Then, mental map in mind, you can navigate the grocery store purposefully, which will make you less tempted by the siren song of enticing but unnecessary purchases.

✔ **Read the unit price labels.** Hmm, there's an 850 gram box of cereal selling for $4.75 and there's a 333 gram bag of the same cereal selling for $1.90. Which is the better deal? Not so easy to figure out without a calculator (and some patience); far easier to look at the unit price label affixed to the shelf and check the per unit cost of an item.

✔ **Buy store-brand goods.** Most large grocery stores carry their own brands. These are typically less expensive than, and just as tasty and nutritious as, name brands. (You might be surprised to know that many store-brand goods are made by the same companies that make name brands; often the only difference is the packaging!)

✔ **Avoid prepared and prepackaged foods.** Prepared rice and pasta dishes, for example, are often higher in calories, sodium, and fat than comparable rice and pasta that you prepare yourself at home. (The recipes in this book are all healthy choices, low in fat and sodium, and are cheaper than prepared foods.)

✔ **Don't be fooled by where the item is located in the store.** Items typically sell better if they are placed in prime locations like the end of an aisle where they are often placed in large stacks, giving the impression that they are on promotion or on sale. This is, in fact, often not the case. Also, more expensive foods are often placed on the shelves at eye level; be sure, therefore, to scan above or below eye level to find less costly items.

✔ **Don't check out the items in the checkout line.** Magazines, chocolate bars, candies, and other non-essentials are invariably placed at the checkout line to encourage impulse buying. Resisting the temptation to buy such items can be tough, especially when you're stuck in a lineup. Tough, yes, but doable.

Buy in bulk

Foods bought in bulk are typically much cheaper on a per unit basis (or per unit of weight basis) than food bought in conventional amounts. If you don't have a place to store bulk purchases or you simply don't have need for bulk purchases, consider partnering with friends and neighbours for these purchases and then divide up the goods (and the savings!). By buying in bulk you will be able to save money on your purchases of chicken, pork, beef, vegetables, and fruits.

Peruse the perishables

Here are some tips about buying perishable foods:

- ✔ **Buy only what you can use.** Rather than buying too much fresh produce only to see it wilt and spoil in your fridge, buy only what you can reasonably expect to use before your next trip to the grocery store.

- ✔ **Check the "best before" date.** The items that have the longest best before date are typically at the back of the shelf, so you may have to reeeaaaach way back for them.

- ✔ **Consider buying frozen vegetables.** Sometimes buying only fresh produce is simply not practical. Having frozen vegetables can be very handy when you want to be able to prepare small quantities.

- ✔ **Purchase your perishable foods last.** That way they'll have the shortest period of time out of the refrigerator as you complete your shopping and then make your way home.

Menu Planning

Planning your meals will help ensure you get the right amounts of the right nutrients. It will also help spare you — or at least help reduce the need for — last-minute scrambling to get a meal together.

When estimating how much food you'll need for an individual meal, use the plate method: half the plate should be vegetables, one quarter should be high fibre grains, and the last quarter should be a lean protein. Accompany the plate with a piece of fruit and a glass of milk or a yogurt and, voilà, balanced to perfection!

As you go about planning your menus, sit down with a piece of paper and write out ideas of what you would like to eat. Look at what you have on hand and in the freezer that needs to be used up and use this as a guide. Also, plan your menus around weekly specials at the grocery store by scanning your flyers or newspapers. Keep a close eye out for discount coupons.

Several helpful resources are available to help you with meal planning, including *Eating Well with Canada's Food Guide* (we discuss this resource in Chapter 2), and the Canadian Diabetes Association's *Just the Basics* and *Beyond the Basics*. And, of course, you can use this book! (Appendix B offers you an entire month of menus.)

Choose a variety of foods from the different food groups. Variety is the secret to eating well and will also help ensure you are getting the whole range of vitamins, minerals, and fibre you require. We encourage you to expand your taste buds' horizons by sampling from the wide range of this book's recipes.

As you go about planning your menus, keep in mind one of Cynthia's favourite maxims: Cook once, eat twice. In other words, plan on doing some "batch cooking" or doubling a recipe. You can freeze the extra food for another day when you're even more rushed than usual or just want a break from cooking. Remember to label and date the items you're storing in the freezer.

Pantry (Non-perishable) Essentials: What to Have on Hand

There are certain non-perishable essentials that most people will want to always have on hand because they're commonly used in recipes. Having them available enables you to make a quick meal. We discuss these non-perishable essentials in this section.

If you have limited kitchen space, keep the extra food in a hall closet in well-sealed containers. Don't have room in your hall closet? Try finding space under your bed.

Frozen and canned fruits and vegetables

Although nothing beats fresh fruits and vegetables, having the following frozen and canned items in your house is helpful:

- ✔ Frozen fruit. In Ian's house, there are often a few leftover bananas in the freezer ready for making banana bread.

- ✔ Canned, unsweetened fruit. Make a point of buying the canned fruit that says "in its own juice" or "no sugar added."

- ✔ Frozen, unsweetened fruit juice

- ✔ Frozen vegetables

- ✔ Canned, low-sodium vegetables

- ✔ Canned, low-sodium vegetable soup

Grains

Here are important grains for you to keep on hand in your home:

- ✔ Oatmeal

- ✔ High-fibre dry cereal

- ✔ Flour

- ✔ Whole-grain bread. Keep this well wrapped (to avoid freezer burn) in your freezer.

- ✔ Whole-grain pasta

- ✔ Other grains, such as rice, couscous, barley, bulgur, and quinoa

Other nutrients

Here are some other non-perishable foods that are good to have in the home:

- ✔ Canned tuna or salmon

- ✔ Canola oil and/or olive oil

- ✔ Dried or canned legumes, lentils, or beans

- ✔ Skim milk powder

- ✔ Peanut butter

Baking and cooking ingredients

Here are some cooking ingredients that are helpful to keep in the home:

- ✔ Baking powder
- ✔ Baking soda
- ✔ Low-sodium broth
- ✔ Cornstarch
- ✔ Pepper
- ✔ Salt
- ✔ Spices and dried herbs you commonly use (these might include cinnamon, thyme, basil, oregano, and others)
- ✔ Sugar
- ✔ Sugar substitute (artificial sweetener)

Reading Labels and Knowing How to Use Them

Nutrition labelling is mandatory in Canada on all packaged foods. Being familiar with nutrition labels is very important as understanding these labels will allow you to make wise food choices.

These are the three components of nutrition labelling:

- ✔ The list of ingredients, which, as you might expect, lists the types of ingredients in a product.
- ✔ The Nutrition Facts table tells you the amounts of certain key ingredients in a product.
- ✔ Nutrition and health claims, which are those brief banners you see on a package that claim the product has a special nutrition or health value.

In the following sections, we look at each of these three important aspects of food labelling.

The list of ingredients

The list of ingredients (see Figure 6-1 for an example of such a list) notes the constituents of a product. (If you're like us, at times you'll find yourself surprised to see how much an otherwise healthy product has of an unexpected ingredient like sugar or oil.)

The items are listed in descending order by weight. Therefore, the first item in the list is present in the product in the greatest amount by weight, the second item in the list is present in the second greatest amount by weight, and so on. In other words, the list of ingredients tells you both the ingredients in a product and their relative amounts.

Although the list of ingredients doesn't tell you the actual (absolute) amount of a product's ingredients (this information is revealed in the Nutrition Facts table, which we discuss in a moment), it does give a pretty good sense of whether the product contains lots or little of a substance. For example, if salt (sodium) is listed as one of the first three ingredients in the list, the product is probably fairly rich in sodium.

Another important role of the list of ingredients is to help people who have food allergies to identify whether a product contains the food they're allergic to. Also, people who avoid certain foods because of religious or other beliefs are able to determine whether the product contains these ingredients.

INGREDIENTS: TOMATOES, TOMATO JUICE, SUGAR, SALT, SEASONING (CONTAINS ONION AND GARLIC POWDERS), CALCIUM CHLORIDE, CITRIC ACID.

Figure 6-1:
An example
of a list of
ingredients.

INGRÉDIENTS: TOMATES, JUS DE TOMATES, SUCRE, SEL, ASSAISONNEMENT (CONTIENT DES POUDRES D'OIGNON ET D'AIL), CHLORURE DE CALCIUM, ACIDE CITRIQUE.

The Nutrition Facts table

The Nutrition Facts table (see Figure 6-2) lists the actual (absolute) amount of calories and 13 core nutrients contained in a product. The Nutrition Facts can be used to compare products, determine the nutrient value of foods, better manage special diets (including a diabetes nutrition program), and help you increase or decrease your intake of a particular nutrient.

Nutrition Facts
Valeur nutritive
Per 125 mL (87 g) / par 125 mL (87 g)

Amount Teneur	% Daily Value % valeur quotidienne
Calories / Calories 80	
Fat / Lipides 0.5 g	1 %
Saturated / saturés 0 g + Trans / trans 0 g	0 %
Cholesterol / Cholestérol 0 mg	
Sodium / Sodium 0 mg	0 %
Carbohydrate / Glucides 18 g	6 %
Fibre / Fibres 2 g	8 %
Sugars / Sucres 2 g	
Protein / Protéines 3 g	
Vitamin A / Vitamine A	2 %
Vitamin C / Vitamine C	10 %
Calcium / Calcium	0 %
Iron / Fer	2 %

Figure 6-2:
An example
of a
Nutrition
Facts table.

Regardless of the product, the table has a consistent look. This is very help-ful as it facilitates comparing the ingredients contained in different products. In this section, we look in detail at the features of the Nutrition Facts table.

Not all foods have a Nutrition Facts table. These are some exempt:

✓ Fresh fruits and vegetables

✓ Raw meat, poultry, fish, and seafood

✓ Foods that are prepared or processed in the store; for example, bakery items and salads

✓ Foods that have very few or no nutrients, such as coffee, tea, and spices

✓ Alcohol-containing beverages

Here's a look at what the listings in the Nutrition Facts table mean, and what you should watch for:

✓ **Serving size:** The serving size is noted immediately under the words "Nutrition Facts." The serving size is *the manufacturer's* estimated amount of the product that one person will eat at one time. This amount may differ significantly from recommendations found in Canada's Food Guide or the Canadian Diabetes Association's *Beyond the Basics* food chart.

If you eat twice the serving size written on the box, then you are, of course, eating twice the amount of *all* the ingredients listed on the Nutrition Facts table for one serving; that is, twice the number of calories, twice the amount of sodium and fibre, and so on.

✔ **% (Percentage) Daily Value:** The % Daily Value lets you quickly see if a product has a little or a lot of a particular nutrient. More specifically, the % Daily Value indicates what percentage of your daily requirements for a given nutrient, based on a 2,000-calorie-per-day diet, is present in one serving. If the percentage of something healthy, like calcium, is high, then, well, that's good. On the other hand, if a product has a high % Daily Value of something you want to minimize, like sodium, then you will want to avoid this product or, at the very least, you will want to consume significantly less than the stated serving size. *Of the 13 core nutrients, 5 percent Daily Value represents a little and 15 percent Daily Value represents a lot of a nutrient.*

Daily values are based on Canadian standards set for overall health outcomes and are aimed at reducing the risk of nutrition-related chronic diseases such as diabetes.

✔ **Calories:** This is the number of calories present in one serving size.

✔ **Fat:** This section notes both the amount of saturated fats and of trans fat (trans fatty acids). If the number of grams of saturated and trans fat do not equal the total fat, then the remainder are polyunsaturated and monounsaturated fats (these don't legally have to be listed on the label). Aim for a % Daily Value of 5 percent or less, signifying a healthier, low fat choice.

✔ **Cholesterol:** A product may or may not have a % Daily Value listed for cholesterol. A product that has a low % Daily Value for saturated fat and trans fat will also have a low % Daily Value for cholesterol. A product with a % Daily Value of 5 percent or less would be considered low in cholesterol.

✔ **Sodium:** A % Daily Value of 5 percent or less for sodium indicates the product is low in sodium.

✔ **Carbohydrates:** This section notes the total amount of carbohydrates in the product, including fibre, sugars, and sugar alcohols. Note these important points about the Nutrition Facts listing for carbohydrates:

   • If you're looking for a cereal with a high fibre content, look for one that has over 15 percent Daily Value listed for fibre (or 4 grams or more of fibre per serving). As we discuss in Chapter 1, although fibre is a carbohydrate, you do not include it in your calculations if you're carbohydrate counting; instead, you subtract the number of grams of fibre from the total number of grams of carbohydrate being ingested. This remainder is called the "available carbohydrate." The recipes in this book list the available carbohydrate per serving.

- The Nutrition Facts table lists sugar available from *all* sources — including both naturally occurring and added sugars. No % Daily Value is listed for sugars because no agreed-upon guidelines exist for the amount that a healthy Canadian population should consume.

- Sugar alcohols, as we discuss in Chapter 3, have no significant effect on raising blood glucose levels.

✔ **Protein:** No % Daily Value is listed for protein. Canadians seldom consume insufficient amounts of protein.

✔ **Vitamin A:** A % Daily Value is listed for vitamin A, but not an absolute amount. A % Daily Value of 15 percent or more for vitamin A indicates that a product contains a high amount of this vitamin.

✔ **Vitamin C:** Like vitamin A, a % Daily Value is listed for vitamin C, but not an absolute amount. A % Daily Value of 15 percent or more indicates that a product is a good source of vitamin C.

✔ **Calcium:** A % Daily Value of 15 percent or more for calcium indicates that the product is a high in calcium.

✔ **Iron:** A % Daily Value is listed for iron, but not an absolute amount. A % Daily Value above 15 percent means a product is a good source of iron.

If a product has a nutrient claim (we discuss nutrient claims in the next section) for an ingredient that is not normally part of the Nutrition Facts table, then the manufacturer must add this other ingredient's name and amount to the table. For example, if a manufacturer stated that a particular product was high in folate, then it would have to list folate on the Nutrition Facts table along with the amount of folate.

For more information on nutrition labelling, talk to your registered dietitian or surf on over to Health Canada (www.hc-sc.gc.ca), the Dietitians of Canada (www.dietitians.ca), or the Canadian Diabetes Association (www.diabetes.ca).

Nutrition and health claims

Nutrition and health claims are those very brief banners or phrases that adorn a package and that state the product offers a special nutritional or health benefit.

Nutrition claims

Nutrition claims typically include words such as

- Free
- Low
- Less
- More
- Reduced
- Lower
- Very high
- Light/lite
- Source of, high source of, good source of, or excellent source of

Nutrition claims are subject to Health Canada regulation. The government currently allows over 40 nutrition claims (including those listed above). If a manufacturer determines that a food meets the government criteria for a nutrition claim, the *manufacturer* then decides whether or not it wants to put the claim on the package. The absence of nutrition claim doesn't necessarily mean that the product doesn't possess these nutrition attributes; it may simply mean that the manufacturer, for whatever reason, elected not to put the claim on the label.

It does not take much stretch of the imagination to conclude that a manufacturer is more likely to put a nutrition claim on a package if it believes the claim will help the product sell.

As Health Canada (www.hc-sc.gc.ca/fn-an/label-etiquet/nutrition/ cons/information_tips-informations_pratiques-eng.php) says — and with which we completely agree — "Use nutrition claims as a starting point, but do not rely only on them to make comparisons. Use the Nutrition Facts to get the full details."

Here are examples that Health Canada helpfully uses to illustrate how to interpret nutrition claims when you are trying to *decrease* the amount of certain nutrients in your diet:

- "Free" means the food contains none or almost none of a nutrient (for example, "sodium-free").
- "Low" means the food contains only a small amount (for example, "low fat").
- "Reduced" means the food contains at least 25 percent less of the nutrient than a similar product (for example, "reduced in calories").

"Light" (or "lite") means, well, we're never really certain what it means. Indeed, it seems to us the term "light" gets thrown around with relative abandon. Heck, sometimes it seems that half the products in the marketplace carry the label "light." Anyhow, Health Canada notes that the word "light" is "only allowed on labels of foods that are 'reduced in fat' or 'reduced in calories'" but that "it could also refer to the sensory characteristics of the food such as "'light in colour.'" When it comes to the word "light" we often feel we're groping in the dark. Our advice: Take the word "light" on a food label with a grain of salt, in a manner of speaking.

Here are examples that Health Canada uses to illustrate how to interpret nutrition claims when you are trying to *increase* the amount of certain nutrients in your diet:

- "Source" means the food contains a useful amount of the nutrient (for example, "source of fibre").

- "High or good source" means the food contains a high amount of the nutrient (for example, "high source of vitamin C").

- "Very high or excellent source" means that the food contains a very high amount of the nutrient (for example, "excellent source of calcium").

Health claims

Health Canada notes (on the same web page we mention in the preceding section) that manufacturers are allowed to place the following health claims on packaging, when appropriate:

- A healthy diet low in saturated and trans fats may reduce the risk of heart disease.

- A healthy diet with adequate calcium and vitamin D, and regular physical activity, help to achieve strong bones and may reduce the risk of osteoporosis.

- A healthy diet rich in vegetables and fruit may help reduce the risk of some types of cancer.

- A healthy diet containing foods high in potassium and low in sodium may reduce the risk of high blood pressure, a risk factor for stroke and heart disease.

Part III
Healthy Eating: Natural, Nutritious Recipes

☺ *Shake Me Up Shake!*

This smoothie can be made in the evening and kept in the refrigerator in a covered bowl or glass for a quick, ready-to-go breakfast the next day. Stir well in the morning.

Preparation Time: *10 minutes*

Yield: *2 servings*

1 cup (250 ml) 1% milk

¾ cup (175 ml) raspberries

½ banana

¼ cup (50 ml) vanilla yogurt, low fat

1 tsp (5 ml) grated lemon zest

1 tbsp (15 ml) ground flaxseed

1½ tsp (7 ml) honey

In a blender, combine the ingredients and mix on high until smooth. If you don't have a blender, use a potato masher to purée the raspberries and banana in a bowl, add the rest of the ingredients to the bowl and mix vigorously with a spoon. For each serving, pour 1 cup (250 ml) into a glass. Enjoy.

Per Serving: *(1 cup/250 ml) Calories 193; Available carbohydrate 26 g; Carbohydrate 34 g; Fibre 8 g; Fat 4 g; Protein 8 g; Cholesterol 8 mg; Phosphorus 220 mg; Potassium 523 mg; Sodium 77 mg.*

1 Serving = 2 Carbohydrate Choices

In this part . . .

Whether you're looking for a quick breakfast before you fly out the door; an exquisite entree for a leisurely, romantic dinner; or anything in between, if it's food and it's tasty and healthy, this is the place you'll discover how to prepare it.

Chapter 7

Rise and Shine with Breakfast

*Y*our mother (or father, of course) was right; breakfast is the most important meal of the day. Breakfast provides you with the fuel your body needs to supply the physical and mental energy you require to start your day. Not surprisingly, eating breakfast improves productivity, whether in the home or in the workplace. As important as breakfast is for adults, it's doubly important for youngsters. Studies have shown that children who eat breakfast have better memory skills, enhanced ability to concentrate, improved school attendance, and better school grades. Children who consistently eat breakfast also do better in physical sports and even have better hand-eye coordination.

Regularly eating a healthy breakfast (not that common Canadian breakfast tradition of a donut or large muffin) makes it more likely that a person will have a healthy body weight. This is an especially important benefit if you have diabetes and also have challenges with overweight.

Another benefit of eating breakfast if you have diabetes is that you'll be less likely to snack excessively, so you're distributing your carbohydrates over three meals, which helps with blood glucose control. Eating breakfast will also make you less likely to have hypoglycemia if you're taking medicine such as insulin or glyburide that has the potential to cause low blood glucose.

Hopefully at this point if you needed any convincing we've won you over and you're now committed to regularly eating a healthy breakfast. Now it's just a matter of figuring out how you're going to fit eating breakfast into your hectic schedule. Fortunately, this *can* be done. In this chapter, we provide some quick and easy breakfast recipes to allow you to get you and your family up and running pronto. We also present some more elaborate breakfast recipes for those occasions when you've got a bit more time available.

Quick, Healthy Breakfast Ideas

When you're on the run and need a quick but nutritious breakfast, here are some healthy options for you to choose:

- A cheese stick, ½ cup (125 ml) grapes, and 1 cup (250 ml) low-fat milk

- 1–2 tbsp (15–30 ml) peanut butter with a small banana in a whole wheat tortilla

- A high-fibre granola bar, a medium apple, and 1 cup (250 ml) of low-fat milk

- ½ cup (125 ml) applesauce, ¼ cup (50 ml) All-Bran Buds, and ¼ cup (50 ml) sliced almonds

- Parfait of ¾ cup (175 ml) artificially sweetened yogurt, ¼ cup (50 ml) high-fibre cereal, and ½ cup (125 ml) fruit

- A medium apple, 1 oz (30 g) low-fat cheddar cheese, and a yogurt drink

- ¼–½ cup (50–125 ml) low-fat ricotta cheese with 1 cup (250 ml) cantaloupe and ¼ cup (50 ml) sliced almonds

- 1 slice whole grain toast with a boiled egg you made last night and stored in the refrigerator and a sliced tomato

- 4 pieces of melba toast, 1–2 tbsp (15–30 ml) peanut butter, and ½ cup (125 ml) probiotic yogurt drink

- A commercially available, diabetes-friendly meal replacement milkshake (We suggest you use these only on occasion.)

Breakfast foods to avoid

As tempting as they sometimes may be, the following breakfast choices are best avoided because they're less nutritious and often provide excess calories and fat compared with the healthier choices we offer in this chapter:

- Large bagels and cream cheese

- Large muffins

- Sausage and egg on tea biscuits

- Sugary cereals lacking in fibre

- Pastries

- Croissants

- Toaster pastries

- Frozen pancakes, French toast, or waffles

Fruit First

A *smoothie* can be a good breakfast choice when time is limited. A smoothie is a thick drink made in the blender from natural ingredients like fresh or frozen fruit, free of additives and preservatives, and resembling a low-fat version of a milkshake. Smoothies have plenty of health benefits; they're

- ✔ Low in calories (depending on how you make it)
- ✔ Full of vitamins and a source of calcium
- ✔ A better source of fibre than juice

Although smoothies can be a good breakfast option, they do have some drawbacks. Smoothies

- ✔ Can be very high in carbohydrate because they typically contain lots of fruit. (Consuming excess carbohydrates will raise your blood glucose — see Chapter 2 for more.)
- ✔ Often contain little protein.
- ✔ May not be as filling as solid foods, and may leave you hungry or consuming too much of the blended drink.

In this section, you find two nutritious and tasty smoothie recipes.

🍅 Mango, Orange, Banana Smoothie

This is a tasty smoothie, but remember that smoothies are generally high in carbohydrates because they're full of fruit, yogurt, and milk.

Preparation Time: *8 minutes*

Yield: *2 servings*

1 banana, small	¼ cup (50 ml) low-fat vanilla yogurt
¼ cup (50 ml) mango	1 tbsp (15 ml) ground flaxseed
⅓ cup (75 ml) orange juice	1 cup (250 ml) 1% milk

In a blender, combine the ingredients and mix on high until smooth. If you don't have a blender, use a potato masher to purée the mango and banana in a bowl, add the other ingredients, and mix vigorously with a spoon. For each serving, pour 1⅛ cup (275 ml) into a glass. Enjoy.

Per Serving: *(1⅛ cup/275 ml) Calories 178; Available carbohydrate 28 g; Carbohydrate 31 g; Fibre 3 g; Fat 4 g; Protein 7 g; Cholesterol 8 mg; Phosphorus 207 mg; Potassium 582 mg; Sodium 77 mg.*

1 Serving = 2 Carbohydrate Choices

⚘ Shake Me Up Shake!

This smoothie can be made in the evening and kept in the refrigerator in a covered bowl or glass for a quick, ready-to-go breakfast the next day. Stir well in the morning.

Preparation Time: *10 minutes*

Yield: *2 servings*

1 cup (250 ml) 1% milk

¾ cup (175 ml) raspberries

½ banana

¼ cup (50 ml) vanilla yogurt, low fat

1 tsp (5 ml) grated lemon zest

1 tbsp (15 ml) ground flaxseed

1½ tsp (7 ml) honey

In a blender, combine the ingredients and mix on high until smooth. If you don't have a blender, use a potato masher to purée the raspberries and banana in a bowl, add the rest of the ingredients to the bowl, and mix vigorously with a spoon. For each serving, pour 1 cup (250 ml) into a glass. Enjoy.

Per Serving: (1 cup/250 ml) Calories 193; Available carbohydrate 26 g; Carbohydrate 34 g; Fibre 8 g; Fat 4 g; Protein 8 g; Cholesterol 8 mg; Phosphorus 220 mg; Potassium 523 mg; Sodium 77 mg.

1 Serving = 2 Carbohydrate Choices

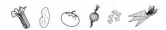

Baked Delights

Baked foods can be healthy breakfast choices so long as they are lower in fat, sugar, and sodium (and, ideally, high in fibre, too). You may choose to have your baked goods only as "treats," reserved for special occasions such as weekend brunches, breakfast in bed, when having company over, and so forth, or you might choose to prepare them in advance, freeze them, and defrost portions as you need them.

When preparing (or, for that matter, buying) baked breakfast goods, be sure to choose those that are high in fibre, and low in sugar and fat.

To ensure your baked goods turn out the way you want, you need to understand how butter functions in baking recipes. The process of *creaming* (or beating) butter with sugar is important to achieving the rising, rich, spongy texture. During the 3 to 5 minutes of beating the sugar into the butter until it is fluffy, the sugar cuts into the butter and aerates the fat. This gives cakes their rich texture and flavour.

TIP

You can easily substitute soft margarine for butter in recipes where the butter must be creamed with sugar; you'll still create a very acceptable product. Cooking oil, however, cannot be substituted for butter in these instances — the final product won't be very good.

⌕ *Banana Bread*

This loaf tastes great but takes an hour to bake, so plan ahead. If you won't eat the whole loaf within a few days, cut it in two and freeze half for another time.

Preparation Time: *20 minutes*

Cooking Time: *60 minutes*

Yield: *1 loaf (12 slices)*

¼ cup (50 ml) soft margarine	¼ tsp (1 ml) salt
¾ cup (175 ml) white sugar	1 tsp (5 ml) baking soda
1 egg, beaten	3 small bananas, mashed
¾ cup (175 ml) white flour	¼ tsp (1 ml) nutmeg
¾ cup (175 ml) whole wheat flour	½ tsp (2 ml) cinnamon
¼ cup (50 ml) ground flaxseed	¼ cup (50 ml) walnuts, chopped

1 Preheat oven to 350 degrees Fahrenheit (175 degrees Celsius).

2 Lightly grease a 4-x-8-inch (10-x-20-cm) loaf pan with canola oil.

3 In a medium-sized bowl, cream the margarine and sugar together with an electric mixer or spatula. Add the egg and mix well.

4 Add the remaining ingredients to the bowl and continue mixing until the batter is smooth. Pour the batter into the pan.

5 Bake for one hour, until a toothpick inserted into the loaf comes out clean, or the loaf starts to slightly pull away from sides of pan. Allow the loaf to cool to room temperature before slicing. Serve and enjoy.

Per Serving: *(1 slice, ¾-inch/1.7 cm, 80 g) Calories 198; Available carbohydrate 28 g; Carbohydrate 31 g; Fibre 3 g; Fat 7 g; Protein 4 g; Cholesterol 18 mg; Phosphorus 76 mg; Potassium 171 mg; Sodium 194 mg.*

1 Serving = 2 Carbohydrate Choices

☺ Raspberry Muffins

Cornmeal gives these treats a satisfying crunch and a different flavour from the average muffin.

Preparation Time: *25 minutes*

Cooking Time: *16 to 18 minutes*

Yield: *12 muffins*

½ cup (125 ml) rolled oats	¼ tsp (1 ml) salt
1 cup (250 ml) 1% milk	½ cup (125 ml) honey
¾ cup (175 ml) white flour	¼ cup (50 ml) canola oil
½ cup (125 ml) cornmeal	2 tsp (10 ml) grated lime zest
¼ cup (50 ml) wheat bran	1 egg, lightly beaten
1 tbsp (15 ml) baking powder	⅔ cup (150 ml) raspberries

1 Preheat oven to 400 degrees Fahrenheit (200 degrees Celsius).

2 Lightly grease a muffin pan with canola oil or line with paper muffin cups.

3 In a large, microwave-safe bowl, combine the oats and milk. Microwave on high for 3 minutes or until the oats are creamy and tender. If you don't have a microwave, place the oats and milk in a pot and cook over medium-high heat for approximately 6 minutes until the oats are creamy and tender.

4 In a large bowl, mix together the flour, cornmeal, wheat bran, baking powder, and salt with a spoon or spatula. Add the honey, canola oil, lime zest, egg, and oat mixture. Stir the ingredients until they are blended but still slightly lumpy.

5 Gently fold in the raspberries.

6 Spoon the batter into the cups of a muffin pan until each cup is two-thirds full.

7 Bake for 16 to 18 minutes or until a toothpick inserted into the centre of a muffin comes out clean.

8 Let the muffins cool in the muffin pan for 2 minutes before removing. Remove the muffins from the pan and place them on a wire rack to cool to room temperature. Serve and enjoy.

Per Serving: (1 muffin, 54 g) Calories 175; Available carbohydrate 27 g; Carbohydrate 29 g; Fibre 2 g; Fat 6 g; Protein 3 g; Cholesterol 19 mg; Phosphorus 1 mg; Potassium 112 mg; Sodium 198 mg.

1 Serving = 2 Carbohydrate Choices

☙ *Baked Homemade Granola*

This recipe yields a large quantity of granola, but it will keep up to three months in a sealed container. You can add the granola to yogurt, eat it as cereal, or simply enjoy it on its own for a snack.

Preparation Time: *20 minutes*

Cooking Time: *30 minutes*

Yield: *7 cups (1,750 ml)*

½ cup (125 ml) warm water	*1 tsp (5 ml) cinnamon*
⅓ cup (75 ml) maple syrup	*½ tsp (2 ml) nutmeg*
½ tsp (2 ml) vanilla	*⅓ cup (75 ml) raisins*
4 cups (1,000 ml) dry rolled oats	*⅓ cup (75 ml) chopped dried apricots*
½ cup (125 ml) slivered almonds	*⅓ cup (75 ml) dried cranberries*
½ cup (125 ml) chopped walnuts	*2 tbsp (30 ml) chopped dates*
¼ cup (50 ml) unsalted sunflower seeds	*¼ cup (50 ml) wheat germ*
2 tbsp (30 ml) roasted pumpkin seeds	*⅓ cup (75 ml) psyllium fibre*
2 tbsp (30 ml) sesame seeds	*¼ cup (50 ml) ground flaxseed*

1 Preheat oven to 300 degrees Fahrenheit (150 degrees Celsius).

2 Use canola oil to lightly grease a jelly roll pan or rimmed cookie sheet.

3 In a small bowl, combine the warm water with the maple syrup and vanilla.

4 In a large bowl, stir together the oats, nuts, seeds, and spices. Slowly add the contents of the small bowl. Continue stirring until evenly mixed.

5 Use a spoon or spatula to evenly spread the oat mixture over the jelly roll pan or cookie sheet.

6 Bake for 30 minutes, stirring every 10 minutes.

7 Remove the granola from the oven, place the tray on a wire cooling rack, and allow to cool to room temperature.

8 Pour the granola into a large bowl and add the dried fruits, wheat germ, psyllium, and flaxseed. Mix well, serve, and enjoy.

*****Per Serving:*** *(¼ cup/50 ml) Calories 125; Available carbohydrate 14 g; Carbohydrate 17 g; Fibre 3 g; Fat 5 g; Protein 4 g; Cholesterol 0 mg; Phosphorus 123 mg; Potassium 153 mg; Sodium 4 mg.*

1 Serving = 1 Carbohydrate Choice

The benefits of flax

Flax is a very healthy food rich in omega-3 fatty acids, fibre, and lignans.

As we discuss in Chapter 2, omega-3 fatty acids are protective against heart disease and there is increasing scientific evidence that ingesting omega-3 fatty acids reduces the risk of various other diseases, including asthma, cancer, depression, and lupus. Consuming fibre helps to improve cholesterol levels, lowers blood glucose, protects against bowel cancer, and helps control your appetite. Flax contains both soluble and insoluble fibre. Lignans have both plant estrogen and antioxidant qualities. Flaxseed contains 75 to 800 times more lignans than other plant foods.

Flax isn't one of those "I know it tastes bad but it's healthy so force yourself to eat it" kinds of food. In fact, flax has a nice, light, nutty taste.

A recommended serving size of ground flaxseed is 1 to 2 tbsp (15 to 30 ml) per day. One tbsp (15 ml) of ground flaxseed contains as much fibre as one slice of whole wheat bread, ¼ cup (50 ml) cooked oat bran, or ½ cup (125 ml) brown rice. Flax contains both soluble and insoluble fibre.

You can purchase flaxseed at the bulk food store. There are two types of flaxseed: brown and golden. They are equal in nutritional value. You'll need to grind the seed (the shells are too hard to chew) in order to release the omega-3 fatty acids. Use a coffee grinder or blender to crush the flaxseed, not a food processor. (Flaxseeds are too small and light to be crushed in a food processor.)

Ground flaxseeds are best stored in the refrigerator in a container that light cannot pass through because the seed is high in oil. *Ground* flax will stay good in your refrigerator for up to three months and *whole* flaxseeds can be stored in the freezer for up to a year.

Flaxseed *oil* can also be consumed, most commonly as an oil in salad dressing, for dipping bread, or for marinades. Compared with ground flaxseed, flaxseed oil has no fibre or lignans. So, use the crushed seeds!

☙ Baked Scone (Aboriginal Bannock)

There are several versions of scones, but this one is Cynthia's favourite. To make the scone healthier, this recipe replaces the traditional lard with soft margarine and combines whole wheat and white flour. For a different twist, try adding ¼ cup (50 ml) of raisins.

Preparation Time: *10 minutes*

Cooking Time: *30 minutes*

Yield: *12 servings*

1 cup (250 ml) white flour

1 cup (250 ml) whole wheat flour

2 tbsp (30 ml) baking powder

½ tsp (2 ml) salt

2 tbsp (30 ml) soft margarine

1 cup (250 ml) 1% milk

2 tsp (10 ml) canola oil (for your hands)

1 Preheat oven to 350 degrees Fahrenheit (175 degrees Celsius).

2 Lightly grease an 8-x-8-inch (20-x-20-cm) pan with canola oil.

3 In a large bowl, stir together the white and whole wheat flour, baking powder, and salt.

4 Mix in the soft margarine with a pastry cutter or fork until small pea-sized lumps form in the flour. Slowly pour the milk into the flour mixture. Stir with a fork until a sticky dough ball is formed.

5 Use the fork to transfer the dough to the pan. Lightly coat your hands with the canola oil. Use your hands (and fork, if necessary) to spread the dough across the pan.

6 Bake for 30 minutes.

7 Place the pan on a wire rack and allow to cool for 20 minutes. Cut each piece away from the sides of the pan using an egg lifter. Serve and enjoy.

Per Serving: (1 piece, 2½-inch x 2-inch/6.5 x 5 cm, 55 g) Calories 102; Available carbohydrate 15 g; Carbohydrate 17 g; Fibre 2 g; Fat 3 g; Protein 3 g; Cholesterol 1 mg; Phosphorus 116 mg; Potassium 83 mg; Sodium 367 mg.

1 Serving = 1 Carbohydrate Choice

Per Serving, with raisins: (1 piece, 2½-inch x 2-inch/6.5 x 5 cm, 57 g) Calories 112; Available carbohydrate 18 g; Carbohydrate 20 g; Fibre 2 g; Fat 3 g; Protein 3 g; Cholesterol 1 mg; Phosphorus 119 mg; Potassium 108 mg; Sodium 367 mg.

1 Serving = 1 Carbohydrate Choice

Go nuts, gently

Nuts are a good food choice, but with nuts you can definitely have too much of a good thing. Nuts are a good source of protein, help raise your good (HDL) cholesterol and lower your bad (LDL) cholesterol, provide phosphorus, are rich in Vitamin E, and contain fibre.

A downside to eating nuts is that they contain lots of calories (¼ cup/50 ml of nuts has 175 calories). That's why you should consume them in limited quantities.

Nuts are a healthier snack alternative to chips or cookies, but only if the portion size is limited and the nuts aren't fried or covered in chocolate, sugar, or salt.

ᓬ *Cranberry Walnut Muffins*

These muffins are very tasty. They are also good to freeze and keep on hand for a later date. You can even pull one out of the freezer in the morning and put it directly in your lunch bag. By lunch time it will be thawed and ready to eat.

Preparation Time: 20 minutes

Cooking Time: 12 to 15 minutes

Yield: 12 muffins

½ cup (125 ml) white sugar

1½ cups (375 ml) white flour

2 tsp (10 ml) baking powder

1 tsp (5 ml) baking soda

¾ tsp (4 ml) cinnamon

1 egg, beaten

½ cup (125 ml) orange juice

¼ cup (50 ml) low-fat sour cream

3 tbsp (45 ml) canola oil

¼ cup (50 ml) chopped walnuts

1 cup (250 ml) chopped fresh or frozen cranberries

1 Preheat oven to 375 degrees Fahrenheit (190 degrees Celsius).

2 Lightly grease a muffin pan with canola oil or line with paper muffin cups.

3 In a medium-sized bowl, combine the sugar, flour, baking powder, baking soda, and cinnamon.

4 In a small bowl, mix the egg, orange juice, sour cream, and oil.

5 Add the liquid mixture to the dry mixture and gently stir together. Fold in the walnuts and the cranberries.

6 Spoon the batter into the cups of the muffin pan until each cup is two-thirds full.

7 Bake for 12 to 15 minutes or until a toothpick inserted in the centre of a muffin comes out clean.

8 Let the muffins cool in the muffin pan for 2 minutes before removing. Remove the muffins from the pan and place them on a wire rack to cool to room temperature. Serve and enjoy.

Per Serving: (1 muffin, 70 g) Calories 173; Available carbohydrate 26 g; Carbohydrate 27 g; Fibre 1 g; Fat 6 g; Protein 3 g; Cholesterol 19 mg; Phosphorus 62 mg; Potassium 133 mg; Sodium 197 mg.

1 Serving = 2 Carbohydrate Choices

Griddle Goodies

If you're like us, when you think of the griddle your mind immediately conjures up a heavenly collection of aromas and tastes. Mmm, mmm.

You can enjoy food from the griddle while avoiding excess fat, carbohydrates, and calories:

- ✔ Some griddles have special non-stick finishes on their surfaces and can be used without any fat or oil source.
- ✔ Use soft margarine instead of butter.
- ✔ Choose "no sugar added" syrups.

One teaspoon (5 ml) of butter, margarine, or cooking oil has the same number of calories (35 to 45) and the same amount of fat (4 g), but not all fat is created equal:

- ✔ Less-healthy fats are solid fats like butter, lard, hydrogenated hard margarines, and shortening. These are all high in saturated fat and cholesterol.
- ✔ Canola oil and soft margarine are healthier choices than solid fats.
- ✔ A good multipurpose olive oil like fine virgin olive oil is a good choice for sautéing, pan frying, or stir frying.

We made all the recipes in this book with soft margarine (except for our Butter Chicken recipe, which was made with, no surprise here, butter), canola oil, or olive oil.

You can also reduce the amount of fat you consume from griddle-prepared meals by using a low-fat cooking spray instead of melting butter on the griddle.

You can make your own cooking spray with canola oil and water:

1. Take 1 cup (250 ml) of water and remove (and discard) 2 tbsp of the water.

2. To the remaining water in the cup, add 2 tbsp (30 ml) of canola oil.

3. Place the canola oil and water mixture in a new plant mister spray bottle and you're all set. Remember to shake well before using.

Cooking oil sprays have many potential uses:

  ✔ Cooking sprays can be used on broiler pans, griddles, and barbecues, before heating.

  ✔ To help prevent sticking, cooking sprays can be used on spatulas, wooden spoons, measuring cups, and skewers.

  ✔ They can be sprayed on skillets, baking pans, casserole dishes, and muffin pans.

Check the manufacturer's recommendations for your baking appliances as cooking spray can ruin some of the new finishes on baking pans and skillets.

Add a little canola oil to a paper towel and, presto, you've got an easy way to coat baking surfaces.

☺ Akoori Scrambled Eggs

These are scrambled eggs with an Indian flair. They can be served with naan bread or plain yogurt if you wish. Naan is a traditional Indian flatbread. It can be purchased at most large grocery store chains.

Preparation Time: *10 minutes*

Cooking Time: *10 minutes*

Yield: *4 servings*

6 eggs	⅔ cup (150 ml) tomato, chopped
2 egg whites	1 tsp (5 ml) fresh ginger, grated
½ tsp (2 ml) pepper	1 green chili, minced (optional)
1 tbsp (15 ml) cilantro or parsley, coarsely chopped	½ tsp (2 ml) cumin
	½ tsp (2 ml) turmeric
2 tsp (10 ml) canola oil	
⅔ cup (150 ml) onion, chopped	

1 Whisk the eggs, egg whites, pepper, and cilantro together in a medium-sized bowl and set aside.

2 In a frying pan, heat the oil over medium heat for 1 minute. Add the onions to the pan. Stir frequently until they are soft (approximately 3 minutes).

3 Use a spatula to stir in the tomatoes, ginger, green chili, cumin, and turmeric. Cook for 1 minute.

4 Slowly pour the egg mixture into the pan with the tomato mixture. Cook and stir the eggs until there is no liquid left in the pan. Serve immediately.

Per Serving: (¼ recipe, 100 g) Calories 154; Available carbohydrate 4 g; Carbohydrate 5 g; Fibre 1 g; Fat 10 g; Protein 12 g; Cholesterol 317 mg; Phosphorus 164 mg; Potassium 263 mg; Sodium 136 mg.

1 Serving = 0 Carbohydrate Choices

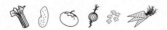

✑ Oatmeal Pancakes

These pancakes are much healthier than conventional pancakes and they taste great too. For added flavour, try them with light pancake syrup or fruit. If you have leftovers, they can be kept covered in the refrigerator and eaten the next day.

Preparation Time: *7 minutes*

Cooking Time: *10 minutes*

Yield: *18 pancakes*

2 cups (500 ml) 1% milk	2 tbsp (30 ml) white sugar
1½ cups (375 ml) large flake oatmeal	½ tsp (2 ml) salt
½ cup (125 ml) whole wheat flour	2½ tsp (12 ml) baking powder
¾ cup (175 ml) white flour	2 eggs, beaten
¼ cup (50 ml) ground flaxseed	½ cup (125 ml) canola oil

1 In a large bowl, mix together the milk and oatmeal with a spoon and let sit for 5 minutes.

2 Combine the other ingredients in a bowl and add to the oatmeal mixture.

3 Lightly grease a frying pan with canola oil and set over medium-high heat for 2 minutes.

4 Drop ¼ cup (50 ml) of batter onto the pan for each pancake. Cook 2 minutes per side or until lightly golden brown. Serve hot.

Per Serving: (1 pancake, 50 g) Calories 144; Available carbohydrate 13 g; Carbohydrate 15 g; Fibre 2 g; Fat 8 g; Protein 4 g; Cholesterol 25 mg; Phosphorus 111 mg; Potassium 108 mg; Sodium 153 mg.

1 Serving = 1 Carbohydrate Choice

☼ Oatmeal Fruit Crepes

These crepes are sweet enough to be eaten for dessert! They can be made in advance and kept in the refrigerator for a day or in the freezer for a month.

Preparation Time: *15 minutes*

Cooking Time: *25 minutes*

Yield: *14 crepes*

Crepes

1 cup (250 ml) quick oats

¼ cup (50 ml) whole wheat flour

1 tbsp (15 ml) white sugar

1 tsp (5 ml) cinnamon

¼ cup (50 ml) orange juice

¼ cup (50 ml) low-fat plain yogurt

½ cup (125 ml) 1% milk

3 eggs

1 tbsp (15 ml) melted soft margarine

Filling

3½ cup (875 ml) low-fat ricotta cheese

1¾ cup (425 ml) strawberries

Sauce

⅓ cup (75 ml) diet strawberry jam

1½ tbsp (22 ml) orange juice

For the crepes:

1 In a blender, mix the oats, flour, sugar, cinnamon, orange juice, yogurt, milk, and eggs on high speed until smooth. If you don't have a blender, use a whisk or fork to mix the ingredients together in a bowl. Let the oat mixture stand for 10 minutes, then add the melted margarine and stir well.

2 Grease a crepe pan or small non-stick frying pan with canola oil and set over medium-high heat.

3 Pour 2 tbsp (30 ml) of batter into the centre of the pan and swirl it around until a thin layer covers the bottom of the pan.

4 Cook each crepe for 1½ minutes per side, until golden brown.

5 Stack the cooked crepes on a plate between layers of wax paper.

For the filling:

6 Place ¼ cup (50 ml) of cheese and 2 tbsp (30 ml) of strawberries in the centre of each crepe. Roll up the crepes so the filling is inside.

For the sauce:

7 In a small bowl, mix together the jam and orange juice. Top each crepe with 1 tbsp (15 ml) of sauce.

Per Serving: (1 crepe with ¼ cup/50 ml cheese, 2 tbsp/25 ml strawberries and 1 tbsp/15 ml sauce, 117 g) Calories 163; Available carbohydrate 15 g; Carbohydrate 16 g; Fibre 1 g; Fat 7 g; Protein 10 g; Cholesterol 65 mg; Phosphorus 188 mg; Potassium 191 mg; Sodium 106 mg.

1 Serving = 1 Carbohydrate Choice

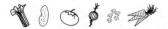

Cottage Cheese Pancakes

These pancakes are an excellent breakfast choice — they're a good source of protein, and they'll keep you energized until lunch. Remember to use light syrup.

Preparation Time: *8 minutes*

Cooking Time: *3 minutes*

Yield: *11 pancakes*

1 cup (250 ml) 1% cottage cheese	*¼ cup (50 ml) ground flaxseed*
1 egg	*½ tsp (2 ml) cinnamon*
2 egg whites	*⅛ tsp (0.5 ml) salt*
3 tbsp (45 ml) wheat germ	*1 tbsp (15 ml) canola oil*
⅓ cup (75 ml) whole wheat flour	

1 Mix together the cottage cheese, egg, and egg whites in a food processor or blender at medium speed. If you don't have a food processor or blender, mix well in a bowl, using a potato masher or fork to break down the cottage cheese.

2 Combine the wheat germ, flour, flaxseed, cinnamon, and salt in a medium-sized bowl and mix well with a spoon or spatula.

3 Add the dry ingredients to the food processor or blender and mix everything together. If you're not using a food processor or blender, mix well by hand.

4 Grease a frying pan with the canola oil and set over medium-high heat for 1 minute.

5 Drop 2 tbsp (30 ml) of batter into the pan for each pancake. Cook for 1½ minutes per side or until golden brown. Serve hot.

Per Serving: (4 pancakes, 160 g) Calories 292; Available carbohydrate 14 g; Carbohydrate 21 g; Fibre 7 g; Fat 14 g; Protein 22 g; Cholesterol 80 mg; Phosphorus 372 mg; Potassium 375 mg; Sodium 404 mg.

1 Serving = 1 Carbohydrate Choice

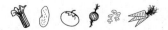

Chapter 8

Savory Soups

In This Chapter

▶ Seeing the clear appeal of broth-based soups

▶ Skimming over creamy soups

*F*ew, if any, foods evoke the warm and cozy, homey feeling that soup creates. Soup reminds people of childhood and simpler times (although we'd be the first to say that whether simpler times ever really existed is arguable).

Think we wax overly poetic? Perhaps. But how about this . . . A number of years ago a well-known soup company, seeking to be contemporary, changed the longstanding, classic appearance of its cans' labels to something modern-looking. It was a dismal marketing failure and sales tanked. Turns out that people didn't want "modern" in their soup; they wanted "traditional."

Well, whether you, too, want something classical or instead are looking for something contemporary, in this chapter you find delectable recipes for all sorts of different types of diabetes-friendly soups.

Making Soups from Leftovers

Don't throw out those leftover meat bones or slightly wilted vegetables! Instead, use these ingredients to make tasty soup. You'll end up with a nutritious product and your economical actions will save you some money at the same time.

To make your soup from leftovers, you will need the following:

✔ A large saucepan

✔ Meat or poultry bones (to make your own broth), or prepared broth

✔ Vegetables, leftover beans, pasta, or rice

✔ Herbs

In the next section, we look at how to make your own broth and then we look at how to add the broth (your own or a prepared one) to the other ingredients to create your pièce de résistance.

Making a basic broth

Making your own broth takes a little work, but it's much tastier and healthier than the commercial alternatives, which are high in sodium. Broth can be refrigerated for two days or stored in the freezer for up to 3 months. Try storing it in ½-cup (125 ml) portions for easy use later in sauces or a stir-fry.

These are the steps to follow to make your own broth:

1. **In a large saucepan, add meat or poultry scraps and leftover bones.**

   Bones can be raw, precooked, or cooked. If using raw meat, baking the bones in the oven at 400 degrees Fahrenheit (200 degrees Celsius) in a roasting pan for 1 hour, turning half way through, will give more flavour to the soup. Don't let the drippings go to waste; add some water to the roasting pan and then add this to the soup pot.

2. **Cover the bones in the pan with cold water until the water comes one inch (2.5 cm) above the bones.** Bring this mixture to a boil over medium-high heat, uncovered, and then reduce the heat to a low simmer.

3. **Add a quartered onion, celery, and carrots to the saucepan.** You could also add a bay leaf, parsley, thyme, celery tops, or a few peppercorns. Make sure the water covers any added vegetables.

4. **Cover and simmer 3 hours for poultry and 4 hours for beef, lamb, or pork.** Skim off any foam that floats to the top of the saucepan during the simmering process.

5. **Remove the bones and vegetables, strain the broth through a fine mesh strainer, and let the broth cool a little.**

   A quick way to cool the broth is to place the cool saucepan in a sink of cold water that comes ¾ of the way up the saucepan.

6. **Refrigerate the broth;** when it's cold, use a spoon to skim off and discard the hardened fat that has risen to the surface.

If you need to use the broth before refrigerating it, you can still remove the fat; try swirling a few ice cubes on the surface of the broth for a minute, then remove. Some fat will have clung to the ice cubes.

The difference between a stock and a broth

Broth (*bouillon* in French) is a clear, savoury combination of meats, vegetables, and herbs that are simmered in water and then strained. *Stock* is made in a similar way to broth but is much more gelatinous. *Consommé* is a completely clear soup similar to broth, but it often has a more intense flavour. Broth and stock are similar enough that they can be used interchangeably in recipes and used for soup, sauces, gravies, or sautés.

Making soup with your homemade broth

With your broth at the ready, these are the next steps to make your soup:

1. Gather all the various ingredients you will be using, including vegetables, rice, pasta, beans, garlic, spices (a bay leaf, parsley, rosemary, marjoram, or thyme), and meat (beef, pork, lamb, or poultry).

2. Chop the vegetables and meat into bite-sized pieces. (For extra flavour you can sauté the vegetables in a bit of olive oil with some garlic or ginger.)

3. Pour the broth into a large saucepan.

4. Add the vegetables, spices, and meat to the saucepan.

5. Bring the mixture to a boil over medium-high heat, then turn down the heat to a low simmer for 1 to 2 hours until the vegetables are tender when pricked with a fork or knife. (Just prior to the vegetables being tender, add the leftover rice, pasta, or beans.)

6. When warm through, ladle into a bowl and serve.

If making your own broth isn't possible, you can use commercial broth bought in a box or can or a cube. Whenever possible, choose a broth that is low in sodium.

Considering Commercially Prepared Soups

Commercially prepared soups (both those in a can and the dry version in a cup) are very handy and can be very tasty, but they're typically high in sodium.

On average 1 cup (250 ml) of commercially prepared soup has 700 to 1,700 mg of sodium; this is 30 to 70 percent of the Daily Value for sodium. (For more about Canada Food Guide's recommendations, see Chapter 2.) In other words, having one cup of soup you buy in a container at the grocery store will provide you with about half of all the sodium you should consume in an entire day!

If you eat soup that's high in sodium, try to make the rest of your day's food choices low in sodium.

Generally, the Nutrition Facts panel lists soup in ½ cup (125 ml) or 1 cup (250 ml) servings. We think the former (that is, the ½ cup listing) is perhaps a bit disingenuous; really now, how many people would think that ½ cup of soup is either sufficient for their desires or represents a full serving of soup? (For more about reading the Nutrition Facts table, refer to Chapter 6.)

To ensure you are not consuming excess sodium, remember to check the Nutrition Facts table for both the serving size and the sodium content per serving size for commercially prepared soup.

Commercial cream soups, like cream of mushroom, are high not only in sodium but in fat, too. A cup (250 ml) of commercial cream soup often contains as much as 1,700 mg or 70 percent of the Daily Value of sodium and 16 g or 24 percent of the Daily Value of fat. Even a cup of "low sodium" cream of mushroom soup can have over 50 percent of the Daily Value for sodium.

Dried soup cups with noodles are also often rich in sodium, with some brands having as much as 61 percent of the Daily Value for sodium.

Broth-Based Soups

For broth-based soups, we recommend using a homemade broth (we show you how to prepare one in the section "Making a basic broth," earlier in this chapter), but you can also use a pre-made broth if you don't have your own on hand. Just remember to go with low-sodium versions.

French Onion Soup

Get your tissues ready — this recipe calls for a lot of onions. Cynthia still hasn't found a way to keep from crying when chopping onions, and she's done a lot of chopping for this book!

Preparation Time: *20 minutes*

Cooking Time: *60 minutes*

Yield: *8 servings*

4 tbsp (60 ml) soft margarine

6 cups (1,500 ml) yellow onions, coarsely chopped

1 tsp (5 ml) sugar

1 tbsp (15 ml) white flour

6 cups (1,500 ml) reduced-sodium beef broth

2 tsp (10 ml) Worcestershire sauce

½ tsp (2 ml) pepper

4 slices whole wheat bread, toasted

1 cup (250 ml) low-fat mozzarella cheese, shredded

1 In a large pot, melt the margarine over medium-high heat. Add the onions, stirring frequently for 10 minutes.

2 Add the sugar and continue stirring until the onions turn a golden colour. Do not let the onions turn brown. Sprinkle the onions with flour and stir for 2 minutes.

3 Slowly add the beef broth to the pot. Mix in the Worcestershire sauce and pepper.

4 Bring the soup to a boil, cover, and let simmer for 15 minutes.

5 Cut the toasted bread into cubes.

6 For each serving, pour 1 cup (250 ml) of soup into a bowl and top with bread cubes (use a half-slice's worth of cubes per serving). Sprinkle 2 tbsp (30 ml) of shredded mozzarella cheese over the bread cubes.

7 Place each bowl in the microwave for 1½ minutes, or until the cheese melts. If you don't have a microwave, pour the soup into ovenproof bowls. Place each bowl under the broiler for 1 minute, until the cheese melts. Remove with oven mitts and serve.

Per Serving: *(1 cup/250 ml) Calories 216; Available carbohydrate 17 g; Carbohydrate 20 g; Fibre 3 g; Fat 10 g; Protein 11 g; Cholesterol 8 mg; Phosphorus 203 mg; Potassium 398 mg; Sodium 270 mg.*

1 Serving = 1 Carbohydrate Choice

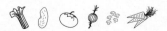

☙ *Veggie Soup*

This soup is easy to make, and it's very colourful and tasty. Remember, vegetables are very low in calories and carbohydrates, so you can enjoy this soup alongside almost any meal. For a vegetarian dish, use vegetable broth instead of chicken.

Preparation Time: *15 minutes*

Cooking Time: *30 to 40 minutes*

Yield: *6 servings*

½ cup (125 ml) carrots, diced

½ cup (125 ml) onion, diced

½ cup (125 ml) celery, diced

½ cup (125 ml) turnip, diced

1 cup (250 ml) chopped tomatoes

1 cup (250 ml) cabbage, shredded

1 clove garlic, minced

4 cups (1,000 ml) reduced-sodium chicken or vegetable broth

½ tsp (2 ml) pepper

¼ tsp (1 ml) basil

¼ tsp (1 ml) oregano

½ cup (125 ml) frozen peas

½ cup (125 ml) parsley, chopped

1 Combine all the ingredients, except for the peas and parsley, in a large pot.

2 Bring the soup to a boil, then reduce the temperature to low heat. Cover the pot and allow the soup to simmer for 30 to 40 minutes, until the vegetables are tender.

3 Add the peas and parsley and let the soup simmer for approximately 5 minutes, until the peas are cooked.

4 For each serving, ladle 1 cup (250 ml) into a bowl. Enjoy.

Per Serving: *(1cup/250 ml) Calories 46; Available carbohydrate 6 g; Carbohydrate 8 g; Fibre 2 g; Fat 0 g; Protein 4 g; Cholesterol 0 mg; Phosphorus 66 mg; Potassium 378 mg; Sodium 411 mg.*

1 Serving = 0 Carbohydrate Choices

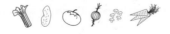

Adobo Soup with Bok Choy

This is the national dish of the Philippines. It is actually more like a stew than a soup and can be made with either chicken or pork. This soup is a high source of potassium and sodium.

Preparation Time: *25 minutes*

Cooking Time: *20 minutes*

Yield: *6 servings*

⅓ cup (75 ml) reduced-sodium soy sauce

⅓ cup (75 ml) rice vinegar

2 cloves garlic, minced

1 bay leaf

1 tsp (5 ml) olive oil

½ cup (125 ml) yellow onions, chopped

4 cups (1,000 ml) reduced-sodium chicken broth

1½ cups (375 ml) cooked chicken or lean pork, cut into bite-sized pieces

½ cup (125 ml) uncooked couscous

8 cups (2,000 ml) bok choy, sliced

2 green onions, chopped

1 In a small pot, combine the soy sauce, vinegar, garlic, and bay leaf. Bring to a boil, then remove from the stovetop and set aside.

2 In a large pot, heat the olive oil for 1 minute over medium-high heat. Add the yellow onions and sauté until they are soft and golden brown, about 6 minutes.

3 Add the chicken stock to the onions and bring the mixture to a boil.

4 Pour the soy sauce mixture into the large pot. Add the chicken or pork and the couscous. Bring the soup to a boil, reduce the heat to low, cover, and simmer for 2 minutes.

5 Add the bok choy and continue to let the soup simmer, covered, for another 2 minutes, until the bok choy is tender.

6 Discard the bay leaf. For each serving, ladle 1 cup (250 ml) into a bowl and top with a few chopped green onions. Enjoy.

Per Serving, with chicken: *(1 cup/250 ml) Calories 198; Available carbohydrate 23 g; Carbohydrate 27 g; Fibre 4 g; Fat 3 g; Protein 19 g; Cholesterol 30 mg; Phosphorus 220 mg; Potassium 975 mg; Sodium 1281 mg.*

Per Serving, with pork: *(1 cup/ 250 ml) Calories 211; Available carbohydrate 22 g; Carbohydrate 26 g; Fibre 4 g; Fat 5 g; Protein 18 g; Cholesterol 27 mg; Phosphorus 223 mg; Potassium 1027 mg; Sodium 1329 mg.*

1 Serving = 1½ Carbohydrate Choices

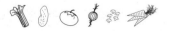

Kale Soup (Portuguese)

Kale is a frilly, dark green plant with a blue, purple, or crimson tinge. It tastes similar to cabbage, but a bit sweeter. When purchasing kale, look for leaves the size of your hand — they will be the most tender and mild tasting. The stems are edible but very fibrous, so they aren't used in this recipe.

Preparation Time: *40 minutes*

Cooking Time: *1 hour 15 minutes*

Yield: *10 servings*

2 tbsp (30 ml) olive oil

2 cups (500 ml) yellow onions, finely chopped

3 cloves garlic, minced

¼ tsp (1 ml) dried chili peppers

1⅓ cups (325 ml) potatoes, diced

6 cups (1,500 ml) reduced-sodium chicken broth

19 oz can (540 ml) red kidney beans

6 cups (1,500 ml) kale leaves, chopped

¾ cup (175 ml) Polish sausage, diced

1 Heat the olive oil in a frying pan on medium-high heat for 1 minute. Add the onions and garlic to the pan and sauté for approximately 5 minutes, until they are soft but not brown.

2 Add the dried chili peppers and diced potatoes to the frying pan. Cook and stir for 2 minutes.

3 In a large pot, combine the onion and potato mixture with the broth and bring to a boil.

4 Add the kale and reduce the heat to low. Cover the pot and allow the soup to simmer for 1 hour.

5 Drain the liquid from the kidney beans in a strainer. Rinse the beans under cold, running water for 2 minutes.

6 Place half of the beans in a medium-sized bowl and mash them with a potato masher.

7 Add the Polish sausage and the beans (both whole and mashed) to the soup and let simmer for another 10 minutes.

8 For each serving, ladle 1 cup (250 ml) into a bowl. Enjoy.

Per Serving: *(1 cup/250 ml) Calories 215; Available carbohydrate 19 g; Carbohydrate 23 g; Fibre 4 g; Fat 11 g; Protein 9 g; Cholesterol 7 mg; Phosphorus 153 mg; Potassium 620 mg; Sodium 319 mg.*

1 Serving = 1 Carbohydrate Choice

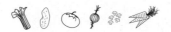

Best Beef Soup

This is one of Cynthia's mother's favourite recipes. Even Cynthia's teenaged son, Jeff, loves it! This soup can be made in advance and kept in the refrigerator overnight — it always tastes better the next day.

Preparation Time: *25 minutes*

Cooking Time: *40 minutes*

Yield: *9 servings*

1 tbsp (15 ml) olive oil	1 cup (250 ml) water
¾ lb (340 g) stewing beef or brisket	14 oz (398 ml) can diced tomatoes
½ cup (125 ml) yellow onion, finely chopped	⅓ cup (75 ml) pearl barley
2 cups (500 ml) carrots, finely chopped	¾ tsp (4 ml) marjoram
1 cup (250 ml) celery, finely chopped	¼ tsp (1 ml) thyme
1 cup (250 ml) parsnip, chopped	1 bay leaf
4 cups (1,000 ml) reduced-sodium beef broth	½ tsp (2 ml) pepper

1 Trim the fat from the beef and cut it into ¼-inch (1 cm) pieces.

2 In a medium-sized frying pan, warm the oil for 1 minute. Add the beef and brown for approximately 5 minutes, until cooked through. Place the beef in a large pot.

3 Place the onions in the frying pan that contained the beef and sauté for 2 to 3 minutes, until they are soft. Add the sautéed onions to the large pot.

4 Place the rest of the ingredients in the pot and bring to a boil. Reduce heat to low, cover, and allow the soup to simmer for 30 to 40 minutes, until the vegetables are tender.

5 For each serving, ladle 1 cup (250 ml) into a bowl. Enjoy.

Per Serving: (1 cup/250 ml) Calories 174; Available carbohydrate 12 g; Carbohydrate 15 g; Fibre 3 g; Fat 7 g; Protein 13 g; Cholesterol 31 mg; Phosphorus 157 mg; Potassium 486 mg; Sodium 139 mg.

1 Serving = 1 Carbohydrate Choice

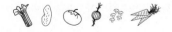

Creamy Soups

Milky and delicious, creamy soups can be particularly comforting, but unfortunately, some can be quite high in fat, too. Happily, the two soups in this section aren't fatty, and in fact, one soup doesn't even include milk at all!

⊙ Broccoli Cheese Soup

Broccoli tastes delicious in this soup and is rich in antioxidants, folate, and vitamins C and E. Antioxidants help protect against cancer and lower the risk of heart disease, stroke, and cataracts. For a vegetarian dish, use vegetable broth instead of chicken.

Preparation Time: *20 minutes*

Cooking Time: *15 minutes*

Yield: *4 servings*

1 tbsp (15 ml) soft margarine	¼ tsp (1 ml) pepper
½ cup (125 ml) yellow onions, chopped	½ tsp (2 ml) salt
1 tbsp (15 ml) flour	1½ cups (375 ml) 1% milk
1½ cups (375 ml) reduced-sodium chicken or vegetable broth	¾ cup (175 ml) low-fat cheddar cheese, grated
4 cups (1,000 ml) broccoli (including peeled stems and stalks), finely chopped	¼ tsp (1 ml) dry mustard
	1 green onion, chopped

1 Melt the margarine in a frying pan and sauté the onions over medium-high heat until tender. Add the flour to the onions and stir for 1 minute.

2 Slowly whisk the broth into the onions. Remove from heat, transfer the mixture to a large pot, and add the broccoli.

3 Bring the soup to a boil. Cover and simmer for 5 to 8 minutes or until the broccoli is tender. If the soup is cooked too long, it will lose its colour. Purée with a hand blender or a potato masher.

4 Add the rest of the ingredients, except the green onions. Heat the soup thoroughly, without bringing to a boil.

5 For each serving, pour 1⅛ cups (275 ml) of soup into a bowl and top with a few chopped green onions. Enjoy.

Per Serving: *(1⅓ cup/275 ml) Calories 153; Available carbohydrate 12 g; Carbohydrate 14 g; Fibre 2 g; Fat 6 g; Protein 13 g; Cholesterol 9 mg; Phosphorus 275 mg; Potassium 504 mg; Sodium 533 mg.*

1 Serving = 1 Carbohydrate Choice

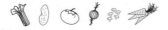

☺ Carrot Parsnip Soup

Carrots are well known as an abundant source of beta carotene, which converts in our bodies to vitamin A. Parsnips are an excellent source of fibre, as well as folate, magnesium, potassium, and vitamins C and E. With both carrots and parsnips, this soup is full of nutrients that will aid in keeping you healthy. For a vegetarian dish, use vegetable broth instead of chicken.

Preparation Time: *15 minutes*

Cooking Time: *30 minutes*

Yield: *5 servings*

1 tbsp (15 ml) soft margarine

1 cup (250 ml) yellow onion, chopped

1 clove garlic, minced

2 cups (500 ml) carrots, chopped

1 cup (250 ml) parsnip, chopped

4 cups (1,000 ml) reduced-sodium chicken or vegetable broth

¼ tsp (1 ml) ginger root, grated

½ tsp (2 ml) salt

¼ tsp (1 ml) pepper

1 green onion

1 Melt the margarine over medium-high heat in a frying pan and add the onions and garlic. Sauté until tender but not brown, then transfer to a large pot.

2 Add the rest of the ingredients to the pot, except for the green onion, and bring the pot to a boil.

3 Cover the pot and simmer on low heat for about 20 minutes or until the vegetables are tender.

4 Purée the soup with a hand blender or potato masher until smooth.

5 For each serving, ladle 1 cup (250 ml) of soup into a bowl and top with a few chopped green onions. Enjoy.

Per Serving: *(1 cup/250 ml) Calories 107; Available carbohydrate 13 g; Carbohydrate 16 g; Fibre 3 g; Fat 4 g; Protein 5 g; Cholesterol 0 mg; Phosphorus 106 mg; Potassium 488 mg; Sodium 350 mg.*

1 Serving = 1 Carbohydrate Choice

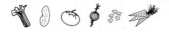

Chapter 9

Snazzy Salads

In This Chapter

▶ Livening up a tossed salad

▶ Getting started with salad

▶ Enjoying salad on the side

▶ Making salad the main attraction

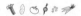

When it comes to salads, how times have changed. Thank goodness! Long gone are the days when "salad" was synonymous with some iceberg lettuce dressed up with a few tomato wedges and thick French dressing. (No wonder salad used to get such a bum rap, especially from us when we were kids.)

Nowadays, so many types of salad are on offer that on some restaurant menus they dwarf the number of different burgers for sale. Hey, now that's progress!

In this chapter, we look at a wide variety of salads, including those eaten at the beginning of a meal (starter salads), with the meal (side salads), and as a meal themselves (main salads). We discuss how you can choose healthy salads when in a restaurant and what to look for in pre-made salads on offer in grocery stores. You'll find salads that work for hot summer days or cold winter nights and everything in between.

Waking Up Tired Tossed Salads

Lettuce wins the popularity contest for the vegetable most likely to be purchased. But as even the hardiest eater knows, lettuce usually needs some help. Eaten alone (no accoutrements, no dressing, no nothin'), lettuce can be at risk of deserving its sometimes maligned status as "rabbit food." On the other hand, when lettuce is a part of dish (salad or otherwise) it takes on a whole new dimension as it blossoms (so to speak) into a tasty food.

In the next few sections, we look at some of the most popular types of lettuce. Following that, we look at how you can make your lettuce come alive!

Getting the lowdown on lettuce

Lettuce is healthy for you; it's low in calories, high in water, and a source of fibre. Romaine lettuce (see later in this section) is the most nutritious of lettuces and is rich in folate, vitamin A, and vitamin C. Other lettuces carry the same nutrients but in lower amounts. Dark green lettuce has a larger amount of beta carotene.

Crisphead lettuce

Crisphead lettuce has a crunch or crispness. The leaves form a compact head that resembles a cabbage. The flavour of crisphead lettuce is mild to bland. Crisphead lettuce can be shredded, cut into wedges, or torn by hand.

Iceberg lettuce, the most famous of crisphead lettuces (well, insofar as lettuce can be famous!), has a very pale green middle and light green outer leaves. Two newly created varieties of iceberg lettuce have red leaves, or red and darker green leaves. Iceberg lettuce is the nutritional loser when it comes to lettuce because it has less fibre and nutrients than other varieties of lettuce. But if iceberg is your favourite, you can always add more healthy toppings to increase the fibre and nutrient content.

Cos lettuce

Cos lettuce has long green, or red and green, thick, crisp leaves that stand upright. The flavour is stronger than other lettuces. Romaine lettuce is the best known and most popular type of cos lettuce and is used in Caesar salad. (Why didn't we ever see Caesar salad around when we were kids? It would have made us into lettuce lovers far earlier.)

Butterhead lettuce

Butterhead lettuce has very soft leaves that are tender and form a loose head. The leaves can be green, red, or bronze. Boston, bibb, and buttercrunch are types of butterhead lettuce. Butterhead lettuce has a soft, buttery texture and a sweet, milky flavour. This lettuce is often mixed with other types of lettuce.

Looseleaf lettuce

Looseleaf lettuce does not form heads and is, you guessed it, a loose bunch of leaves. Oakleaf; dark red, frilly Lollo Rosso; arugula; and tubular Deer Tongue are (colourfully named) types of looseleaf lettuce. A mesclun mix is often a mixture of these types of lettuce.

Looseleaf lettuce comes in a variety of colours (including pale to darker green, red, and bronze) and flavours (ranging from mild to woody to sweet). Arugula, with the shape of an oak leaf, has a very distinct nutty to bitter, peppery taste.

Adding life to salad

Using lettuce as your base ingredient, you can create lively, tasty, nutritious salads; here's how: Add

- ✔ Other vegetables like red onion, mini corn on the cob, pea pods, Chinese napa cabbage, broccoli, cauliflower, watercress, sprouts, spinach, or blanched asparagus

- ✔ Fruit such as mandarin oranges, raisins, dried cranberries, berries, grapefruit, apple, avocado, or mango

- ✔ A protein-rich ingredient like grated low-fat cheddar cheese, goat cheese, low-fat feta cheese, blue cheese, low-fat mozzarella cheese cubes, boiled egg, nuts, seeds, leftover roast beef, chicken, pork, fish, shrimp, crab, or beans (chickpeas, kidney beans, and so forth)

- ✔ Fresh herbs such as parsley, cilantro, mint, dill, or basil

Be careful when choosing toppings (like crumbled bacon, for instance) and dressings: These can be very high in fat.

Storing lettuce

Lettuce tends to spoil quite easily, but here are a few simple measures to keep your lettuce healthy longer:

- ✔ Remove any bands holding the lettuce together. Bands tend to bruise the lettuce.

- ✔ Remove any bruised or wilted leaves. They promote spoiling of the other, still healthy leaves.

- ✔ Don't cut, tear, or shred the unused lettuce leaves. Leaving the leaves intact until you

are ready to use them will help the lettuce retain its nutrients and will help prevent the leaves from turning brown.

- ✔ Dry the leaves before storing them. A salad spinner is a particularly effective way to dry lettuce leaves.

- ✔ To extend their shelf life, wrap the leaves in a paper towel or a clean cloth and place them in a perforated plastic bag in the vegetable crisper of the refrigerator.

Giving salads zip with a homemade vinaigrette

Store-bought salad dressings are notoriously rich in calories. You can avoid these extra calories by making your own salad dressing. Here's a recipe for a homemade low-calorie vinaigrette:

Mix together:

- ✔ ¼ cup (50 ml) balsamic vinegar
- ✔ 1 tbsp (15 ml) plus 1 tsp (5 ml) olive oil
- ✔ 1 tbsp (15 ml) water
- ✔ 2 tsp (10 ml) honey
- ✔ 2 tsp (10 ml) Dijon mustard
- ✔ 1 clove garlic, minced

That's it!

One tablespoon of this vinaigrette (15 ml) provides 33 calories, 2 g fat, 3 g carbohydrate, and 16 mg sodium.

Think of salad dressing as you think of perfume: It should enhance, not overpower!

Choosing store-bought salad dressings

Grocery store shelves feature a seemingly limitless number and variety of salad dressings. These dressings vary greatly in their content of calories, fat, and sodium so you must carefully read the Nutrition Facts table to see what the product contains before you buy it. Keeping a couple of general principles in mind will help you choose the best dressing:

- ✔ A vinaigrette is often the lowest in calories. Be careful when it comes to oil and vinegar dressings; they can have more calories, fat, and sodium than some brand-name ranch dressings!

- ✔ When choosing a creamy dressing, select a low-fat version. (If you have diabetes, a low-fat version is also typically a better choice than an "ultra low-fat" version. Ultra low-fat salad dressings do, as advertised, have very little fat, but to maintain taste they typically contain more sugar.)

Whatever product you buy, remember to keep tabs on portion size. A "low calorie" dressing may not end up being so low in calories if — as can easily happen if you're not paying attention when pouring the sometimes watery contents from the bottle — you inadvertently end up putting on three servings' worth!

Making sure the lettuce is dry before adding it to your salad will help the dressing cling to it.

Starter Salads

In this section, we look at salads that serve as a fitting introduction to the meal to follow. The Tomato Cucumber Salad is a nice beginning to a light lunch or a dinner on a hot day. Classic Caesar Salad is a welcome start to a lovely Italian meal. Fruity Spinach Salad and Marinated Mushroom Salad are a great way to begin a lunch with friends. And Pecan, Mango, and Brie Salad — Ian's favourite of the bunch — is a scrumptious and relatively easy way to set the groundwork for a gourmet meal.

◌ Tomato Cucumber Salad

This recipe is quick and easy — perfect for when company arrives unexpectedly! It's even more delicious when made with fresh, in-season tomatoes.

Preparation Time: 15 minutes

Yield: 5 servings

1½ cups (375 ml) tomatoes, chopped into chunks

2 tbsp (30 ml) red onion, chopped into chunks

1 cup (250 ml) cucumber, chopped into chunks

2 tbsp (30 ml) parsley, coarsely chopped

2 tbsp (30 ml) olive oil

1½ tbsp (22 ml) red wine vinegar

¼ tsp (1 ml) salt

⅛ tsp (0.5 ml) pepper

1 tsp (5 ml) fresh oregano, finely chopped

1 tbsp (15 ml) fresh basil, finely chopped

1 Mix together the tomato, onion, cucumber, and parsley in a medium-sized bowl.

2 In a second smaller bowl, whisk together the oil, vinegar, salt, and pepper. Pour over the vegetables.

3 Add the herbs to the bowl, toss, and serve.

Per Serving: (½ cup/125 ml) Calories 64; Available carbohydrate 2 g; Carbohydrate 3 g; Fibre 1 g; Fat 6 g; Protein 1 g; Cholesterol 0 mg; Phosphorus 21 mg; Potassium 179 mg; Sodium 121 mg.

1 Serving = 0 Carbohydrate Choices

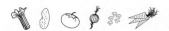

Classic Caesar Salad

This Caesar salad dressing is modified from one created by Cynthia's sister-in-law, Cindy Payne. The recipe is likely much thicker than you're used to eating. This recipe makes 1 cup (250 ml) of dressing, but if you want to double it to make more for later, it will keep well in the refrigerator up to two days.

Preparation Time: *10 minutes*

Yield: *8 servings*

2 egg yolks	*¼ tsp (1 ml) pepper*
2 cloves garlic, minced	*⅛ tsp (0.5 ml) salt*
¾ cup (175 ml) canola oil	*¼ cup (50 ml) low-fat Parmesan cheese*
1 tbsp (15 ml) lemon juice	*8 cups (2,000 ml) romaine lettuce, washed and dried*
½ tsp (2 ml) red wine vinegar	
1 tsp (5 ml) white vinegar	*½ cup (125 ml) croutons*
½ tsp (2 ml) oregano	*6 tbsp (90 ml) reduced-sodium bacon bits (about 3 slices of bacon, chopped)*
¼ tsp (1 ml) dry mustard	

1 To make the dressing, beat the egg yolks with a whisk or fork in a small bowl until they are thick. Add the garlic and mix well.

2 Very slowly add the oil, while continuing to whisk the mixture so it doesn't separate. Add the lemon juice, vinegars, spices, and Parmesan cheese, and mix well. If the dressing is too thick, more lemon juice can be added. But add it sparingly — the dressing is supposed to be thick.

3 Remove the stalks of the romaine lettuce, as well as any brown pieces. Break the lettuce into bite-sized pieces and place in a salad bowl. Pour on the dressing and mix well.

4 Add the croutons and bacon bits, toss, and serve.

Per Serving: *(1 cup/250 ml) Calories 240; Available carbohydrate 3 g; Carbohydrate 5 g; Fibre 2 g; Fat 24 g; Protein 3 g; Cholesterol 58 mg; Phosphorus 75 mg; Potassium 224 mg; Sodium 177 mg.*

1 Serving = 0 Carbohydrate Choices

☕ *Fruity Spinach Salad*

This is a quick and tasty salad — Cynthia's never served it to anyone who's disliked it, and it's also good for you! Spinach is an excellent source of vitamin A, folate, iron, magnesium, potassium, and riboflavin (vitamin B$_2$).

Preparation Time: *15 minutes*

Yield: *8 servings*

½ cup (125 ml) slivered almonds	*¼ cup (50 ml) olive oil*
2 tbsp (30 ml) sesame seeds	*¼ cup (50 ml) cider vinegar*
2 tbsp (30 ml) white sugar	*1 tbsp (15 ml) poppy seeds*
1½ tbsp (22 ml) red onion, chopped	*9 cups (2,250 ml) fresh spinach*
¼ tsp (1 ml) Worcestershire sauce	*1 cup (250 ml) sliced strawberries*
¼ tsp (1 ml) paprika	

1 Place the almonds in a dry frying pan over medium-high heat. Stir the almonds frequently for 3 to 5 minutes, until they are lightly toasted. Watch the almonds closely because they can burn easily. Remove the almonds from the frying pan and allow them to cool. Repeat with the sesame seeds.

2 To make the dressing, combine the sugar, onion, Worcestershire sauce, paprika, oil, and vinegar in a small bowl. Mix vigorously with a whisk or fork.

3 Mix together the almonds, sesame seeds, poppy seeds, spinach, and strawberries in a salad bowl. Pour the dressing on the salad, toss, and serve immediately.

Per Serving: (1 cup/250 ml) Calories 167; Available carbohydrate 6 g; Carbohydrate 9 g; Fibre 3 g; Fat 14 g; Protein 4 g; Cholesterol 0 mg; Phosphorus 97 mg; Potassium 323 mg; Sodium 65 mg.

1 Serving = 0 Carbohydrate Choices

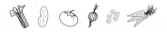

↻ *Marinated Mushrooms with Herbs*

Mushrooms are low in calories and a very good source of pantothenic acid (vitamin B$_5$). For enhanced flavour, prepare this recipe a day in advance to allow the mushrooms plenty of time to marinate. This is a revised recipe from Cynthia's sister-in-law, Roberta Payne.

Preparation Time: *10 minutes*

Cooking Time: *8 minutes*

Yield: *6 servings*

3 cups (750 ml) small, whole mushrooms	*¼ tsp (1 ml) dried thyme*
½ cup (125 ml) olive oil	*¼ tsp (1 ml) dried basil*
2 tbsp (30 ml) lemon juice	*1 clove garlic, minced*
2 tbsp (30 ml) white vinegar	*¼ cup (50 ml) red onion, chopped*
½ tsp (2 ml) salt	*2 tbsp (30 ml) red pepper, chopped*
½ tsp (2 ml) pepper	*2 tbsp (30 ml) green onion, chopped*
1 tsp (5 ml) dried tarragon	

1 Clean the mushrooms and place them in a medium-sized saucepan with the oil, lemon juice, vinegar, herbs, spices, and garlic. Simmer over low heat for 8 minutes.

2 Remove the saucepan from the heat and add the peppers and onion. Mix well with a spoon.

3 Place the salad in a medium-sized bowl, cover, and place in the refrigerator overnight. Stir the salad occasionally to prevent the marinade from settling at the bottom of the bowl.

4 When you're ready to eat, remove the mushrooms from the refrigerator, give them a good stir, and serve.

Per Serving: *(½ cup/125 ml) Calories 105; Available carbohydrate 2 g; Carbohydrate 3 g; Fibre 1 g; Fat 12 g; Protein 1 g; Cholesterol 0 mg; Phosphorus 35 mg; Potassium 152 mg; Sodium 197 mg.*

1 Serving = 0 Carbohydrate Choices

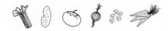

ℰ *Pecan, Mango, and Brie Salad*

This salad is easy to prepare, but serve it to your friends and family and they'll think you've been taking gourmet cooking classes. When picking mangoes, choose ones that are slightly soft to the touch and have no black spots.

Preparation Time: *12 minutes*

Yield: *8 servings*

½ cup (125 ml) mango, washed, peeled and cubed (for dressing)

1 large mango, washed, peeled and cubed (for salad)

1 small shallot, peeled and finely chopped

¼ cup (50 ml) white wine vinegar

½ cup (125 ml) olive oil

2 tbsp (30 ml) maple syrup

¼ tsp (1 ml) salt

¼ tsp (1 ml) pepper

⅛ tsp (0.5 ml) curry powder

½ cup (125 ml) halved pecans

8 cups (2,000 ml) mixed baby greens

6 oz (128 g) brie cheese, chopped into small cubes

1 For the dressing, place the ½ cup (125 ml) of cubed mango, shallot, vinegar, oil, maple syrup, salt, pepper, and curry powder into a blender and purée. If you don't have a blender, use an electric hand mixer or a potato masher to make the dressing as smooth as possible.

2 Lightly toast the pecans by placing them in a dry frying pan over medium-high heat. Stir frequently for 3 to 5 minutes, until the pecans are lightly toasted. Watch the pecans closely because they can burn easily.

3 In a salad bowl, mix together the baby greens, remaining mango cubes, toasted pecans, and brie. Pour on the dressing, toss, and serve.

Per Serving: *(1 cup/250 ml) Calories 287; Available carbohydrate 11 g; Carbohydrate 13 g; Fibre 2 g; Fat 25 g; Protein 6 g; Cholesterol 21 mg; Phosphorus 81 mg; Potassium 298 mg; Sodium 224 mg.*

1 Serving = ½ Carbohydrate Choice

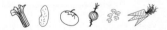

Side Salads

Side salads are those salads that are eaten with the rest of a meal (as opposed to starter salads which are eaten before the rest of the food is served). Side salads can be made ahead of time; a very helpful feature because the advance preparation allows you to spend more time with your company — and feel less harried after they arrive.

☙ Chunky Apple Coleslaw

Cabbage is an excellent source of antioxidants and is very affordable. Store it in a perforated plastic bag in the crisper of the refrigerator.

Preparation Time: *20 minutes*

Yield: *9 servings*

3 cups (750 ml) green cabbage, finely chopped	*2 tsp (10 ml) Dijon mustard*
½ cup (125 ml) carrot, grated	*½ tsp (2 ml) celery seed*
½ cup (125 ml) celery, chopped	*¼ tsp (1 ml) salt*
½ cup (125 ml) apple, diced	*¼ tsp (1 ml) pepper*
¼ cup (50 ml) red onion, chopped	*¼ cup (50 ml) light mayonnaise*
¼ cup (125 ml) red pepper, diced	*½ cup (125 ml) low-fat plain yogurt*
2 tbsp (30 ml) parsley, chopped	

1 Combine the vegetables, apple, and parsley in a large bowl.

2 For the sauce, mix together the mustard, celery seed, salt, pepper, mayonnaise, and yogurt.

3 Add the sauce to the vegetables and mix well with a fork until the sauce evenly covers the vegetables. Serve.

Per Serving: *(½ cup/125 ml) Calories 48; Available carbohydrate 5 g; Carbohydrate 6 g; Fibre 1 g; Fat 2 g; Protein 1 g; Cholesterol 2 mg; Phosphorus 36 mg; Potassium 149 mg; Sodium 132 mg.*

1 Serving = 0 Carbohydrate Choices

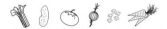

☙ Beet and Feta Salad

This vibrant salad offers a new way to eat beets and is ready in a flash.

Preparation Time: *15 minutes*

Yield: *4 servings*

14 oz (398 ml) can of small, whole, rosebud beets	*⅛ tsp (1 ml) pepper*
2 tbsp (30 ml) olive oil	*¼ cup (50 ml) red onion, chopped*
2 tbsp (30 ml) red wine vinegar	*½ cup (125 ml) low-fat feta cheese, cubed*
⅛ tsp (1 ml) salt	*2 tbsp (30 ml) fresh mint, chopped*

1 Empty the can of beets into a strainer, rinse with cold water, and let drain.

2 Cut the beets into quarters and place in a medium-sized bowl.

3 In a small bowl, whisk together the oil, vinegar, salt, and pepper. Pour over the beets.

4 Just before serving, add the onion, feta, and mint. Gently toss and serve.

Per Serving: *(½ cup/125 ml) Calories 78; Available carbohydrate 5 g; Carbohydrate 6 g; Fibre 1 g; Fat 7 g; Protein 3 g; Cholesterol 15 mg; Phosphorus 78 mg; Potassium 130 mg; Sodium 398 mg.*

1 Serving = 0 Carbohydrate Choices

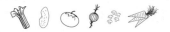

Pre-made and deli salads

If you need a salad in a pinch, you can pop into the grocery store and grab a bag of pre-washed salad greens, salad blends, or spinach. These pre-made salads are more expensive than making salad yourself, but the time saved may be worth it for you. Remember to check the "best before" date on the bag before you buy the salad. Resealing the bag and keeping it in your refrigerator's vegetable crisper will help to keep it fresh for a while longer. Some pre-made salads come complete with a small bag of croutons and dressing. Having these on the side can be helpful to help you limit the number of croutons and the amount and type of dressing on your salad. Think of it as undressing your salad!

Grabbing a pre-made, pre-dressed salad at a fast-food chain is not necessarily as healthy a choice as you might think. You may be surprised to hear that sometimes a burger has fewer calories and less fat than some of the salads on offer at these restaurants! The best thing to do, when possible, is to order the salad without dressing and to add the dressing yourself, in small quantities. Even better, ask for the nutritional analysis guide for the restaurant's foods and check out what the salad (or the burger, for that matter) contains.

Deli salads (that is, those pre-made salads like potato, macaroni, broccoli and raisin, chickpea,

seven grain, and so forth that you buy at the deli) are useful in a pinch when unexpected company arrives or you just need a break from preparing food. Be careful when choosing these salads as they can be a dietary minefield, festooned with fat, sodium, and calories.

Here are some ways to have a healthier deli salad:

✔ Ask the deli staff for the salad with the least dressing or with low-fat dressing. Even better, whenever possible, ask for the dressing to be given to you in a separate small dish or on the side of your plate. Dip the tongs of your fork in the dressing and then spear your salad morsel, with the little bit of dressing coming along for the ride to your mouth.

✔ Choose salads with broccoli, spinach, mixed greens, or romaine lettuce — the darker the colour, the better. (Dark green vegetables are often rich in calcium, iron, potassium, magnesium, vitamin A, beta-carotene, and folate.)

✔ Avoid salads with fried noodles and regular mayonnaise.

✔ Pick salads that are a good source of fibre, like whole wheat pasta, bulgur, seven grain, whole wheat couscous, or barley.

Washing your salad

To avoid ingesting contaminated salad, washing your greens (even those in "pre-washed" salad bags) is wise. Here is the most effective way to wash your greens:

✔ Wash your sink, your hands, and any container you will use.

✔ Rinse the greens under running water, gently rubbing the leaf surface with your hands.

✔ Place greens in a clean colander, salad spinner, or rack.

✔ Blot dry with a paper towel.

The drying step is important. Research shows that more bacteria is removed from the leaf when it is towel dried rather than air dried. Use a clean cloth towel or, better yet, a single use paper towel as it will not have been contaminated by previous use.

🍎 Light Potato Salad

This potato salad is much lighter than the traditional creamy type. It can be served warm or chilled — you choose.

Preparation Time: *15 minutes*

Yield: *4 servings*

3 medium-sized red potatoes, unpeeled (about 2 cups/500 ml)

1 tbsp (15 ml) Dijon mustard

1 tbsp (15 ml) grainy mustard

2 tbsp (30 ml) rice vinegar

2 tsp (10 ml) red wine vinegar

2 tbsp (30 ml) shallot, minced

1 tbsp (15 ml) olive oil

2 tbsp (30 ml) parsley, chopped

½ tsp (2 ml) salt

¼ tsp (1 ml) pepper

1 Place the unpeeled potatoes in a medium-sized pot. Fill the pot with enough water to cover the potatoes.

2 Bring the potatoes to a boil. Reduce the heat to medium and cook, uncovered, for approximately 20 minutes, until the potatoes are tender.

3 Drain the potatoes, rinse with cool water, drain again, and let the potatoes sit until they are cool enough to handle.

4 Cut the potatoes into 1 inch (2.5 cm) cubes and place in a medium-sized bowl.

5 For the dressing, whisk together the mustards, vinegars, and shallot in a small bowl. Slowly add the oil to the mustard mixture while continuing to whisk. Add the parsley, salt, and pepper and mix well.

6 Pour the dressing over the potatoes and mix gently until they are evenly coated. Serve warm or chilled.

Per Serving: (½ cup/125 ml) Calories 105; Available carbohydrate 13 g; Carbohydrate 14 g; Fibre 1 g; Fat 5 g; Protein 2 g; Cholesterol 0 mg; Phosphorus 56 mg; Potassium 384 mg; Sodium 221 mg.

1 Serving = 1 Carbohydrate Choice

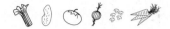

Asian Noodle Salad

This unique peanut-flavoured salad is a refreshing alternative to traditional North American salads. Chow mein noodles are long, thin, yellow noodles. They can be found in vacuum-sealed packages in the produce department of most grocery stores. This salad can be kept covered in the refrigerator for up to three days.

Preparation Time: *25 minutes*

Yield: *5 servings*

2½ tbsp (37 ml) reduced-sodium soy sauce	1 tbsp (15 ml) canola oil
2 tbsp (30 ml) lime juice	½ cup (125 ml) snow peas, cut in half
1½ tsp (7 ml) ginger, minced	¾ cup (175 ml) carrots, cut into fine strips
1 clove garlic, minced	2 green onions, chopped into ½-inch (1.25 cm) pieces
2 tbsp (30 ml) tahini	
1 tbsp (15 ml) honey	½ cup (125 ml) sweet red pepper, chopped
1½ tsp (7 ml) hoisin sauce	⅛ tsp (0.5 ml) salt
½ tsp (2 ml) red pepper flakes	⅛ tsp (0.5 ml) pepper
½ tsp (2 ml) sesame oil	¼ cup (50 ml) unsalted roasted peanuts, chopped
8 oz (250 g) chow mein noodles, uncooked	

1 For the dressing, mix together the soy sauce, lime juice, ginger, garlic, tahini, honey, hoisin sauce, red pepper flakes, and sesame oil in a bowl.

2 Place the chow mein noodles in a large pot. Add enough boiling water to cover the noodles in 1 inch (2.5 cm) of water. Stir gently, cover, and let sit for approximately 5 minutes, until the noodles are tender.

3 Drain the noodles in a strainer, then transfer them to a large salad bowl. Add the canola oil and toss.

4 Fill a small saucepan with water and bring to a boil. Add the snow peas and cook for 1 minute. Place the peas in a strainer and rinse them well with cold running water. Allow the peas to drain thoroughly and cool to room temperature.

5 Combine the salad ingredients in the bowl. Add the dressing, mix thoroughly, and serve.

Per Serving: (1 cup/250 ml) Calories 362; Available carbohydrate 33 g; Carbohydrate 37 g; Fibre 4 g; Fat 22 g; Protein 7 g; Cholesterol 0 mg; Phosphorus 152 mg; Potassium 265 mg; Sodium 605 mg.

1 Serving = 2 Carbohydrate Choices

Main Salads

A main salad is a salad that constitutes the entirety of a meal; that is, the salad *is* the meal.

Eating a salad as a meal is perfectly appropriate for anyone, but if you have diabetes you should ensure your main salad contains a protein source and a carbohydrate source. (If you have diabetes and you're taking certain types of blood glucose–lowering medication — like glyburide or insulin — and your meal doesn't contain carbohydrate, you'll be at risk of developing low blood glucose.)

The salads in this section contain protein and carbohydrate.

☼ Mixed Bean Salad

Try this bean salad for lunch instead of the same old sandwich. Beans are low in fat and are an excellent source of carbohydrates, protein, and fibre.

Preparation Time: *15 minutes*

Yield: *6 servings*

¼ cup (50 ml) canola oil	19 oz (540 ml) can of mixed beans
¼ cup (50 ml) red wine vinegar	⅓ cup (75 ml) red pepper, chopped
2 tbsp (30 ml) white sugar	½ cup (125 ml) celery, chopped
½ tsp (2 ml) salt	¼ cup (50 ml) red onion, chopped
¼ tsp (1 ml) pepper	¼ cup (50 ml) parsley, chopped

1 For the dressing, whisk together the oil, vinegar, sugar, salt, and pepper in a small bowl.

2 Drain the canned beans in a strainer and rinse under cold running water for 2 minutes.

3 Place the drained beans into a medium-sized bowl and add the dressing. Add the red pepper, celery, onion, and parsley. Stir well and serve.

Per Serving: *(½ cup/125 ml) Calories 228; Available carbohydrate 18 g; Carbohydrate 24 g; Fibre 6 g; Fat 10 g; Protein 7 g; Cholesterol 0 mg; Phosphorus 94 mg; Potassium 322 mg; Sodium 480 mg.*

1 Serving = 1 Carbohydrate Choice

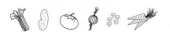

☺ *Bulgur and Chickpea Salad with Lemon Dressing*

Bulgur is whole wheat that has been cooked, dried, and broken into angular fragments. It is similar in nutritional value to whole wheat and is often used as an alternative to rice.

Preparation Time: 30 minutes

Cooking Time: 15 minutes

Yield: 8 servings

1 cup (250 ml) reduced-sodium vegetable broth	¼ tsp (1 ml) pepper
1 cup (250 ml) dry bulgur	¼ cup (50 ml) lemon juice (juice of one large lemon)
19 oz (540 ml) can of chickpeas	3 cloves garlic, minced
½ cup (125 ml) red onion, chopped	1 tbsp (15 ml) lemon zest
2 tbsp (30 ml) sun-dried tomatoes, chopped	1 tsp (5 ml) cumin
2 tbsp (30 ml) black olives, sliced	½ tsp (2 ml) paprika
2 tbsp (30 ml) cilantro, chopped	½ tsp (2 ml) ground coriander
¼ tsp (1 ml) salt	2 tbsp (30 ml) olive oil

1 Pour the broth into a small saucepan and bring to a boil.

2 Add the bulgur to the broth, stir, remove from heat, cover, and let sit for 15 minutes. The bulgur will absorb the broth and become tender.

3 Drain the canned chickpeas in a strainer and rinse well under cool running water for 2 minutes.

4 In a large bowl, mix together the chickpeas, onion, tomatoes, olives, cilantro, salt, and pepper. Add the bulgur and stir.

5 In small bowl, whisk together the lemon juice, garlic, lemon zest, cumin, paprika, and coriander. Slowly add the oil to the mixture while continuing to whisk.

6 Pour the lemon mixture into the bulgur mixture, toss well, and serve.

Per Serving: (½ cup/125 ml) Calories 140; Available carbohydrate 17 g; Carbohydrate: 21 g; Fibre 4 g; Fat 4 g; Protein 5 g; Cholesterol 0 mg; Phosphorus 86 mg; Potassium 221 mg; Sodium 326 mg.

1 Serving = 1 Carbohydrate Choice

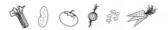

☙ Couscous Chickpea Salad

This salad may take longer to prepare than other main salads, but it's well worth the extra effort. Chickpeas are low in fat and an excellent source of carbohydrates, protein, and fibre, so this salad will satisfy your hunger. This salad will keep in the refrigerator for two days.

Preparation Time: *30 minutes*

Yield: *6 servings*

2 cloves garlic, minced	1 medium tomato, chopped
2 tsp (10 ml) soft margarine	½ cup (125 ml) red pepper, chopped
¾ cup (175 ml) water	⅓ seedless cucumber, diced
¼ tsp (1 ml) salt	1 tbsp (15 ml) lemon juice
½ cup (125 ml) dry couscous	1 tsp (5 ml) olive oil
1½ cups (375 ml) canned chickpeas	1 tsp (5 ml) cumin
⅓ cup (75 ml) cilantro, chopped	⅓ cup (75 ml) low fat feta cheese
2 tbsp (30 ml) fresh mint, chopped	⅛ tsp (0.5 ml) pepper
2 green onions, chopped	

1 In a medium pot, sauté the garlic in the margarine over medium heat for 2 to 3 minutes. Add the water and salt to the pot and bring to a boil. Remove the pot from the heat, add the couscous, stir, cover, and let sit for 5 minutes.

2 Drain the canned chickpeas in a strainer and rinse under cold running water for 2 minutes.

3 Combine the chickpeas and remaining ingredients in a large bowl. Fluff the couscous with a fork and add to the bowl. Stir well and serve.

Per Serving: *(¾ cup/175 ml) Calories 180; Available carbohydrate 24 g; Carbohydrate 28 g; Fibre 4 g; Fat 5 g; Protein 7 g; Cholesterol 6 mg; Phosphorus 125 mg; Potassium 267 mg; Sodium 386 mg.*

1 Serving = 1½ Carbohydrate Choices

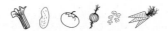

Walnut, Pear, and Chicken Salad

Walnuts are good for you because they contain healthy fats — so good, in fact, that some heart experts suggest we eat ten every day! Bear in mind, however, that nuts have calories. One ounce of walnuts (14 halves) has 166 calories, 18 g of fat, of which 13 g are the healthy polyunsaturated type.

Preparation Time: *20 minutes*

Yield: *6 servings*

⅓ cup (75 ml) olive oil	⅛ tsp (0.5 ml) pepper
3 tbsp (45 ml) apple cider vinegar	⅓ cup (75 ml) walnuts
3 tbsp (45 ml) white sugar	6 cups (1,500 ml) mixed baby greens
1 tsp (5 ml) celery seed	1 pear, diced
¼ tsp (1 ml) salt	1½ cups (375 ml) cooked chicken, diced

1 For the dressing, combine the oil, vinegar, sugar, celery seed, salt, and pepper in a small bowl. Mix well with a fork, making sure the sugar is dissolved.

2 Place the walnuts in a dry frying pan over medium-high heat, stirring frequently for 3 to 5 minutes, until the walnuts are lightly toasted. Let cool for 1 minute.

3 Combine the ingredients in a large bowl, toss, and serve immediately.

Per Serving: *(1 cup/250 ml) Calories 258; Available carbohydrate 12 g; Carbohydrate 14 g; Fibre 2 g; Fat 18 g; Protein 12 g; Cholesterol 29 mg; Phosphorus 119 mg; Potassium 242 mg; Sodium 130 mg.*

1 Serving = 1 Carbohydrate Choice

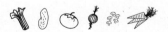

Chapter 10

Appealing Appetizers

In This Chapter

▶ Whipping up appetizers in a hurry

▶ Serving up classy hors d'oeuvres

▶ Pleasing party guests with fun finger foods

*W*e love appetizers. An appetizer is an opening act, an introduction to a meal if you will. Appetizers provide lovely esthetics, can have wonderful aromas, are typically scrumptious to eat, take an edge off a voracious appetite, and provide a hint of the undoubtedly great meal to follow. Sort of a food to get you ready for more food.

Another important role appetizers play is to provide casual food that your family, friends, and other guests can nibble on while you're making your last-minute preparations for the meal to come.

Appetizers are often too high in calories, fat, and salt, but they don't have to be. When you're in charge of preparation, you can take steps to ensure you cook up appetizers that are not only healthy and diabetes-friendly, but are fast and easy to make at the same time. In this chapter, we show you how.

Just in the Nick of Time: Fast, Easy Appetizers

If you're like most people, you likely find that entertaining often feels like a juggling act as you try to prepare the food to be ready at the right time and in the right order. We can't completely eliminate your acrobatics (or your stress), but you may find life is easier the next time company is coming over if you prepare one or more of these quick and easy appetizers:

- Bocconcini balls (small) with grape tomatoes and fresh basil leaves held together by toothpicks
- Bread sticks with hummus or guacamole dip
- Cream cheese (light, ½ to 1 block) topped with canned crab meat and cocktail sauce. Serve with crackers.
- Endive leaves with a spoon of goat's cheese or hummus
- Kabobs of cheese, olives, and meat, or fruit and cheese
- Prosciutto wrapped around a cube of honeydew or cantaloupe
- Pumpernickel bread spread with light cream cheese, a sprinkle of dill, and a slice of smoked salmon, topped with capers
- Sardines and light cream cheese on high-fibre crackers or pumpernickel bread

Elegant Starters

Appetizers are a staple at parties, and they can be a part of a light nibble or a "theme" meal or a nice treat when Saturday night rolls around and you're relaxing in front of the television (one of the few exceptions we make in our households to our "no eating in front of the TV" policy).

Shanghai Dumplings

Don't be afraid of this recipe. It's quick and easy to make, especially if you have a food processor or blender. Leftover dumplings can be kept in the refrigerator for two days or frozen for up to one month. It's best to store them in a sealable container between layers of wax paper. Extra sauce will keep in the refrigerator for ten days.

Preparation Time: *25 minutes*

Cooking Time: *20 minutes*

Yield: *6 servings*

½ lb (225 g) lean ground pork, uncooked

⅓ cup (75 ml) green onion, chopped

1 tbsp (15 ml) reduced-sodium soy sauce

1 tsp (5 ml) garlic, minced

1 tsp (5 ml) ginger, minced

1 tsp (5 ml) sesame oil

½ tsp (2 ml) salt

¼ tsp (1 ml) pepper

18 wonton wrappers

1½ tbsp (22 ml) plum sauce

1 tbsp (15 ml) grainy mustard

1½ tsp (7 ml) rice vinegar

1 Place the pork, onion, soy sauce, garlic, ginger, oil, salt, and pepper in a blender or food processor. Pulse the blender or food processor at medium speed until the mixture is smooth. If you don't have a blender or food processor, use a hand mixer or mix vigorously by hand.

2 Spoon 1½ tsp (7 ml) of the filling into the centre of a wonton wrapper.

3 Moisten the edges of the wrapper with cold water and fold to meet over the centre of the wonton. Press the seams firmly together.

4 Fill a wok or pot with 1 inch (2.5 cm) of water and bring to a boil.

5 Spray or rub a bamboo steamer, metal vegetable steamer, or cooling rack with cooking oil and place in the wok or pot over the water. Place the wontons on the rack, cover, and steam for 10 minutes.

6 For the sauce, whisk together the plum sauce, mustard, and vinegar in a small bowl.

7 Remove the wontons from the steamer or rack and serve with the sauce.

Per Serving: *(3 dumplings and ½ tsp/2 ml sauce) Calories 200; Available carbohydrate 16 g; Carbohydrate 17 g; Fibre 1 g; Fat 10 g; Protein 10 g; Cholesterol 32 mg; Phosphorus 100 mg; Potassium 158 mg; Sodium 500 mg.*

1 Serving = 1 Carbohydrate Choice

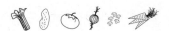

Sushi

Sushi isn't as difficult to prepare as you might think, and it will really impress your guests!

Preparation and Cooking Time: *1 hour*

Yield: *9 servings*

1 cup (250 ml) short-grain white rice

1 cup (250 ml) water

3 tbsp (45 ml) rice vinegar

1½ tsp (7 ml) white sugar

½ tsp (2 ml) salt

3 tbsp (45 ml) low-fat mayonnaise

1½ tsp (7 ml) wasabi paste

1 egg

6 nori sheets (sheets of seaweed)

1 cup (250 ml) crab or imitation crab

¼ English cucumber, thinly sliced lengthwise

1 small avocado, thinly sliced lengthwise and sprinkled with 1½ tsp (7 ml) lemon juice to prevent browning

¼ red pepper, thinly sliced lengthwise

½ cup (125 ml) carrots, grated

1 green onion, thinly sliced lengthwise

6 tbsp (90 ml) reduced-sodium soy sauce, for dipping

Pickled ginger, as an accompaniment

1 Place the rice in a strainer. Rinse well with cold water and stir until the water runs clear. Place the rinsed rice in a medium-sized saucepan, cover with cold water, and let soak for 30 minutes.

2 Drain the rice in the strainer. Return the rice to the saucepan, add 1 cup (250 ml) of water, and bring to a boil. Cover and simmer for 12 minutes.

3 Remove the rice from the heat, but do not remove the lid. Let the rice stand for 10 minutes.

4 Use a fork to spread the rice in a thin layer over a plastic tray to cool. Keep the rice moist by covering it with a damp paper towel.

5 In a saucepan, whisk together the vinegar, sugar, and salt. Heat over medium-low heat until the sugar is dissolved. Remove from the heat and allow the mixture to cool to room temperature.

6 Mix together the mayonnaise and wasabi in a small bowl and set aside.

7 In a bowl, beat the egg with a fork. Pour into a non-stick frying pan and fry over medium heat until the egg is firm. Remove the egg from the frying pan, place on a cutting board, and cut the egg into thin strips.

8 Spoon the rice from the plastic tray into a medium-sized bowl. Sprinkle the vinegar mixture over the rice and mix gently.

9 Place one nori sheet, shiny side down, on a cutting board or bamboo mat in front of you. Using a wet spoon, spread ½ cup (125 ml) of rice in an even layer over the nori sheet. Do not cover the 1½ inches (4 cm) of nori along the edge that is farthest from you.

10 Spread 2 tsp (10 ml) of the wasabi mixture in a narrow, lengthwise strip 2 inches (5 cm) from the edge of the nori that is closest to you. On top of the wasabi, layer 3 tbsp (45 ml) of crab, a small amount of egg, cucumber, avocado, red pepper, carrots, and green onion.

11 With a clean, wet finger, moisten the bare strip of nori. Fold the edge of the nori that is closest to you around the ingredients, and roll as tightly as you can. Seal by pressing the moistened strip against the outside of the roll. Repeat steps 9 through 11 for the other five nori.

12 Wrap each nori in plastic wrap and place in the refrigerator to chill for at least 2 hours.

13 After 2 hours, remove the nori from the refrigerator. Gently remove the plastic wrap and, using a wet knife, slice each roll into 6 pieces. Serve with soy sauce and pickled ginger.

Per Serving: (4 pieces and 2 tsp/10 ml soy sauce) Calories 158; Available carbohydrate 23 g; Carbohydrate 25 g; Fibre 2 g; Fat 4 g; Protein 5 g; Cholesterol 31 mg; Phosphorus 80 mg; Potassium 203 mg; Sodium 695 mg.

1 Serving = 1½ Carbohydrate Choices

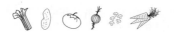

☙ Goat Cheese and Sun-Dried Tomato Mushroom Caps

When purchasing the mushrooms for this appetizer, choose the ones that are medium-small in size, enough for a one- or two-bite appetizer.

Preparation Time: *20 minutes*

Cooking Time: *20 minutes*

Yield: *10 servings*

20 medium-small mushrooms

2 tsp (10 ml) canola oil

5 oz (150 g) goat cheese

½ of a 250 g package of light cream cheese, softened

⅓ cup (75 ml) oil-packed sun-dried tomatoes, finely chopped

2 tbsp (30 ml) parsley, chopped

1 tbsp (15 ml) lemon juice

¼ tsp (1 ml) pepper

1 Heat oven to 400 degrees Fahrenheit (200 degrees Celsius).

2 Remove the stems from the mushrooms to create space for the filling. Brush the tops of the mushrooms with oil and place, hollow side down, on a baking sheet lined with parchment paper or foil.

3 Bake for 6 to 8 minutes, until the mushrooms are slightly soft. Remove from the oven and let them cool and drain on the tray for 5 minutes.

4 Reduce the oven temperature to 375 degrees Fahrenheit (190 degrees Celsius).

5 Place the mushrooms, hollow side up, on a baking sheet lined with a new sheet of parchment paper or foil.

6 In a small bowl, mix together the cheeses, tomatoes, parsley, lemon juice, and pepper.

7 Spoon the filling into the mushroom caps and bake for 10 minutes, until the cheese is slightly bubbling. Remove from the oven and serve.

Per Serving: *(2 mushrooms, 65 g) Calories 100; Available carbohydrate 3 g; Carbohydrate 4 g; Fibre 1 g; Fat 6 g; Protein 6 g; Cholesterol 18 mg; Phosphorus 109 mg; Potassium 225 mg; Sodium 148 mg.*

1 Serving = 0 Carbohydrate Choices

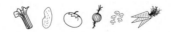

Party Pleasers

Party food is rich in taste and rich in fun. Party food is also often rich in sugar, fat, and calories. Oh darn! But hey, who says you can't have it all? In this section, we provide recipes for party food that has lots of the good stuff and goes easy on the bad.

☙ Feta Bruschetta

Bruschetta, an Italian favourite, has tomato as its main ingredient. (Trivia alert: Is tomato a fruit or a vegetable? Botanically speaking, the tomato is a fruit — a berry, to be precise. Legally speaking, however, the tomato is a vegetable — more than one hundred years ago, a court legally declared it so!)

Preparation Time: *15 minutes*

Cooking Time: *2 minutes*

Yield: *6 servings*

6 slices French bread	*¼ cup (50 ml) fresh basil or parsley, chopped*
1½ tbsp (22.5 ml) olive oil	*⅓ cup (75 ml) low-fat feta cheese, crumbled*
1 clove garlic, sliced in half	*⅛ tsp (0.5 ml) pepper*
2 cloves garlic, minced	
2 cups (500 ml) Roma tomatoes, chopped and drained	

1 Grill or toast bread on both sides until golden brown.

2 Brush one side of each slice with oil and rub with the halved garlic clove.

3 In a bowl, gently combine the minced garlic, tomatoes, basil or parsley, feta, and pepper.

4 Spoon ⅓ cup (75 ml) of the tomato mixture over the bread. Serve and enjoy.

Per Serving: (1 slice, 80 g) Calories 121; Available carbohydrate 19 g; Carbohydrate 21 g; Fibre 2 g; Fat 3 g; Protein 6 g; Cholesterol 6 mg; Phosphorus 83 mg; Potassium 208 mg; Sodium 306 mg.

1 Serving = 1 Carbohydrate Choice

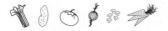

Dilly Shrimp Cucumber Bites

With savoury shrimp and cool cucumber, this appetizer is both flavourful and refreshing.

Preparation Time: *10 minutes*

Draining Time: *30 minutes*

Yield: *12 servings*

2 English cucumbers (each approximately 12-inch/30 cm long)

1 tsp (5 ml) salt

12 medium-sized shrimp, cooked and diced

2 tbsp (30 ml) light mayonnaise

1 tbsp (15 ml) fresh dill, chopped

1 tsp (5 ml) lemon zest

2 tsp (10 ml) lemon juice

⅛ tsp (0.5 ml) pepper

1 Cut off the ends of the cucumbers. To create a striped effect, cut thin, lengthwise strips of peel from the cucumber using a vegetable peeler. Cut the cucumbers into 24 1-inch (2.5 cm) slices.

2 Using a melon baller or small spoon, scoop out 1 tsp (5 ml) from the centre of each cucumber slice, leaving the bottom of each slice intact. Sprinkle the hollowed side of the slices with salt and place upside down on sheets of paper towel to drain for 30 minutes.

3 For the filling, mix together the remaining ingredients in a bowl.

4 With a spoon, place 1 to 2 tsp (5 to 10 ml) of the filling into the hollowed cucumbers. To garnish, place a small piece of dill on top of each slice. Serve and enjoy.

Per Serving: (2 cucumber slices) Calories 21; Available carbohydrate 2 g; Carbohydrate 2 g; Fibre 0 g; Fat 1 g; Protein 2 g; Cholesterol 11 mg; Phosphorus 20 mg; Potassium 75 mg; Sodium 244 mg.

1 Serving = 0 Carbohydrate Choices

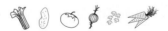

The Devilish Egg

Devilish eggs are a great classic that can be made up to two days in advance and kept in the refrigerator — if they don't get eaten first!

Preparation Time: *20 minutes*

Cooking Time: *22 minutes*

Yield: *12 servings*

6 eggs	*2 dashes pepper*
2 dashes salt	*3 tbsp (45 ml) light mayonnaise*
½ tsp (2 ml) dry mustard	*1 tsp (5 ml) white vinegar*
Sprinkle of paprika	

1 Place the eggs in a saucepan and fill with cold water until the eggs are covered by 1 inch (2.5 cm) of water.

2 Bring the water to a boil, then remove the saucepan from the heat, cover, and let stand. After 22 minutes, remove the eggs from the saucepan and place them immediately in cold water to cool.

3 Gently tap each cooled egg to crack its shell. Peel the shells gently under cold running water.

4 Cut eggs in half lengthwise with a sharp knife and gently scoop out the yolks with a teaspoon. Place the yolks in a bowl.

5 To create the filling, mash the yolks with a fork or potato masher, then add the salt, mustard, pepper, mayonnaise, and vinegar. Mix well.

6 Spoon the filling into the hollowed egg whites and arrange on a platter and sprinkle each egg with paprika. Serve and enjoy.

Per Serving: (½ egg) Calories 49; Available carbohydrate 1 g; Carbohydrate 1 g; Fibre 0 g; Fat 4 g; Protein 3 g; Cholesterol 107 mg; Phosphorus 49 mg; Potassium 36 mg; Sodium 27 mg.

1 Serving = 0 Carbohydrate Choices

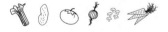

◌ *Toasted Walnut Hummus*

With savoury garlic and a hint of orange, this nutritious dip makes a great snack or light meal.

Preparation Time: *10 minutes*

Cooking Time: *5 minutes*

Yield: *8 servings*

½ cup (125 ml) walnut pieces	⅓ cup (75 ml) orange juice
3 tbsp (45 ml) olive oil	¼ tsp (1 ml) salt
1 clove garlic, minced	⅛ tsp (0.5 ml) pepper
19 oz (540 ml) can of chickpeas	1 tbsp (15 ml) parsley, chopped
1 tsp (5 ml) grated orange rind	

1 Place the walnuts in a dry frying pan and set over medium-high heat. Stir often, until the walnuts are lightly toasted, about 5 minutes. Let cool for 5 minutes.

2 Pour the chickpeas into a strainer and rinse under cool running water until it runs clear. Allow the chickpeas to drain.

3 In a food processor or blender, combine the walnuts, oil, and garlic. Purée until smooth.

4 Add the chickpeas, orange rind, juice, salt, and pepper. Blend until the ingredients become smooth in consistency, about 2 minutes.

5 Spoon the hummus into a bowl and garnish with parsley. Serve with raw veggies or with crackers, pita, or melba toast. Don't forget to count any extra carbohydrates.

Per Serving: (¼ cup/50 ml) Calories 179; Available carbohydrate 14 g; Carbohydrate 18 g; Fibre 4 g; Fat 5 g; Protein 5 g; Cholesterol 0 mg; Phosphorus 89 mg; Potassium 174 mg; Sodium 275 mg.

1 Serving = 1 Carbohydrate Choice

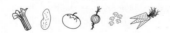

⬠ *Black Bean Salsa*

Here's a Mexican recipe that's a snap to make and can be eaten as either a snack or a lunch. It can also be used as a topping over fish or chicken.

Preparation Time: *10 minutes*

Yield: *6 servings*

19 oz (540 ml) can of black beans	*3 tbsp (45 ml) lime juice*
¾ cup (175 ml) canned corn kernels	*4 tbsp (60 ml) cilantro, finely chopped*
1½ cup (375 ml) tomato, diced small	*1 clove garlic, minced*
1 tbsp (15 ml) olive oil	*⅛ tsp (0.5 ml) pepper*

1 Place the black beans in a strainer and rinse under cool, running water until it runs clear. Allow the black beans to drain.

2 Drain the corn and tomato in another strainer.

3 Combine the ingredients in a medium-sized bowl and gently toss with a spatula or spoon.

4 Serve with baked tortilla chips, crackers, or melba toast. Alternatively, you can stuff the salsa into a ½ pita with shredded cheese and lettuce for a fast lunch. Don't forget to count the extra carbohydrates.

Per Serving: (⅔ cup/150 ml) Calories 130; Available carbohydrate 14 g; Carbohydrate 21 g; Fibre 7 g; Fat 3 g; Protein 7 g; Cholesterol 0 mg; Phosphorus 122 mg; Potassium 430 mg; Sodium 347 mg.

1 Serving = 1 Carbohydrate Choice

Store-Bought Dips

Over the past few years, we've seen a veritable explosion in the number and variety of dips and spreads available at the grocery store. Many of these, however, aren't particularly healthy food choices due to their high sodium, fat, and calorie content. As with other foods, use a product's Nutrition Facts table (see Chapter 6) to help guide your selection.

Here are a few tips on dips:

- ✔ Of the various prepared dips and spreads you can find in the store, hummus is often lower in calories and fat.
- ✔ Compared with cheddar cheese–based products, those made with a goat cheese base are often lower in calories, fat, and sodium.
- ✔ For a quick dip, try low-fat sour cream or plain yogurt mixed with dried onion soup mix or dried vegetable soup mix.
- ✔ A great dip for fruits is plain yogurt mixed with some diet Jello powder.
- ✔ Prepared spinach dip is very high in calories, fat, and sodium.

As we say many times in this book, no food is forbidden, and that includes store-bought dips. Even a very "rich" dip is okay to eat; just watch your portions.

Chapter 11

Creative Carbohydrate Concoctions

In This Chapter

▶ Dishing out great potato plates

▶ Doing right by rice

▶ Pleasing with pasta

▶ Bursting with beans

arbohydrates are an essential nutrient. As we discuss in Chapter 2, carbohydrates provide the energy your body (including your brain) requires to function normally. Also, carbohydrate in the form of fibre helps control blood glucose, lowers cholesterol, and helps prevent constipation.

Carbohydrates (with the exception of fibre) also raise blood glucose, so you need to keep the amount of carbohydrates you consume in check. The Canadian Diabetes Association recommends that carbohydrates make up between 45 to 60 percent of your daily calorie intake.

Because carbohydrates raise blood glucose, many people have come to believe that carbohydrates are, in some way, "bad" for you and should be severely restricted. The truth of the matter is that carbohydrates are a key nutrient (as we just described) and, as long as you eat the appropriate amount, they will not only not hurt your health, they will enhance it.

Carbohydrate-based dishes can range from the simple to the complex. And you can make even the most seemingly mundane of carbohydrate dishes come alive, with just a little effort. Think your rice looks boring? Try adding some finely chopped vegetables. Baked potato seems dull? Try topping it with some light sour cream and chives, low-fat cheddar cheese, or even salsa or baked beans. In this chapter, we provide a wide variety of carbohydrate-based recipes for you to enjoy.

Potato, Please!

Potatoes are part of a healthy diet for people living with diabetes. (And they are part of a healthy living for many Canadian farmers, too. Canada is one of the largest potato producers in the world.) In addition to providing energy, potatoes are a good source of potassium and vitamins (including vitamin B_6 and vitamin C), and potato skin provides fibre.

Popular *baking potatoes* like russet are light, fluffy, and creamy and are ideal for baking, mashing, and French fries.

Popular *boiling potatoes* like White, Red, and Ruby Crescent, are great for soups, casseroles, salads, roasting, and barbecuing because of their tendency to hold their shape. (They can be mashed, but will result in thick and lumpy potatoes.)

These are some other types of potatoes:

- Yukon Gold potatoes are moister than the baking variety and will hold together during boiling. They can be used for roasting, pan frying, stews, soups, and gratins. They can be also used for baking, mashing, and frying, but will not produce the quality that baking potatoes can.

- New potatoes are immature, small potatoes of any variety.

- Sweet potatoes grow on a vine above the ground and actually have no real relation to the white potato. Sweet potato is rich in beta carotene, vitamin C, and vitamin E.

- Yams are native to Africa and are larger than sweet potatoes and have fewer nutrients. (Yams are often mixed up with sweet potatoes in the grocery store, but fortunately, both can be used interchangeably in recipes.)

☺ *Greek Potatoes*

This easy recipe adds a Mediterranean twist to traditional oven-baked potatoes.

Preparation Time: *15 minutes*

Cooking Time: *1 hour*

Yield: *6 servings*

3 cups (458 g) red potatoes

⅓ cup (75 ml) fresh lemon juice

3 tbsp (45 ml) olive oil

2 cloves garlic, minced

½ tsp (2 ml) salt

⅛ tsp (0.5 ml) pepper

1 tsp (5 ml) Italian seasoning

¼ tsp (1 ml) paprika

Boiling water, approximately 2½ cups (625 ml)

1 Preheat oven to 400 degrees Fahrenheit (200 degrees Celsius).

2 Clean and lightly scrub the potatoes in cool water. Cut the potatoes into pieces, no greater than 1½ inches (4 cm) thick, and place in a medium-sized casserole dish.

3 In a small bowl, mix together the lemon juice, oil, garlic, salt, pepper, and spices with a whisk or fork. Pour this mixture over the potatoes, and, using a spoon, toss until the potatoes are coated.

4 Add enough boiling water to just cover the potatoes, then bake uncovered for 1 hour. Stir the potatoes every 20 minutes.

5 The potatoes are done when most of the water has evaporated and the potatoes are soft when pierced with a knife. Serve and enjoy.

Per Serving: *(½ cup/125 ml, 72 g) Calories 118; Available carbohydrate 12 g; Carbohydrate 14 g; Fibre 2 g; Fat 7 g; Protein 2 g; Cholesterol 0 mg; Phosphorus 49 mg; Potassium 367 mg; Sodium 199 mg.*

1 Serving = 1 Carbohydrate Choice

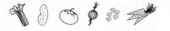

☙ *Potato Latkes*

These little potato pancakes are often described as Jewish soul food. Here is the recipe for all to enjoy.

Preparation Time: *30 minutes*

Cooking Time: *2 to 3 minutes per side*

Yield: *9 pancakes*

4 medium-large Yukon Gold potatoes, peeled	*½ tsp (2 ml) cayenne pepper*
3 large eggs	*1 green onion, finely chopped*
¼ cup (50 ml) all-purpose flour	*1 medium onion, finely chopped*
2 tsp (10 ml) baking powder	*½ cup (125 ml) canola oil*
½ tsp (2 ml) salt	*Low-fat sour cream, if desired*

1 Using a food processor or hand grater, finely grate the potatoes.

2 Place the grated potatoes in a strainer and press out as much liquid as you can.

3 Transfer the potatoes onto a clean tea towel and use it to again squeeze as much moisture from the potatoes as you can. Set the potatoes aside, covered with the tea towel.

4 In a small bowl, whisk together the eggs, flour, baking powder, salt, and pepper.

5 Place the potatoes in a large bowl with the onions and egg mixture. Mix together with a spoon.

6 Cover the bottom of a large frying pan with ⅛ inch (0.3 cm) of canola oil. Heat over medium-high heat.

7 Add ½ cup (125 ml) of the potato mixture to the hot frying pan, flattening into a pan-cake form with a spatula. Cook for 2 to 3 minutes per side, until the pancake is golden brown. Repeat until you have used all the grated potatoes.

8 Serve the latkes warm with low-fat sour cream, if desired.

Per Serving: *(1 pancake, 117 g) Calories 218; Available carbohydrate 18 g; Carbohydrate 20 g; Fibre 2 g; Fat 14 g; Protein 4 g; Cholesterol 70 mg; Phosphorus 113 mg; Potassium 432 mg; Sodium 267 mg.*

1 Serving = 1 Carbohydrate Choice

Selecting and storing potatoes

Choose firm, dry potatoes that are free of cracks, cuts, blemishes, or sprouts. If a potato has a green tinge, avoid it. For even cooking, try to choose potatoes that are the same size.

Store your potatoes in paper bags in a cool spot (near an outside wall or in the cold cellar) that is dark, dry, and well ventilated. Don't store onions near the potatoes. The onions give off a gas that can cause potatoes to decay more quickly. Store an apple in the bag with the potatoes; the apple will stop the potatoes from sprouting! (The only type of potato that can be stored in the refrigerator are new potatoes, which can be stored in a plastic bag in the fridge for up to one week.)

⟶ Sweet Potato Fries

These sweet potato fries are a much healthier alternative to deep-fried French fries — and they taste yummy too!

Preparation Time: *10 minutes*

Cooking Time: *20 minutes*

Yield: *3 servings*

2 medium (350 g) sweet potatoes, peeled	⅛ tsp (0.5 ml) garlic powder
2 tsp (10 ml) canola oil	⅛ tsp (0.5 ml) pepper
¼ tsp (1 ml) paprika	

1 Preheat oven to 400 degrees Fahrenheit (200 degrees Celsius).

2 Lightly grease a cookie sheet with canola oil or cover with parchment paper.

3 Cut the sweet potatoes lengthwise into thin, fingerlike pieces.

4 In a large bowl, mix together the oil and spices, add the potatoes, and toss to coat.

5 Spread out one even layer of the potatoes onto the cookie sheet.

6 Bake for about 20 minutes, turning once, until the fries are soft when pierced with a fork. Serve and enjoy.

Per Serving: (about 12 fries, 130 g) Calories 106; Available carbohydrate 17 g; Carbohydrate 19 g; Fibre 2 g; Fat 3 g; Protein 1 g; Cholesterol 0 mg; Phosphorus 43 mg; Potassium 271 mg; Sodium 2 mg.

1 Serving = 1 Carbohydrate Choice

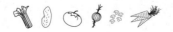

⟳ *Garlic Mashed Potatoes*

This garlicky potato dish is a treat for potato lovers looking to add variety to their meals.

Preparation Time: *10 minutes*

Cooking Time: *15 to 20 minutes*

Yield: *5 servings*

2 medium-large Yukon Gold potatoes	*1 tbsp (15 ml) soft margarine*
1 garlic clove, sliced in half	*¼ tsp (1 ml) salt*
¼ cup (50 ml) 1% milk, warm	*⅛ tsp (0.5 ml) pepper*

1 Peel the potatoes and cut into 2-inch (5-cm) pieces.

2 Place the potatoes and garlic in a medium saucepan and add just enough water to cover them.

3 Place a lid on the saucepan and bring to a boil over high heat.

4 When the potatoes have started to boil, take the lid partially off to prevent the water from boiling over. Continue to cook for about 15 minutes or until the potatoes are soft and can easily be pierced with a fork. Turn the burner off.

5 Drain the potatoes and garlic well in a strainer. Return the potatoes to the saucepan and place over the burner. Even though the burner is now off, its remaining warmth will help excess water to evaporate. Add the milk, margarine, salt, and pepper.

6 Mash the potatoes well with a potato masher until smooth and fluffy. Serve warm.

Per Serving: (½ cup/125 ml, 127 g) Calories 92; Available carbohydrate 14 g; Carbohydrate 16 g; Fibre 2 g; Fat 2 g; Protein 2 g; Cholesterol 1 mg; Phosphorus 61 mg; Potassium 380 mg; Sodium 147 mg.

1 Serving = 1 Carbohydrate Choice

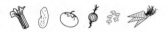

Rice Is Right

Rice is a healthy, easy-to-prepare, very convenient food that has no fat, cholesterol, or sodium. If you need to follow a gluten-free diet (as you would if you have a bowel disorder called *celiac disease*), rice fits well because it doesn't contain gluten. (For more about celiac disease, check out *Celiac Disease For Dummies* [Wiley], a book that Ian co-wrote.) Rice is an incredibly versatile food that can be used in dishes ranging from appetizers to soups, main dishes, side dishes, and even desserts. Rice can be eaten for breakfast, lunch, or dinner; it always pays to have some rice handy in your pantry.

Exploring the different types of rice

There are three main types of rice (long grain, medium grain, and short grain). In Table 11-1, we look at some of the main features of these three types of rice and some other varieties that are popular in Canada.

Table 11-1		Types of Rice	
Type of Rice	*Examples*	*Characteristics*	*Uses*
Long grain	White	Separate grains	Casseroles
	Basmati	Fluffy	Salads
	Jasmine	Least sticky	Side dishes
Medium grain	Arborio	Plumper and shorter than long grain	Salads
	Calrose		
		Moist	Side dishes
		Tender	Soup
Short grain	Arborio	Short	Pudding
		Plump	Risotto
		Sticky	Sushi
Parboiled	Converted	Firm	Pilafs
		Not very sticky	Side dish
		Fluffy	Good for general use
Brown rice	Medium and short grain	Chewy	Side dish
		Nutty flavour	Salads

Parboiled rice originated in India. It is prepared by having steam pass through grains that have their husks on. By keeping the husks on during steaming, nutrients stay within the grain during and after processing; this makes parboiled rice more nutritious than white rice.

Wild rice has a nutty flavour, is chewy, and is excellent in soup, rice pudding, stuffing, and mixed with rice. (Despite its name, wild rice is not a rice at all; it's a grass seed native to North America.)

Instant rice is pre-cooked, dehydrated, white or brown rice that can be cooked in just a few minutes as it simply requires re-hydrating and warming.

Cooking rice right

When it comes to cooking rice there isn't a single, "best" way because, just like art and music, there are different strokes for different folks. How you go about cooking rice will depend on several factors, including the type of rice used, the cooking method used, and, importantly, your personal preferences. For instance, if you like your rice soft and moist, you'll cook your rice with more water than if you prefer your rice firm and dry, in which case you'd use less water.

If you don't have a lot of experience cooking rice, just go ahead and follow the directions on the rice package.

Before cooking rice, rinse the rice in cold water, using a fine strainer, until the water runs clear. (This doesn't apply to instant rice.) Also, when cooking rice be sure to use a tight-fitting lid and don't remove the lid from the pot while the rice is cooking. After the rice has finished cooking, continue to keep the lid on the pot for at least 10 minutes until the rice has sat. At that point, you can remove the lid and fluff the rice using a chopstick or fork.

In the next few sections, we look in detail at several ways to cook one cup of uncooked rice, yielding 3 to 4 cups (750–1,000 ml) as outlined in Table 11-2.

Stove-top method

To cook rice on a stove-top:

1. Combine 1 cup (250 ml) rice, liquid measured according to Table 11-2 (see page 159), ½ tsp (2 ml) salt (optional), and 1 tbsp (15 ml) margarine (optional) in a medium saucepan.

2. Bring the mixture to a boil, stirring once or twice.

3. Reduce the heat to a low simmer and cover with a tight-fitting lid.

4. Cook according to the time indicated in Table 11-2. If the rice is not quite tender or the liquid is not absorbed, cover with the lid and cook 2 to 4 minutes longer. Remove the rice from the heat and let sit covered for 10 minutes. Fluff with a chopstick or fork and serve.

Table 11-2	Stove-top Rice Cooking Times		
Type of Uncooked Rice (1 cup / 250 ml)	*Liquid*	*Cooking Time*	*Yield*
Long grain	1¾ cups (425 ml)– 2 cups (500 ml)	15 min	3 cups (750 ml)
Medium grain	1½ cups (375 ml)	15 min	3 cups (750 ml)
Brown rice	2 cups (500 ml)– 2½ cups (625 ml)	45–50 min	3–4 cups (750–1,000 ml)
Parboiled/ converted	2 cups (500 ml)– 2½ cups (625 ml)	20–25 min	3–4 cups (750–1,000 ml)

Oven-baked method

Using the quantities listed in Table 11-2, place measured, boiling water in an oven-proof casserole dish with a lid. Stir and cover tightly, then bake at 350 degrees Fahrenheit (175 degrees Celsius) for 25 to 30 minutes (30 to 40 minutes for parboiled/converted rice and 1 hour for brown rice). Let sit for 10 minutes, covered. Fluff with a chopstick or fork before serving.

Microwave method

Follow the stove-top measurements and use a medium microwave safe dish with a lid. Cover and cook on high for 5 minutes or until boiling then reduce to medium (50% power) and cook 15 minutes more. Let sit 10 minutes, covered. Fluff with a chopstick or fork. (For parboiled/converted rice, cook 20 minutes and, for brown rice, 30 minutes.)

Storing rice

Once its container has been opened, most types of uncooked rice can be stored for up to a year in a sealed container in a cool, dry place.

The exception is uncooked brown rice, which has a shorter shelf life (due to the bran and oil) than other forms of rice. It needs to be stored differently. After you open a bag of brown rice, store it in a sealed container in the refrigerator, where you can keep it for up to six months.

Cooked rice can be refrigerated for up to seven days or frozen for six months.

Reheating rice

Leftover rice needn't go to waste. To reheat rice, place one cup (250 ml) cooked rice in a covered saucepan with 3 tbsp (45 ml) of water. Warm over low heat for about five minutes and it will be hot and fluffy. For 2 cups (500 ml) cooked rice, use 5 tbsp (75 ml) water. You can also reheat rice on low in the microwave or in the oven with low heat, using the above amounts.

⌖ *Vegetable Fried Rice*

For a fluffier dish, we recommend using long grain rice and cooking it a day in advance. Typically, fried rice is very high in fat and sodium, but this Chinese version uses healthy oil and reduced-sodium soy sauce.

Preparation Time: 10 minutes

Cooking Time: 10 minutes

Yield: 5 servings

1 tbsp (15 ml) canola oil

½ cup (125 ml) onions, finely chopped

¼ cup (50 ml) carrots, finely chopped

¼ cup (50 ml) celery, finely chopped

¼ cup (50 ml) red pepper, finely chopped

½ cup (125 ml) frozen peas

1 cup (250 ml) long grain rice, cooked a day in advance

1 egg

1 tbsp (15 ml) reduced-sodium soy sauce

¼ tsp (1 ml) salt

1 green onion, chopped

1 Heat the oil in a large frying pan or wok, over medium-high heat. Add the onions and sauté for 2 to 3 minutes, until they are soft.

2 Add the carrots and celery to the onion and sauté for another 2 to 3 minutes, until they are slightly soft. Add the red pepper and peas, and sauté for another 2 to 3 minutes, until the red pepper and peas are slightly soft as well.

3 Add the rice and stir for 1 minute, until thoroughly mixed.

4 In a small bowl, mix together the egg, soy sauce, and salt with a whisk or fork. Pour this mixture into the rice and vegetables, and stir constantly for 2 to 3 minutes until the egg is cooked. Add the green onion, stir for 1 minute. Serve warm and enjoy.

Per Serving: (½ cup/125 ml, 82 g) Calories 107; Available carbohydrate 12 g; Carbohydrate 14 g; Fibre 2 g; Fat 4 g; Protein 4 g; Cholesterol 42 mg; Phosphorus 60 mg; Potassium 132 mg; Sodium 311 mg.

1 Serving = 1 Carbohydrate Choice

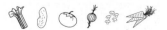

♻ *Saffron Almond Rice*

Saffron is the world's most expensive spice. Each purple crocus flower produces only three saffron stigmas (threads) that must be hand-picked. Heat releases saffron's flavour and colour. This Indian dish goes exceptionally well with the Saffron Fish and Tandoori Chicken recipes we offer in Chapters 13 and 14, respectively.

Preparation Time: 20 minutes

Cooking Time: 23 minutes

Yield: 5 servings

⅔ cup (150 ml) basmati rice	1 cinnamon stick
½ tsp (2 ml) saffron threads	3 green cardamom pods
5 tsp (25 ml) warm water	1¼ cups (300 ml) water
1½ tsp (7 ml) canola oil	⅛ tsp (0.5 ml) salt
1 tbsp (15 ml) almonds, sliced	

1 Place the rice in a strainer and rinse with cool running water until it runs clear. Allow the rice to drain.

2 Crumble the saffron threads into small chunks between your fingers and add them to 5 teaspoons (25 ml) of warm water. Set aside for at least 20 minutes (or for best results, 12 hours).

3 Add the oil to a medium-sized pot with a lid. Place the pot over medium-high heat. When the oil is warm, add the almonds, cinnamon stick, and cardamom pods to the pot. Stir for about 2 minutes, until the almonds become slightly brown.

4 Add the rice to the pot and sauté, stirring constantly, for 1 minute. Pour in the saffron and water mixture, add 1¼ cups (300 ml) of water, and bring to a boil over high heat.

5 Add the salt, cover the pot, and simmer over low heat for about 20 minutes, until no water remains in the saucepan and the rice is tender.

6 Remove the rice from the heat. Leave the lid on the pot and allow the rice to sit for 4 minutes. Fluff the rice with a fork and serve.

Per Serving: (½ cup/125 ml, 72 g) Calories 109; Available carbohydrate 19 g; Carbohydrate 20 g; Fibre 1 g; Fat 2 g; Protein 2 g; Cholesterol 0 mg; Phosphorus 34 mg; Potassium 38 mg; Sodium 59 mg.

1 Serving = 1 Carbohydrate Choice

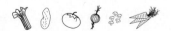

Plenty of Pasta

Pasta is a perennial favourite, and it's so versatile. It can be made for a quick weekday supper or as part of a special Sunday feast. In this section, we offer some tips on preparing pasta and share some of our favourite recipes.

Cooking pasta to perfection

To make perfect pasta follow these steps:

1. Fill a large saucepan with water; the more the better. (Pasta will stick if not enough water is used.) Add two dashes of salt to help prevent the water from boiling over. Cover the saucepan with a lid and heat to a rolling boil.

2. Add the pasta to the boiling water and stir often to prevent sticking.

3. When the water starts to boil again, start timing. Most pastas cook in 8 to 12 minutes. Check the package directions. Pasta is best if cooked to *al dente* — firm but still tender.

4. Drain the pasta in a strainer or colander as soon as the pasta is done.

   If pasta sits in hot water past its cooking time it will go soggy.

If using the pasta to make a hot dish, don't rinse it because then the sauce won't stick as well. If you're using the pasta to make a cold dish, rinse with cool water so that the pasta won't stick together.

Knowing how much pasta to prepare

Cooking usually makes pasta double in size.

When preparing long pasta, measure around the bundle of pasta with a measuring tape to calculate the amount you need for a serving using the following guidelines:

- 2½ inches (6 cm) is 3 oz (90 g) = about 1 serving
- 4½ inches (11 cm) is 8 oz (250 g) = about 2 to 3 servings
- 5¼ inches (12.5 cm) is 12 oz (375 g) = about 4 servings

Past-a its prime: Storing tips

Commercial dry pasta should be stored in an air-tight container or in its resealed box in a cool, dry place. It can be kept for up to one year.

Commercial fresh pasta should be stored in a well-sealed container or bag in the refrigerator and used by the "best before" date indicated by the manufacturer on the package.

Homemade pasta is best cooked and eaten as soon as it is prepared; otherwise, uncooked pasta should be stored in the refrigerator in a well-sealed container for up to two days.

☙ Cheesy Noodles with Nuts

This traditional Hispanic dish is made with walnuts — tasty and good for your heart health!

Preparation Time: *10 minutes*

Cooking Time: *16 minutes*

Yield: *4 servings*

1 cup (250 ml) dry whole wheat, penne pasta

¼ cup (50 ml) soft margarine

3 tbsp (45 ml) walnuts, finely chopped

1 tbsp (15 ml) parsley, chopped

⅛ tsp (0.5 ml) salt

½ cup (125 ml) low-fat mozzarella cheese, shredded

1 In a medium-sized saucepan, bring 3 cups (750 ml) of water to a boil over high heat. Add the pasta and stir. Cook for 13 minutes, stirring occasionally. Drain in a strainer and cover to keep warm.

2 Melt the margarine in a medium-sized frying pan set over medium heat. Add the walnuts and stir constantly until they are golden brown, about 3 minutes. Make sure the walnuts don't burn — scorched nuts will taste bitter.

3 Add the parsley and salt, and remove from heat. Add the pasta to the frying pan and toss until it is coated in the walnut mixture. Sprinkle the dish with the cheese. Serve and enjoy.

Per Serving: *(½ cup/125 ml, 87 g) Calories 292; Available carbohydrate 17 g; Carbohydrate 23 g; Fibre 6 g; Fat 18 g; Protein 9 g; Cholesterol 8 mg; Phosphorus 135 mg; Potassium 75 mg; Sodium 410 mg.*

1 Serving = 1 Carbohydrate Choice

☙ Pasta Primavera

A great, colourful dish that can be made at anytime of the year and, of course, Cynthia has made this a low-fat, high-fibre version!

Preparation Time: *25 minutes*

Cooking Time: *16 minutes*

Yield: *8 servings*

¼ lb (100 g) dry whole wheat spaghettini	1 medium tomato, chopped
1 tbsp (15 ml) olive oil	3 cups (750 ml) baby spinach
½ cup (125 ml) onion, chopped	¼ cup (50 ml) parsley, chopped
1 clove garlic, minced	¼ tsp (1 ml) salt
1 cup (250 ml) celery, chopped diagonally	¼ tsp (1 ml) pepper
1 cup (250 ml) snow peas, topped and tailed	½ cup (125 ml) 1% milk
1 large red pepper, thinly sliced	1 tsp (5 ml) dried basil
1 cup (250 ml) mushrooms, sliced	½ cup (125 ml) low-fat Parmesan cheese

1 In a medium-sized saucepan, bring 4 cups (1,000 ml) of water to a boil over high heat. Add the pasta and stir. Cook for 8 minutes, stirring occasionally. Drain in a strainer and set aside.

2 In a large frying pan, warm the oil over medium heat and add the onion, garlic, and celery. Sauté for 3 minutes, stirring occasionally with a spatula or wooden spoon.

3 Add the snow peas, pepper, and mushrooms and sauté for another 3 minutes.

4 Add the tomatoes and spinach to the frying pan and sauté for 2 minutes.

5 Stir in the remaining ingredients, saving ¼ cup (50 ml) of the cheese for the topping.

6 Remove from the heat and serve, topped with the remaining Parmesan cheese. Enjoy.

Per Serving: *(⅔ cup/150 ml, 85 g) Calories 113; Available carbohydrate 14 g; Carbohydrate 16 g; Fibre 2 g; Fat 4 g; Protein 5 g; Cholesterol 6 mg; Phosphorus 132 mg; Potassium 320 mg; Sodium 201 mg.*

1 Serving = 1 Carbohydrate Choice

☞ Quinoa Risotto

Quinoa (pronounced keen-wa) is a grain that originates in the Andes Mountains of South America. It has a nutty flavour, is gluten-free, and easily digested, and is a breeze to prepare. For a vegetarian dish, use vegetable broth instead of chicken.

Preparation Time: *25 minutes*

Cooking Time: *14 minutes*

Yield: *8 servings*

1 cup (250 ml) quinoa

2 tsp (10 ml) canola oil

½ cup (125 ml) onion, chopped

1 clove garlic, minced

2¼ cups (550 ml) reduced-sodium chicken or vegetable broth

2 cups (500 ml) arugula, chopped

¼ cup (50 ml) carrot, shredded

¾ cup (175 ml) shiitake mushroom, sliced

¼ cup (50 ml) low-fat Parmesan cheese, grated

¼ tsp (1 ml) salt

¼ tsp (1 ml) pepper

1 Place the quinoa in a strainer and rinse thoroughly under cool water for 3 minutes. Drain.

2 In a large saucepan, heat the oil over medium heat and add the onion. Sauté until the onion is soft and translucent, about 3 minutes. Add the garlic and quinoa and cook for 1 minute, stirring occasionally.

3 Add the broth to the frying pan with the quinoa and bring to a boil. Reduce the heat to low, cover, and simmer for about 12 minutes, until the quinoa is almost tender, but slightly hard in the centre. There should still be lots of unabsorbed broth in the mixture.

4 Stir in the arugula, carrots, and mushrooms, and simmer until the quinoa has turned from white to translucent, about 2 minutes.

5 Mix in the Parmesan cheese, salt, and pepper. Serve immediately.

Per Serving: (½ cup/125 ml, 14 g) Calories 119; Available carbohydrate 15 g; Carbohydrate 17 g; Fibre 2 g; Fat 4 g; Protein 6 g; Cholesterol 3 mg; Phosphorus 158 mg; Potassium 259 mg; Sodium 147 mg.

1 Serving = 1 Carbohydrate Choice

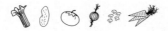

⌖ Spinach Mushroom Lasagna

This hearty main dish can be prepared ahead of time, refrigerated, and baked the next day. Substituting ready-to-bake lasagna noodles for the regular variety will cut 15 minutes off the preparation time. For a vegetarian dish, use vegetable broth instead of chicken.

Preparation Time: *60 minutes*

Cooking Time: *35 minutes (plus 10 minutes to cool)*

Yield: *9 servings*

1 tbsp (15 ml) canola oil

2 tbsp (30 ml) flour

2 cloves garlic, minced

1 cup (250 ml) 1% milk

1 cup (250 ml) reduced-sodium chicken or vegetable broth

2 green onions, chopped

½ cup (125 ml) dry-packed sun-dried tomatoes, chopped, and rehydrated

2 tsp (10 ml) canola oil

2¼ cups (550 ml) shiitake mushrooms, sliced

1 shallot, chopped

3 tbsp (45 ml) parsley, chopped

⅓ cup (75 ml) ground flaxseed

¼ tsp (1 ml) salt

1 tsp (5 ml) canola oil

12 cups (3,000 ml) baby spinach

2 cups (500 ml) low-fat ricotta cheese

¾ cup (175 ml) low-fat Parmesan cheese, grated

1 egg white

12 sheets spinach lasagna noodles, cooked

1 In a large saucepan, heat 1 tbsp (15 ml) of oil over medium-high heat. Whisk in the flour and stir constantly for 1 minute.

2 Add the garlic and stir for 30 seconds. Whisk in the milk and broth. Cook and stir with a whisk or spatula for about 4 minutes, until the mixture thickens slightly. Remove the saucepan from the heat and mix in the green onion and sun-dried tomatoes, then set aside.

3 In a large frying pan, heat 2 teaspoons (10 ml) oil over medium-high heat. Add the mushrooms and shallot, and sauté for about 8 minutes, until the mushrooms and shallots are lightly browned. Remove the pan from the heat, mix in the parsley, flaxseed, and salt. Transfer this to a large bowl and set aside.

4 Using the same frying pan, heat the remaining teaspoon (5 ml) of oil over medium-high heat. Add the spinach and stir until it is slightly wilted and bright green. Remove the pan from the heat and let the spinach cool slightly.

5 In another large bowl, mix together the ricotta, ½ cup (125 ml) of the Parmesan cheese, and the egg white with a large spoon. Add the spinach and stir until the mixture is well blended.

6 Lightly grease a 9–x-13-inch (20-x-30-cm) baking dish with canola oil. With a spatula, spread ½ cup (125 ml) of sauce over the bottom of the baking dish and cover with 3 sheets of pasta. Spoon half the spinach mixture over the pasta and spread evenly with a spoon. Cover with 3 more pasta sheets and then top with another ½ cup (125 ml) of sauce. Evenly distribute a thin layer of mushrooms over the sauce. Cover the layer of mushrooms with ½ cup (125 ml) of sauce and 3 more pasta sheets. Spoon the remaining spinach filling over the pasta and then add the last 3 pasta sheets. Top with the remaining sauce and ¼ cup (50 ml) of Parmesan cheese.

7 When you are ready to bake the lasagna, preheat your oven to 375 degrees Fahrenheit (190 degrees Celsius).

8 Cover the lasagna with foil and bake for 25 minutes. Remove the foil and allow the dish to bake for another 10 minutes or so, until it is golden brown. Let the lasagna cool for 10 minutes before serving. Enjoy.

Per Serving: (1 slice, 3 x 4¼ inch/6.5 cm x 10 cm, 197 g) Calories 288; Available carbohydrate 27 g; Carbohydrate 32 g; Fibre 5 g; Fat 12 g; Protein 17 g; Cholesterol 26 mg; Phosphorus 353 mg; Potassium 669 mg; Sodium 558 mg.

1 Serving = 2 Carbohydrate Choices

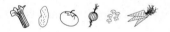

Szechuan Noodles

A must at Chinese celebrations isn't cake, but noodles! The long Chinese noodle signifies long, unbroken life — the trick is to slurp with dignity.

Preparation Time: *25 minutes*

Cooking Time: *20 minutes*

Yield: *8 servings*

Marinade:

1 tsp (5 ml) rice vinegar

1 tsp (5 ml) reduced-sodium soy sauce

1 tsp (5 ml) cornstarch

Sauce:

½ cup (125 ml) reduced-sodium chicken broth

1 tsp (5 ml) chili pepper paste

½ tsp (2 ml) sugar

1 tsp (5 ml) sesame oil

2 tsp (10 ml) cornstarch

Noodles:

½ lb (225 g) chicken breast, cut into strips

6 oz (175 g) fresh chow mein noodles

1 tbsp (15 ml) canola oil

½ cup (125 ml) shrimp, shelled and cleaned

½ cup (125 ml) onion, chopped

1 clove garlic, minced

3 cups (750 ml) bok choy, cut into bite-sized pieces

1 cup (250 ml) carrots, chopped diagonally

1 cup (250 ml) broccoli florets

2 tbsp (30 ml) canola oil

1 tbsp (15 ml) reduced-sodium soy sauce

For the marinade:

1 In a medium bowl, use a whisk or fork to mix together the marinade ingredients. Add the chicken to the bowl and stir with a large spoon until the chicken is coated. Set the bowl aside for at least 20 minutes to allow the chicken to marinate.

For the sauce:

2 In a small bowl, mix together all the sauce ingredients with a whisk or fork. Set aside.

For the noodles:

3 Fill a large pot with water and bring to a boil over high heat. (Make sure there is enough water to completely cover the noodles.) Once the water has reached a boil, add the chow mein noodles and remove the pot from the heat. Stir the noodles, cover the pot, and let it sit for 5 minutes, until the noodles are tender. Toss with a fork to loosen the noodles and then drain in a strainer. Cover the noodles and set them aside.

4 Add 1 tbsp (15 ml) oil to a wok or large frying pan and set over medium-high heat. Add the marinated chicken and stir-fry for 5 minutes. Remove the chicken from the frying pan and place in a medium-sized bowl.

5 Add the shrimp to the wok or frying pan and stir-fry over medium-high heat for 3 minutes. Add the shrimp to the bowl with the chicken and cover to keep warm.

6 Add another tablespoon (15 ml) of oil to the wok or frying pan and set over medium-high heat. Add the onion, garlic, bok choy, carrots, and broccoli and stir-fry until the vegetables are tender crisp, about 4 minutes. Set aside.

7 Warm 2 tbsp (30 ml) of oil in the wok or frying pan and place over medium heat. Add the noodles and toss to separate them. Add the soy sauce and toss again over the heat for 1 minute.

8 Combine the chicken, shrimp, and vegetables in a large bowl. Add the sauce and mix thoroughly. Add this mixture to the wok with the noodles, toss until the ingredients are thoroughly mixed. Serve and enjoy.

Per Serving: (¾ cup/175 ml, 175 g) Calories 280; Available carbohydrate 16 g; Carbohydrate 19 g; Fibre 3 g; Fat 16 g; Protein 17 g; Cholesterol 47 mg; Phosphorus 178 mg; Potassium 444 mg; Sodium 429 mg.

1 Serving = 1 Carbohydrate Choice

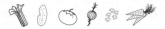

Bountiful Beans

Beans and legumes are very economical and are very versatile in recipes. Buy them dry, frozen, or canned. Frozen and canned beans make for quick meals.

Beans and legumes are a great source of protein, carbohydrate, and fibre. They are low in fat and free of cholesterol. Beans are a source of B vitamins, calcium, iron, phosphorus, potassium, and zinc. Beans and legumes are also gluten-free. In addition to their myriad health benefits, beans and legumes are also tasty. Don't believe us? Then you have to try some of the recipes in this section; that will make a believer out of you!

Store dried beans for up to one year in air-tight containers. Cooked beans can be stored in plastic bags or containers in the refrigerator for up to 5 days and in the freezer for up to 6 months. Canned beans can be stored in a cool, dry place for up to one year.

☙ Dal

There are many versions of this Indian dish. This authentic recipe comes from one of Cynthia's friends, Dr. Nita Rajesh, who let Cynthia into her kitchen for close observations!

Preparation Time: *10 minutes*

Cooking Time: *30 minutes*

Yield: *3 servings*

½ cup (125 ml) yellow lentils

2 cups (500 ml) water

½ tsp (2 ml) salt

¼ tsp (1 ml) turmeric

1 tbsp (15 ml) ghee-clarified butter (or use canola oil)

½ cup (125 ml) onion, finely chopped

1 clove garlic, minced

¼ tsp (1 ml) cumin powder

⅛ jalapeño pepper, chopped

⅛ tsp (0.5 ml) asafoetida spice, optional

1 tbsp (15 ml) cilantro, chopped

1 Check the lentils for stones and remove any you may find. Place the lentils in a strainer and rinse with cool running water until it runs clear. Allow the lentils to drain.

2 Place the lentils in a medium-sized saucepan. Add 2 cups (500 ml) water, salt, and turmeric. Cover the pot with a lid and bring to a boil over high heat. Cook for 5 minutes.

3 Reduce the heat to low and simmer, with the lid on, for 25 minutes, until the lentils are soft and have become a souplike mixture.

4 While the lentils are cooking, add the ghee to a medium-sized frying pan. Place over medium heat and add the onions, garlic, and cumin. Stir constantly until the onions are soft and translucent, about 2 minutes.

5 Add the jalapeño and asafoetida and stir for 1 minute. Remove from heat.

6 Add the onion mixture to the lentils and mix well.

7 Serve hot, topped with cilantro.

Per Serving: (⅔ cup/150 ml) Calories 165; Available carbohydrate 12 g; Carbohydrate 22 g; Fibre 10 g; Fat 5 g; Protein 9 g; Cholesterol 11 mg; Phosphorus 156 mg; Potassium 366 mg; Sodium 396 mg.

1 Serving = 1 Carbohydrate Choice

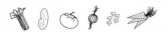

✿ *Mango Bean Mix*

This recipe is quick and colourful, and the beans are a great source of protein, carbohydrate, and fibre.

Preparation Time: *10 minutes*

Yield: *4 servings*

10 oz (270 ml) canned black beans	*⅛ cup (25 ml) lime juice (1 lime)*
½ mango, peeled and diced	*1 tbsp (15 ml) olive oil*
1 small red pepper, finely chopped	*1½ tsp (7 ml) reduced-sodium soy sauce*
1 green onion, chopped	*⅛ cup (25 ml) cilantro, chopped*

1 Place the beans in a strainer and rinse with cool running water until it runs clear. Allow the beans to drain.

2 In a medium-sized bowl, combine the beans, mango, red pepper, and onion.

3 To make the dressing, whisk together the lime juice, oil, and soy sauce.

4 Add the dressing to the bean mixture and toss with a spoon. Add the cilantro and toss again.

5 Serve as a side dish, on its own, or with mini nachos. (Remember 12 mini nachos will add a second Carbohydrate Choice to this dish.)

Per Serving: *(½ cup/125 ml) Calories 119; Available carbohydrate 12 g; Carbohydrate 18 g; Fibre 6 g; Fat 4 g; Protein 8 g; Cholesterol 0 mg; Phosphorus 87 mg; Potassium 316 mg; Sodium 289 mg.*

1 Serving = 1 Carbohydrate Choice

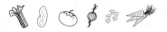

Taking the gas out of beans

Many people who otherwise like beans shy away from them because of concerns over bloating, burping, or flatulence. You can, however, minimize gaseousness. Without, ahem, getting long-winded about it, here are some tips to help you avoid problems with gas from eating beans or other forms of fibre:

- When first adding (or increasing the amount of) fibre (like beans) to your diet, always start with small portions and gradually increase your portion size.

- Drink plenty of fluids when you add extra fibre to your diet.

- For canned beans (except baked beans in sauce), drain the beans in a strainer or colander under cool running water for 2 minutes. An additional benefit of doing this is that it will reduce the amount of sodium present.

- Soak dried beans in cool water for 4 to 12 hours, depending on the type of bean (check the package directions). After a few hours, drain the beans and add fresh water. When ready to cook, drain the water off again, add fresh water and simmer the beans gently until softened. Some people say that adding ⅛ teaspoon (0.5 ml) of baking soda to the soaking water helps reduce gas, but this is controversial.

- Rinse legumes. (They don't have to be soaked.)

- Try not to eat other famous gas-producing foods (such as broccoli, cauliflower, cabbage, and Brussels sprouts) at the same meal as beans.

If none of these tips helps, you can always resort to that old tried and true remedy: Simply be "loud and proud." Not genteel perhaps, but, well, like we said elsewhere in this chapter, different strokes for different folks.

⟳ Chickpea Curry

Flavourful, easy, and quick to prepare, here is another true Indian dish. This one comes from one of Cynthia's dietetic interns, Ruby Ubhi.

Preparation Time: *15 minutes*

Cooking Time: *20 to 25 minutes*

Yield: *4 servings*

19 oz (540 ml) can of chickpeas	*½ tsp (2 ml) garam masala*
3 cloves garlic, minced	*1 tsp (5 ml) chana masala*
1½ tbsp (22 ml) canola oil	*½ tsp (2 ml) turmeric*
1 medium onion, finely chopped	*1 tsp (5 ml) paprika*
1 tsp (5 ml) ginger, grated	*¾ cup (175 ml) water*
1 large tomato, chopped	*⅓ cup (75 ml) cilantro, chopped*
⅛ tsp (0.5 ml) salt	

1 Pour the chickpeas into a strainer and rinse under cool running water until it runs clear. Allow the chickpeas to drain.

2 Heat the oil in a medium-sized frying pan over medium heat. Add the garlic and onion and sauté for 2 minutes, until the onion becomes soft.

3 Add the ginger, tomato, and spices. Stir for another 2 minutes.

4 Add the chickpeas to the frying pan with ¾ cup (175 ml) of water. Cover and let simmer on medium-low heat for 15 minutes. More water can be added if you prefer a souplike curry.

5 Remove from the heat and serve, sprinkled with cilantro. (This curry can be served with brown rice, basmati rice, or naan bread, but remember that these additions will increase the carbohydrates.)

Per Serving: *(¾ cup/175 ml) Calories 273; Available carbohydrate 34 g; Carbohydrate 42 g; Fibre 8 g; Fat 9 g; Protein 8 g; Cholesterol 0 mg; Phosphorus 168 mg; Potassium 489 mg; Sodium 510 mg.*

1 Serving = 2 Carbohydrate Choices

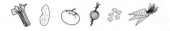

☉ Curried Chickpeas in Tomato Cups

You will look like a true gourmet when you present these tasty tomatoes to dinner guests! This dish can be made in advance and kept refrigerated until your guests arrive. Leftover curried chickpeas can be kept covered in the fridge for two days.

Preparation Time: *15 minutes*

Cooking Time: *20 minutes*

Yield: *8 servings*

¾ cup (175 ml) water	*2 tbsp (30 ml) curry powder*
½ cup (125 ml) dry bulgur	*¼ cup (50 ml) water*
8 firm medium tomatoes	*1 cup (250 ml) baby spinach*
1 cup (250 ml) canned chickpeas	*¼ cup (50 ml) basil, finely chopped*
1 tsp (5 ml) canola oil	*½ cup (125 ml) low-fat plain yogurt*
1 clove garlic, minced	*¼ tsp (1 ml) salt*
1 small onion, chopped	*⅛ tsp (0.5 ml) sugar*

1 Fill a large saucepan with water and bring to a boil over high heat. Stir in the bulgur and boil for 1 minute. Remove from heat, cover, and let sit for 15 minutes until the bulgur has absorbed most of the water.

2 Slice off the top ½ inch (1.25 cm) of each tomato. Remove the stems, and coarsely chop the tomato tops.

3 Using a spoon, gently scoop out the inside of the tomato and discard. Place the tomatoes, upside down, on paper towels to drain.

4 Pour the canned chickpeas into a strainer and rinse under cool water for 2 minutes. Drain.

5 Add the oil to a large frying pan and place over medium heat. Add the garlic and onion, and stir for 2 minutes, until the onion starts to soften. Add the curry powder and continue to stir for 20 seconds.

6 Add the water and chopped tomato tops to the frying pan. Mix well for 4 minutes over medium heat.

7 Add the chickpeas, spinach, basil, yogurt, salt, and sugar to the frying pan. Stir well until the ingredients are evenly mixed.

8 Add the bulgur to the frying pan and stir well with a spatula for 1 minute.

9 Using a spoon fill each tomato cup with ⅓ cup (75 ml) of the bulgur mixture. Serve right away or place in the fridge until your guests arrive. Hot or cold, these stuffed tomatoes are delicious!

Per Serving: *(1 tomato with ⅓ cup/75 ml filling, 180 g) Calories 113; Available carbohydrate 15 g; Carbohydrate 20 g; Fibre 5 g; Fat 2 g; Protein 5 g; Cholesterol 1 mg; Phosphorus 119 mg; Potassium 482 mg; Sodium 146 mg.*

1 Serving = 1 Carbohydrate Choice

Chapter 12

Don't Forget Your Veggies!

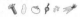
Although vegetables are nutritious and an essential part of any healthy diet, most Canadians don't consume enough of them. Health Canada's Eating Well with Canada's Food Guide (www.healthcanada.gc.ca/foodguide) recommends at least seven servings of fruits and vegetables per day for people 14 years of age and older; most Canadians consume only about two-thirds that amount.

If you don't get enough veggies in your diet because you find them bland or boring, not varied enough, or just not to your liking, we've got three words for you: Read This Chapter. In this chapter are tasty recipes for those vegetables that are available seasonally and those that are available all year long. We also offer cooking tips to help you ensure you derive the maximum health benefit from your produce.

Be Veggie Savvy

Vegetables are inherently rich in nutrients, but to derive the maximum benefit that veggies can offer, you need to be aware of some important points, including how best to cook them. In this section, we look at how to prepare vegetables. We also discuss the benefits of buying your vegetables locally.

Is local produce more nutritious than imported produce?

Although locally grown vegetables are fresher and often taste better than remotely grown (and transported) produce, local vegetables are — popular wisdom to the contrary — not necessarily more nutritious than imported produce. Many factors influence the nutritional content of produce, including the type of food in question, how it is grown, its ripeness when harvested, how it is stored, and how it is processed and packaged. Every step from the seed in the ground to the mature vegetable on your kitchen table can affect the food's nutritional value. This is true for both local produce and imported produce. All of which is to say that the blanket statement that "local equals good and remote equals bad" doesn't necessarily hold true. (However, this statement does in fact apply to a group of vegetables. Broccoli, green beans, kale, tomatoes, red peppers, peaches, and apricots all lose nutrients when harvested and transported for longer distances, so in general you should make a special point of buying these items locally whenever possible.)

Buying locally, in season

Many of the vegetables on your corner grocery store's shelves are likely better travelled than you are. With modern storage and transportation techniques, foods that were formerly seldom available in Canada — especially when out of season — are now available year-round. This availability is wonderful in that it allows for more food choices, more diverse menu planning, and so forth, but it does come at a price. In addition to the higher cost of foods that have been shipped great distances, certain environmental issues must also be considered. For example, many vegetables for sale in Canada — especially when local produce is not available — come from the southern U.S. and beyond. To get them to Canada requires, of course, transportation (truck, rail, ship, and so forth), which requires fuel, generates carbon, and has other affects on the environment.

When you buy food grown locally, you support local farmers, their families, and your community's economy. Purchasing locally means less fossil fuel is used for — and less greenhouse gas created from — transportation. Also, locally produced foods are usually fresher because they're harvested when ripe and immediately ready to enjoy instead of being shipped from afar and needing to then ripen during transportation or on supermarket shelves. (Having said all this, we wouldn't want to leave the impression that this is a black-and-white issue. Some contrarians point out the benefits of choosing more remotely grown produce, including the efficiencies of farming in southern climes where a greater number of crops per year can be harvested. In our opinion, however, the many pros of buying locally grown produce outweigh the cons.)

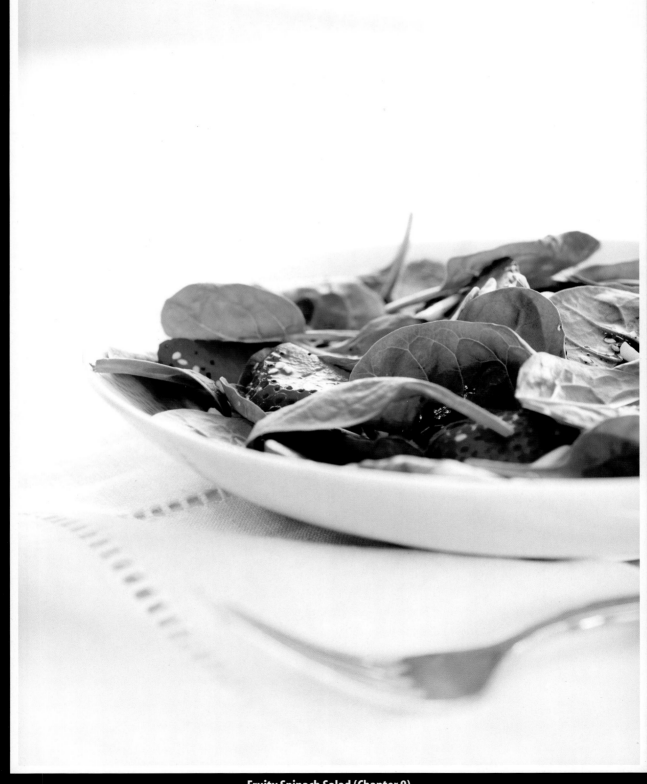

Fruity Spinach Salad (Chapter 9)

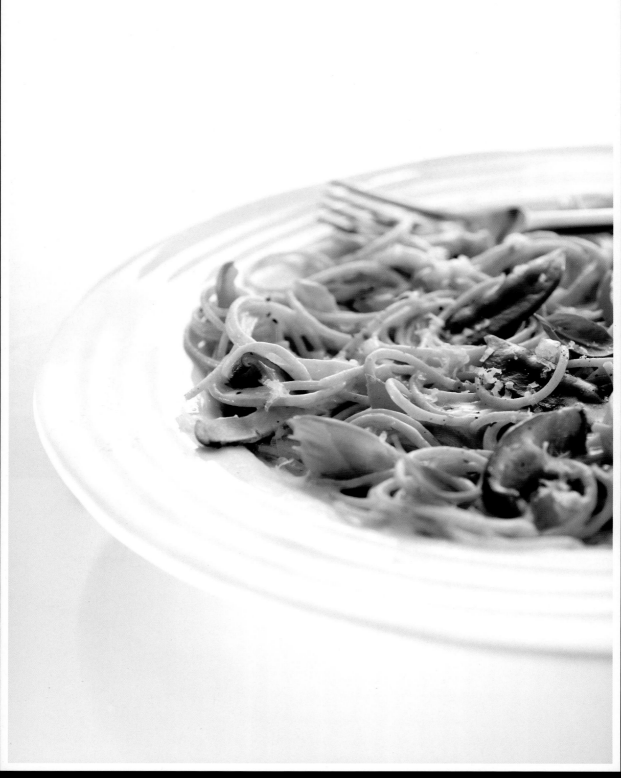

Pasta Primavera (Chapter 11)

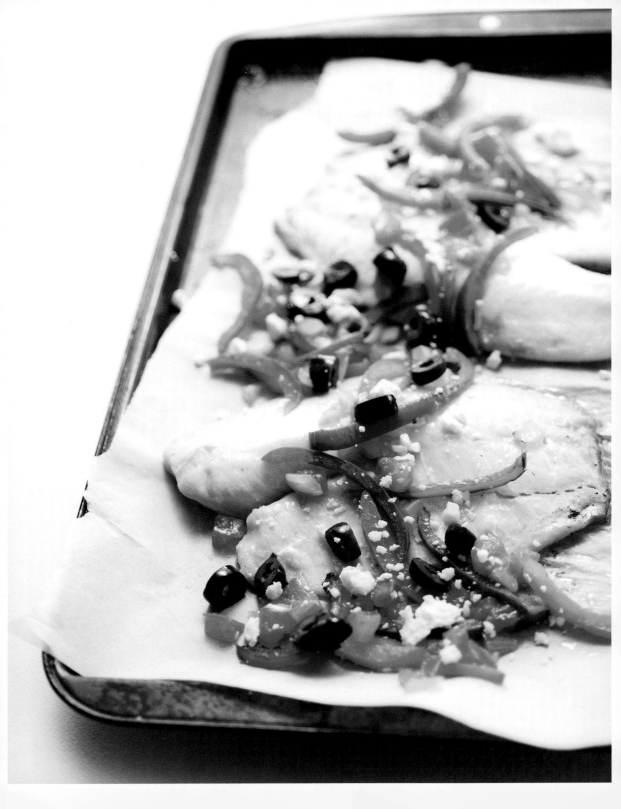

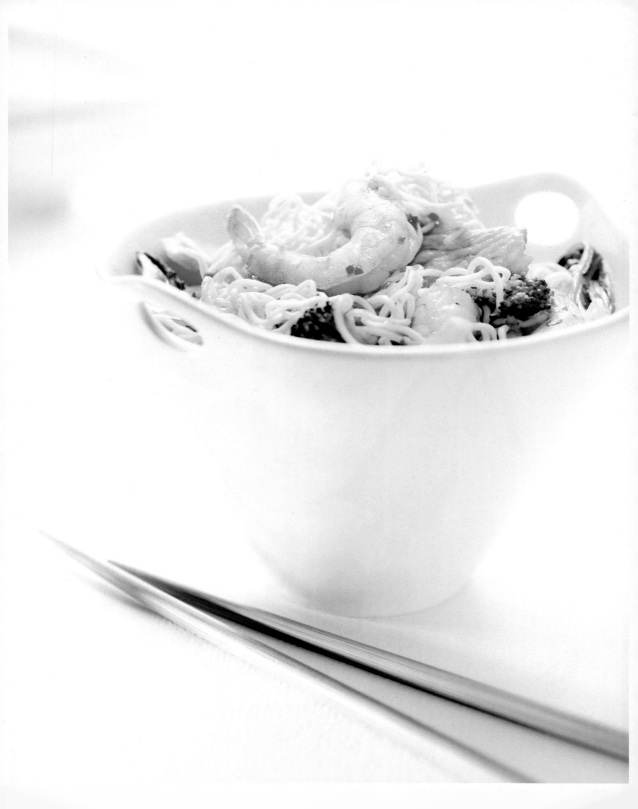

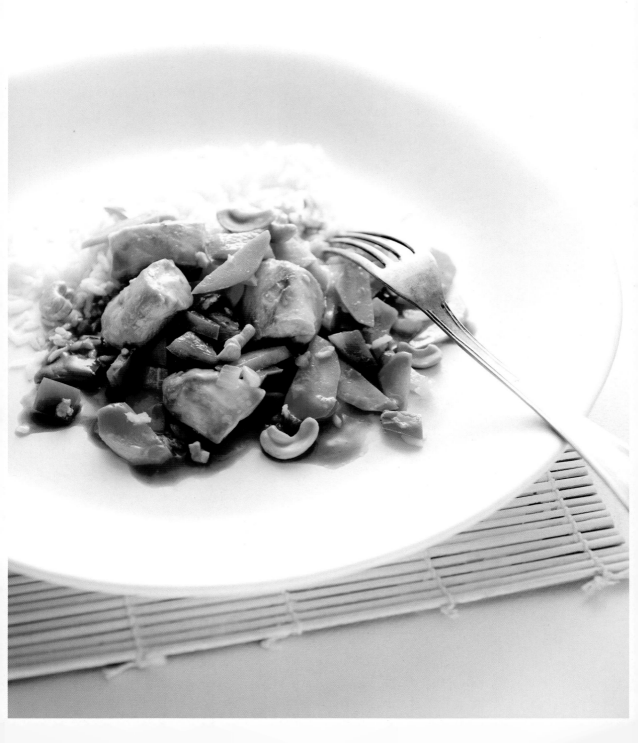

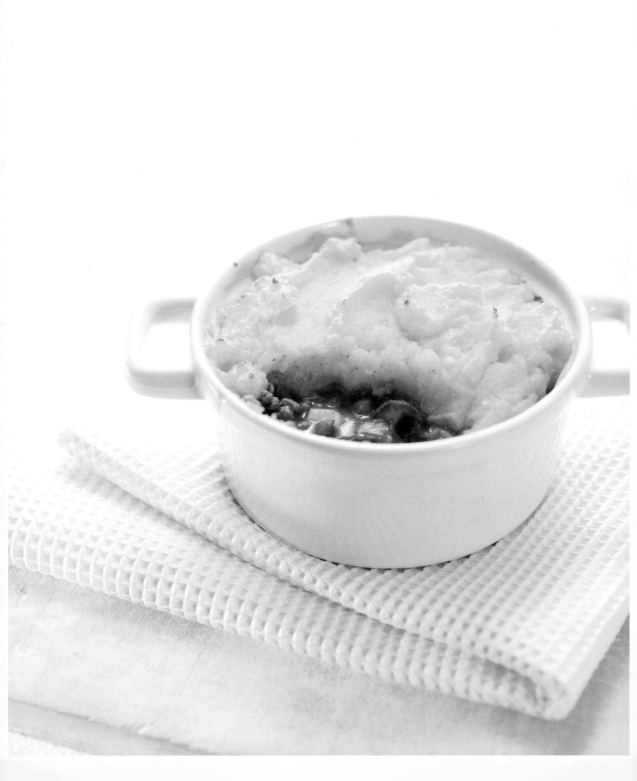

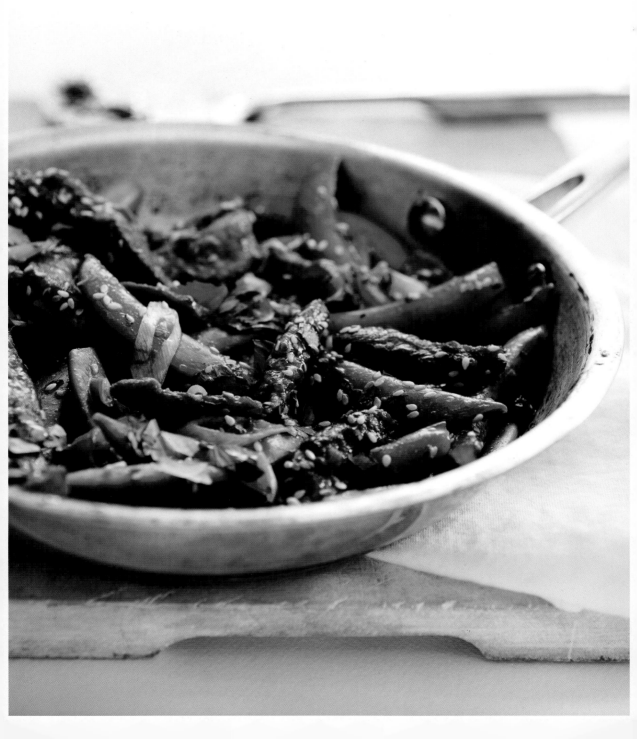

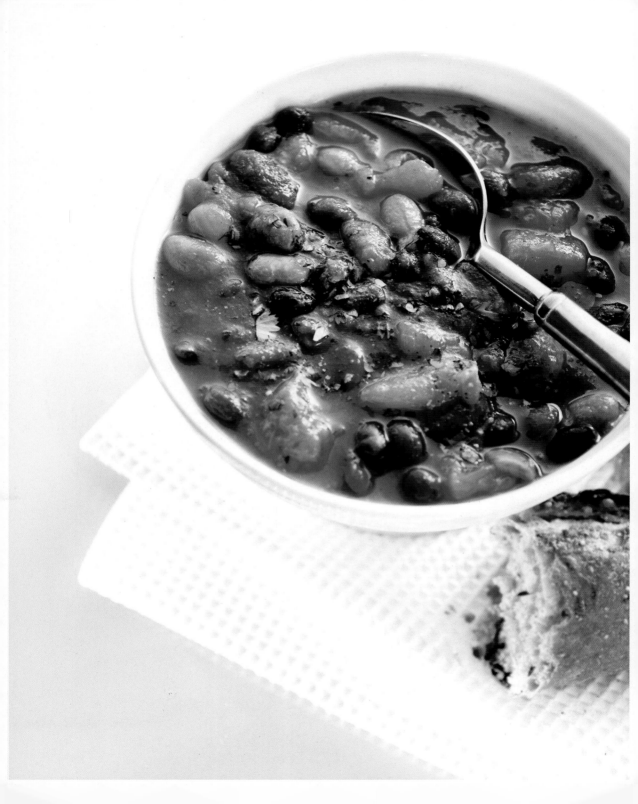

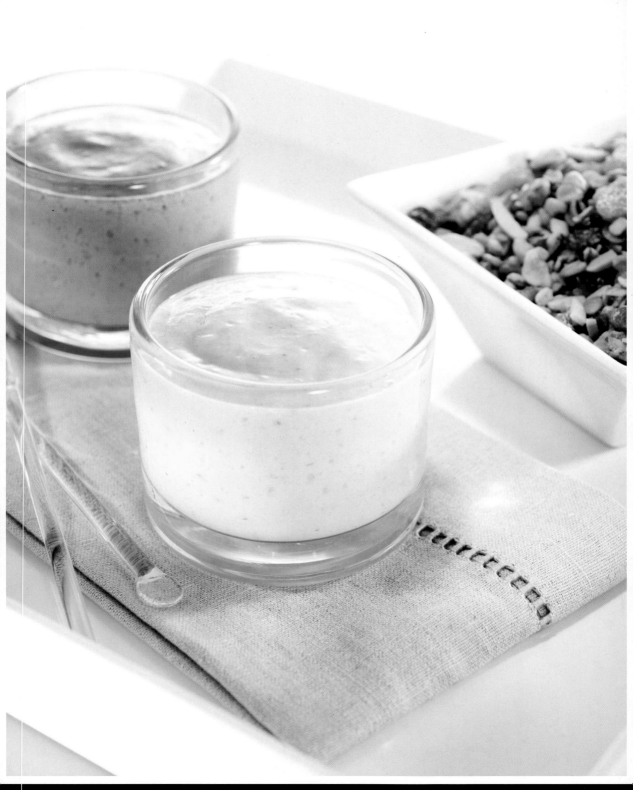

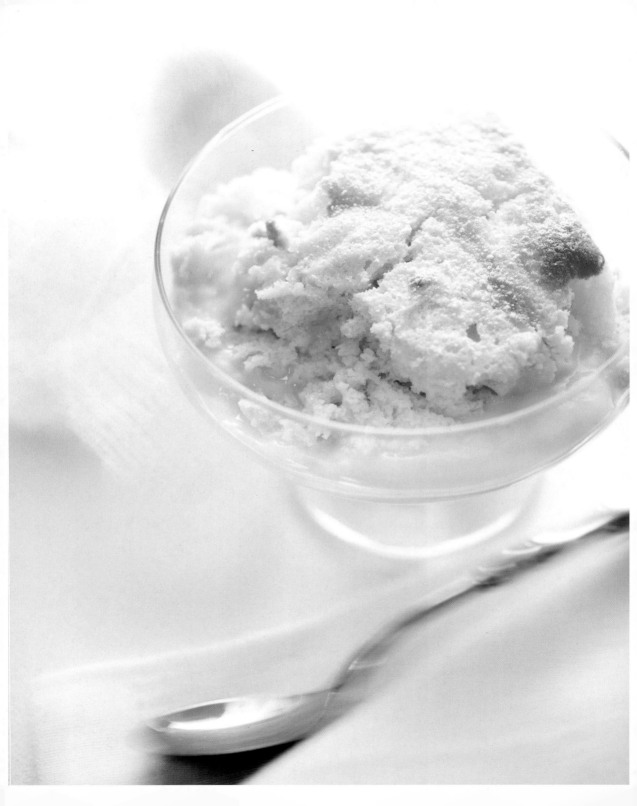

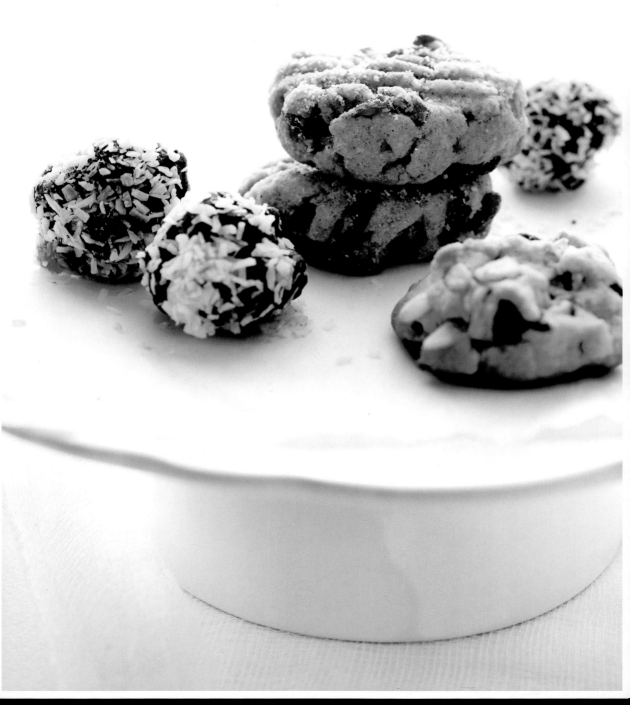

Snickers Cookies, Chocolate Chip Cookies, and Rocky Road Balls (Chapter 17)

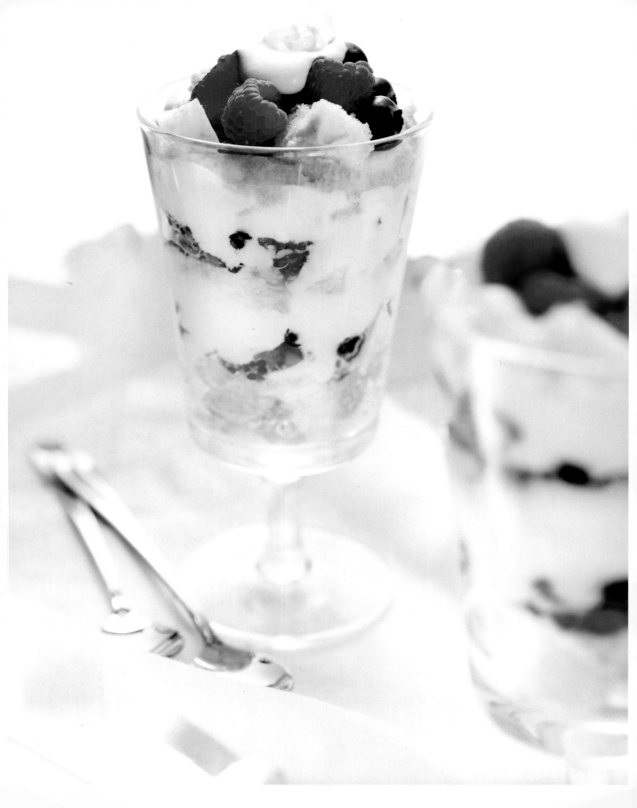

The Canadian Produce Marketing Association's Availability Guide (www.cpma.ca/en_serv_available.asp) lists seasonally available produce and when it can be found.

Maintaining your veggies' nutrients

The best way to ensure you get all the nutrients in vegetables is to eat your vegetables raw. Even though we enjoy the crunch of a carrot stick as much as anyone else, we do love the variety that cooking can impart to vegetables. So, here are some tips that help you retain those essential nutrients without having to give up your stove and oven.

These are measures you can take to retain as much nutrient value as possible when cooking vegetables:

- ✔ Keep the skins intact. The skins contain valuable nutrients and also help protect the nutrients inside the vegetable from escaping.

- ✔ Avoid cutting raw vegetables into small pieces prior to cooking. Small pieces of vegetables are more prone to losing nutrients into the cooking water. Try to cook vegetables in pieces as large as is practical.

- ✔ Don't overcook your vegetables. Cooking vegetables until they are tender-crisp — that is, tender but firm — allows them to retain their characteristic colour and flavour.

- ✔ Avoid cooking at overly high temperatures. Higher temperatures will lead to greater nutrient loss.

- ✔ Use the least amount of water necessary. The more water you cook with, the more nutrients are lost.

- ✔ If boiling vegetables, add vegetables to a small amount of boiling water, bring them back to the boil, and then simmer over medium heat.

- ✔ Microwave your vegetables rather than boiling them on your stove. Put your vegetables in a microwave-safe container and add a minimal amount of water, then cover. Cooking your vegetables in this way will help conserve their nutrient value and will also reduce cooking time.

- ✔ Stir-fry your vegetables. If stir-frying, cook the vegetables until they are tender-crisp.

- ✔ Steaming vegetables takes a little longer than boiling, but it has the advantage of conserving nutrients and retaining the shape of the vegetables.

- ✔ Cook under pressure with a pressure cooker; it's the shortest method of cooking vegetables.

Frozen vegetables are a convenient and economical option to fresh vegetables. Frozen vegetables are picked at their peak and flash-frozen to retain their nutrients. Also, cooking with frozen vegetables can be time-saving as they are pre-chopped. Avoid frozen vegetables in sauces, however; these are usually higher in calories, fat, and salt.

Anytime Veggies

Many vegetables are available to enjoy year-round; anytime veggies, if you will. In this section, we look at some great recipes (sorry to brag) that use anytime veggies. The recipes in this section don't take long to prepare and can open up new ideas for some of the "same old" vegetables.

☙ Ethiopian Cabbage

This traditional African dish is easy to make and packed with flavour.

Preparation Time: *20 minutes*

Cooking Time: *8 minutes*

Yield: *7 servings*

2 tbsp (30 ml) olive oil	¼ tsp (1 ml) salt
2 ½ cups (625 ml) yams, sliced into ½-inch (1.25 cm) slices	¼ tsp (1 ml) pepper
1 cup (250 ml) carrots, thinly sliced	1½ tsp (7 ml) ground cumin
½ medium onion, thinly sliced	1 tsp (5 ml) turmeric
	3 cups (750 ml) cabbage, shredded

1 Add the oil to a large frying pan and set over medium heat.

2 Add the yams and cook for 3 minutes, stirring occasionally with an egg lifter. Add the carrot and onion, and cook another 2 minutes.

3 Add the spices and cabbage, cover, and let cook for 5 minutes, stirring occasionally, until the vegetables are soft. Serve warm as a side dish.

Per Serving: *(½ cup/125 ml, 92 g) Calories 116; Available carbohydrate 15 g; Carbohydrate 19 g; Fibre 4 g; Fat 4 g; Protein 2 g; Cholesterol 0 mg; Phosphorus 48 mg; Potassium 569 mg; Sodium 107 mg.*

1 Serving = 1 Carbohydrate Choice

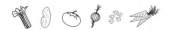

☝ *Broccoli with Feta and Roasted Peppers*

When choosing broccoli, look for a bunch that is firm, crisp, and deep green. The head should be tightly budded and the stem should be slender.

Preparation Time: *12 minutes*

Cooking Time: *5 minutes*

Yield: *4 servings*

1 head of broccoli, about 4 cups (1,000 ml), cut into bite-sized pieces

¾ cup (175 ml) bottled roasted red peppers

⅓ cup (75 ml) low-fat feta

2 tbsp (30 ml) sun-dried tomato, chopped

1 tbsp (15 ml) oil from roasted red pepper jar

1 Place the broccoli in a large saucepan, cover with water, and bring to a boil over high heat. Boil the broccoli for 3 to 4 minutes, until it is slightly soft. Leave the saucepan uncovered, so the broccoli remains bright green in colour.

2 Using a strainer, drain the water from the broccoli.

3 In a large bowl, mix together the remaining ingredients with a spoon or spatula. Add the broccoli, mix well, and serve.

Per Serving: *(1 cup/250 ml, 123 g) Calories 77; Available carbohydrate 5 g; Carbohydrate 9 g; Fibre 4 g; Fat 4 g; Protein 4 g; Cholesterol 2 mg; Phosphorus 78 mg; Potassium 378 mg; Sodium 376 mg.*

1 Serving = 0 Carbohydrate Choice

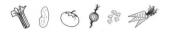

☞ Stir-Fried Snow Peas

Snow peas are a staple in Chinese cooking. They have flat, tender pods covering the tiny, immature peas inside. Both the bright green peas and pods are edible.

Preparation Time: *15 minutes*

Cooking Time: *8 minutes*

Yield: *3 servings*

1 tbsp (15 ml) olive oil

1 small clove garlic, minced

1 tbsp (15 ml) green onion, chopped

¾ cup (175 ml) shiitake mushrooms, thinly sliced

1½ cup (375 ml) snow peas

¼ cup (50 ml) water chestnuts, sliced

1 Add the oil to a wok or medium-sized frying pan and place over medium-high heat.

2 Add the garlic and onion, and stir for about 2 minutes with a spatula, until the onions are soft and translucent.

3 Add the remaining ingredients and stir-fry for about 6 minutes until the mushrooms are browned. Serve and enjoy.

Per Serving: (½ cup/125 ml, 67 g) Calories 76; Available carbohydrate 6 g; Carbohydrate 7 g; Fibre 1 g; Fat 5 g; Protein 2 g; Cholesterol 0 mg; Phosphorus 53 mg; Potassium 205 mg; Sodium 3 mg.

1 Serving = 0 Carbohydrate Choice

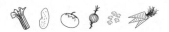

◌ Swiss Chard and Pine Nuts

Swiss chard has long, flat, celery-like stalks that can be wide or narrow, depending on the variety. Always separate the leaves from the stems before cooking — the stems take longer to cook.

Preparation Time: *10 minutes*

Cooking Time: *7 minutes*

Yield: *3 servings*

6 cups (1,500 ml) Swiss chard

1½ tbsp (22 ml) raisins

1 tbsp (15 ml) olive oil

1 clove garlic, minced

⅛ tsp (0.5 ml) salt

2 tsp (10 ml) red wine vinegar

2 tbsp (30 ml) pine nuts

1 Thoroughly wash the Swiss chard in cool water. Remove the stalks from the leaves and set them aside. Chop the stalks into ½-inch (1.25 cm) pieces.

2 Place 1 cup (250 ml) of water in a large saucepan and bring to a boil over medium heat. Add the stalks and cook for about 4 minutes, until they are tender, stirring occasionally with a large spoon.

3 Add the chopped Swiss chard leaves and raisins and cook for another 3 minutes, stirring occasionally, until the leaves are wilted. Drain.

4 In a wok or large frying pan, heat the oil over medium heat and add the garlic. Sauté for 1 minute. Add the Swiss chard, raisins, and salt and then remove from the heat.

5 Add the vinegar and stir well with a large spoon.

6 Sprinkle with pine nuts and serve.

Per Serving: (½ cup/125 ml, 88 g) Calories 107; Available carbohydrate 5 g; Carbohydrate 7 g; Fibre 2 g; Fat 8 g; Protein 2 g; Cholesterol 0 mg; Phosphorus 72 mg; Potassium 345 mg; Sodium 251 mg.

1 Serving = 0 Carbohydrate Choice

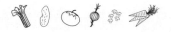

Springtime Veggies

As Canadians emerge from our collective cocoons after yet another long winter, one thing to look forward to is the emergence of local, springtime vegetables (and putting away the snow shovels, packing away the winter coats, hats and gloves, having a clean car . . . the list is endless).

○ Zesty Asparagus

Green asparagus is a good source of folate, vitamin C, vitamin A, iron, phosphorus, and potassium — and it's low in calories to boot!

Preparation Time: *20 minutes*

Cooking Time: *10 minutes*

Yield: *4 servings*

4 cups (1,000 ml) asparagus	*¼ tsp (1 ml) lemon zest*
3 tbsp (45 ml) sliced almonds	*2 tsp (10 ml) fresh lemon juice*
1 clove garlic, minced	*2 tsp (10 ml) olive oil*
1 tbsp (15 ml) parsley, chopped	*½ tsp (2 ml) salt*

1 Clean the asparagus and break off the tough ends by bending the asparagus in your hands. (Hold the asparagus at the centre of the stalk with one hand and use your other hand to gently bend the base of the stalk until it snaps off.) Discard the ends.

2 Bring 1 cup (250 ml) of water to boil in a medium-sized saucepan. Add the asparagus and boil uncovered for 4 to 6 minutes, until tender crisp. Drain the asparagus in a strainer.

3 Toast the almonds by placing them in a dry frying pan and setting it over medium-high heat. Stir the almonds often, for about 5 minutes, until they are lightly browned.

4 In a large bowl, combine all ingredients and toss well. Serve hot.

Per Serving: (½ cup/125 ml, 100 g) Calories 80; Available carbohydrate 4 g; Carbohydrate 7 g; Fibre 3 g; Fat 5 g; Protein 4 g; Cholesterol 0 mg; Phosphorus 94 mg; Potassium 302 mg; Sodium 149 mg.

1 Serving = 0 Carbohydrate Choice

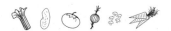

⟳ Asparagus Cheddar Quiche

Look for straight, crisp asparagus with nicely rounded spears and closed, deep green or purplish tips. Asparagus is grown in sandy soil, so wash it well in cool running water to get rid of the grit.

Preparation Time: *30 minutes*

Cooking Time: *50 to 60 minutes*

Yield: *6 servings*

9-inch (22.5 cm) frozen deep dish pie shell	¾ cup (175 ml) 1% milk
1½ cups (375 ml) asparagus	1 tsp (5 ml) dried dill (or 2 tbsp/30 ml fresh)
1 tbsp (15 ml) Dijon mustard	¼ tsp (1 ml) salt
1½ tsp (7 ml) soft margarine	⅛ tsp (0.5 ml) pepper
½ cup (125 ml) onion, chopped	⅛ tsp (0.5 ml) nutmeg
1 cup (250 ml) low-fat cheddar, grated	⅛ tsp (0.5 ml) cayenne pepper
2 eggs	

1 Preheat the oven to 375 degrees Fahrenheit (190 degrees Celsius).

2 Thaw the frozen pie shell for 10 to 15 minutes.

3 Clean the asparagus and break off the tough ends by bending the asparagus in your hands. (Hold the asparagus at the centre of the stalk with one hand and use your other hand to gently bend the base of the stalk until it snaps off.) Discard the ends.

4 Bring about 1 cup (250 ml) of water to boil in a medium-sized saucepan. Add the asparagus and boil uncovered for 4 to 6 minutes, until it becomes tender crisp. Drain the asparagus in a strainer and allow it to cool. When the asparagus is cool to touch, cut it into 1-inch (2.5-cm) pieces.

5 With a fork, prick the base of the pie shell in several places. Bake for 10 minutes then remove from the oven. Cover the bottom of the pie shell with a thin layer of the Dijon mustard.

6 Melt the margarine in a large frying pan and sauté the onion for 2 minutes or until soft.

7 In a medium-sized bowl, combine the onion, asparagus, and cheese. Stir thoroughly. Spread the mixture evenly over the bottom of the pie shell.

8 In a medium-sized bowl, beat the eggs. Add the milk and spices, and mix well. Pour this mixture into the pie shell as well.

9 Bake for 40 to 50 minutes. The quiche is done when a knife inserted in the centre comes out clean.

10 Allow the quiche to cool for 10 minutes before serving. Enjoy!

Per Serving: *(⅙ quiche, 117 g) Calories 251; Available carbohydrate 19 g; Carbohydrate 20 g; Fibre 1 g; Fat 15 g; Protein 10 g; Cholesterol 76 mg; Phosphorus 199 mg; Potassium 239 mg; Sodium 560 mg.*

1 Serving = 1 Carbohydrate Choice

☺ *Green Pea, Cauliflower, and Tomato Curry*

This classic Indian curry is quick and easy to prepare. Serve with grilled meats, chicken, or fish, and a bowl of brown rice.

Preparation Time: *15 minutes*

Cooking Time: *20 minutes*

Yield: *6 servings*

2½ cups (625 ml) cauliflower florets	*½ tsp (2 ml) ground cardamom*
1 tbsp (15 ml) soft margarine	*⅓ cup (75 ml) light coconut milk*
1 medium onion, finely chopped	*2 medium tomatoes, chopped*
1 clove garlic, minced	*½ tsp (2 ml) sugar*
1 tsp (5 ml) fresh ginger, grated	*⅛ tsp (0.5 ml) salt*
1½ tsp (7 ml) ground coriander	*⅛ tsp (0.5 ml) pepper*
1½ tsp (7 ml) curry powder	*¾ cup (175 ml) frozen peas*
½ tsp (2 ml) turmeric	

1 Add 1 cup (250 ml) of water to a large pot. Bring the water to boil over high heat. Add the cauliflower and cook for about 8 minutes, until tender. Drain in a strainer.

2 Melt the margarine in a large frying pan over medium-high heat and add the onion. Stir occasionally until the onion is translucent. Add the garlic and ginger and sauté for 1 minute. Add the spices and continue to sauté for another minute.

3 Stir in the coconut milk, tomatoes, sugar, salt, and pepper. Cover the frying pan with a lid and simmer on low heat for 5 minutes.

4 Add the cauliflower and peas. Cover and simmer for another 4 minutes. Serve hot.

Per Serving: *(½ cup/125 ml, 84 g) Calories 64; Available carbohydrate 6 g; Carbohydrate 9 g; Fibre 3 g; Fat 3 g; Protein 3 g; Cholesterol 0 mg; Phosphorus 65 mg; Potassium 335 mg; Sodium 102 mg.*

1 Serving = 0 Carbohydrate Choice

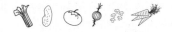

Going organic

Organic farming is farming without the use of chemical pesticides or fertilizers, genetically modified organisms, growth hormones, or antibiotics.

Although "organic" is often considered to be synonymous with "healthy," and conventionally grown food as being "less healthy," the truth of the matter is that — at least at the present time — there is insufficient scientific evidence to justify this claim. Many factors affect the nutritional quality of food, including the quality of the soil, the weather, the light available during the growing season, the type of seed planted (or, in the case of livestock, the breed of the animal), the planting and harvesting dates, the way the product is stored and transported, and so on. Based on these factors, some organic foods, compared with conventionally grown foods, may have more nutritional value, the same nutritional value, or even less nutritional value.

As for the absence of chemical pesticides, growth hormones, and so forth, although it intuitively makes sense that avoiding these substances would be better, there is much variation in the way these products are used and at the present time there is insufficient scientific literature — one way or the other — to make a blanket statement about possible detrimental effects of these products. Therefore, at least for now, one cannot make a blanket statement that avoiding non-organically grown products is always best.

Like purchasing anything, buying organic food is a personal choice that can depend on food availability, appearance, taste, price, and personal values.

If you do choose organic foods, look for the new mandatory logo attesting to a food being produced organically.

Fall Harvest Vegetables

We have mixed feelings about fall. The air is fresh, the humidity less, the leaves a painter's pallet of colours . . . But fall also brings heating bills that climb, leaves that need raking, and snow that falls before we've finished the raking. (Rats! You'd think we'd have learned from last year's experience.) But we put our ambivalence aside when it comes to the availability of fall harvest vegetables, one of our favourite types of food.

In this section, we look at some great ways to prepare meals with fall vegetables.

☺ Grilled Vegetables

Unless you're very carefully monitoring your carbohydrate, phosphorus, and potassium intake, you can substitute a variety of vegetables for this recipe — just watch that they all cook in the same time. For more about carb counting, refer to Chapter 1.

Preparation Time: *20 minutes, plus 1 hour for the vegetables to marinate*

Cooking Time: *8 to 10 minutes*

Yield: *6 servings*

1 cup (250 ml) zucchini, cut into ¼-inch (6 mm) slices	*1 cup (250 ml) whole cherry tomatoes*
1 large red pepper, cut into chunks	*½ cup (125 ml) balsamic vinegar*
1 cup (250 ml) whole mushrooms	*2 cloves garlic, minced*
½ medium onion, cut into wedges	*½ cup (125 ml) olive oil*
½ cup (125 ml) snow peas	*1 tbsp (15 ml) black pepper, coarsely ground*
	1 tsp (5 ml) salt

1 In a large bowl, mix together the vinegar, garlic, oil, pepper, and salt with a whisk or fork.

2 Add the vegetables to the bowl and mix with a large spoon until the vegetables are coated with the marinade. Cover the bowl and place it in the fridge for at least 1 hour to marinate, stirring occasionally.

3 Drain the vegetables, place them in a grill basket, and set the basket on the barbecue over medium-high heat for 8 to 10 minutes. Turn the vegetables frequently, until they are cooked. If you don't have a grill basket, substitute an aluminum pie plate, but watch the vegetables closely so they don't burn. You can also cook the vegetables in a large frying pan on your stove top for 8 to 10 minutes, until they are tender. Serve hot.

Per Serving: (⅔ cup/150 ml, 108 g) Calories 206; Available carbohydrate 7 g; Carbohydrate 9 g; Fibre 2 g; Fat 18 g; Protein 2 g; Cholesterol 0 mg; Phosphorus 46 mg; Potassium 273 mg; Sodium 399 mg.

1 Serving = 0 Carbohydrate Choice

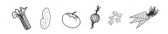

☺ Squash Apple Bake

A butternut squash is a yellowish tan and is shaped like a bowling pin, with a bulbous end and a narrow neck. It is easier to peel than most squashes. The flavour is fruity and sweet.

Preparation Time: *20 minutes*

Cooking Time: *17 to 19 minutes*

Yield: *10 servings*

1 medium-sized butternut squash, peeled, seeded, and cut into 1-inch (2.5 cm) cubes

1 tbsp (15 ml) brown sugar

3 tbsp (15 ml) soft margarine

1½ tsp (7 ml) flour

½ tsp (2 ml) salt

¼ tsp (1 ml) cinnamon

2 medium apples, peeled, cored, and cut into ½-inch (1.25 cm) wedges

1 In a large microwave-safe casserole dish, combine the brown sugar, margarine, flour, salt, and cinnamon. Microwave* on medium power for 30 seconds. Stir with a spatula or spoon.

2 Add the squash to the casserole dish, mix, and cover with a lid. Microwave on high for 10 minutes.

3 Add the apple to the squash, stir, and microwave, covered, for an additional 7 to 9 minutes or until the squash is soft enough to pierce with a fork.

* If you don't have a microwave, combine the ingredients, toss, and place in a covered casserole dish in an oven heated to 350 degrees Fahrenheit (175 degrees Celsius) for 30 minutes.

Per Serving: (½ cup/125 ml, 93 g) Calories 91; Available carbohydrate 14 g; Carbohydrate 16 g; Fibre 2 g; Fat 3 g; Protein 1 g; Cholesterol 0 mg; Phosphorus 33 mg; Potassium 328 mg; Sodium 150 mg.

1 Serving = 1 Carbohydrate Choice

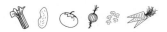

↻ Orange-Glazed Carrots

When choosing carrots avoid the ones with cracks (this usually indicates a woody core) or green around their tops (this usually means the carrot is bitter). Carrots are an excellent source of beta carotene, which our bodies convert into vitamin A.

Preparation Time: *15 minutes*

Cooking Time: *5 to 6 minutes*

Yield: *3 servings*

2 tbsp (30 ml) orange juice

1 tbsp (15 ml) honey

1 tsp (5 ml) cornstarch

1 tbsp (15 ml) soft margarine

½ tsp (2 ml) lemon zest

⅛ tsp (0.5 ml) salt

⅛ tsp (0.5 ml) nutmeg

2 cups (500 ml) carrots, sliced into coins ¼-inch (6 mm) wide

1 In a large, microwave-safe* casserole dish, combine all the ingredients except the carrots. Mix well with a large spoon.

2 Add the carrots, mix well, and cover with a lid. Microwave on high for 3 minutes. Stir the carrots again and microwave for an additional 3 minutes, until the carrots are tender crisp.

3 Leave covered for 3 minutes, stir, and serve.

* If you don't have a microwave, place the carrots in a medium-sized saucepan with 1 cup (250 ml) of water and boil for about 10 minutes, until the carrots are tender crisp. Drain the water from the carrots. Add the remaining ingredients and stir constantly for 2 minutes over medium heat. Serve and enjoy.

Per Serving: *(⅔ cup/150 ml, 83 g) Calories 99; Available carbohydrate 13 g; Carbohydrate 16 g; Fibre 3 g; Fat 4 g; Protein 1 g; Cholesterol 0 mg; Phosphorus 32 mg; Potassium 296 mg; Sodium 190 mg.*

1 Serving = 1 Carbohydrate Choice

☼ *Balsamic Brussels Sprouts*

When choosing Brussels sprouts, it's best to pick ones of similar size, so they will cook evenly in the same time. Eat Brussels sprouts within two days of purchase — the longer you wait, the stronger they will taste.

One way to reduce the bitter taste of Brussels sprouts is to soak them in water with a touch of lemon juice for half an hour before cooking.

Preparation Time: *7 minutes*

Cooking Time: *5 minutes*

Yield: *5 servings*

3 cups (750 ml) Brussels sprouts	*2 tbsp (30 ml) balsamic vinegar*
1 tbsp (15 ml) soft margarine	*½ tsp (2 ml) sugar*

1 Clean the Brussels sprouts and remove the stems and any wilted outer leaves.

2 To make sure the Brussels sprouts cook evenly, use a sharp knife to cut an ⅛-inch (3 ml) X in the bottom of each one.

3 Cover the bottom of a medium-sized saucepan with 1-inch (2.5 cm) of water and place over high heat. Place a steamer over the water. Put the Brussels sprouts in the steamer and cook for about 5 minutes, until the sprouts are tender and emerald green.

4 Melt the margarine in a medium-sized saucepan set over low heat. Add the vinegar and sugar. Stir until the sugar is dissolved.

5 Add the sprouts to the saucepan and stir with a spoon or spatula until they are evenly coated with the vinegar mixture. Serve and enjoy.

Per Serving: (½ cup/125 ml, 90 g) Calories 50; Available carbohydrate 4 g; Carbohydrate 6 g; Fibre 2 g; Fat 2 g; Protein 2 g; Cholesterol 0 mg; Phosphorus 38 mg; Potassium 213 mg; Sodium 35 mg.

1 Serving = 0 Carbohydrate Choice

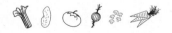

Chapter 13

Fishing for the Right Dish: Fish and Seafood Entrées

In This Chapter

▶ Getting tips on buying and cooking fish

▶ Preparing delicious fish

▶ Serving up succulent seafood

Because fish are so nutritious (hey, they're so nutritious that even fish eat other fish), *Eating Well with Canada's Food Guide* — the Canadian bible when it comes to healthy eating — recommends eating two servings of fish each week.

As we discuss in Chapter 2, certain types of fish are rich in omega-3 fatty acids, which makes them an important food source. Strong scientific evidence links the ingestion of omega-3 fatty acids with a reduced risk of a variety of serious health problems, including cancer, arthritis, depression, lupus, and asthma.

When selecting your omega-3-rich fish, you also want to choose fish that is low in mercury (ingesting mercury is, as you likely know, unhealthy). These are fish that are rich in omega-3 fatty acids and low in mercury: anchovy, Atlantic mackerel, capelin, char, hake, herring, mullet, salmon, smelt, pollock (Boston bluefish), rainbow trout, and lake whitefish. Certain types of seafood are also rich in omega-3 fatty acids (and low in mercury), such as clams, blue crab, mussels, oysters, and shrimp.

Fish that is cooked using a low-fat method (such as poaching or broiling) is a great protein replacement for red meat, because the total fat content is lower and you get a plate full of omega-3 fatty acids to boot.

In addition to their benefits as a source of omega-3 fatty acid and protein, fish are also a significant source of B vitamins, vitamin D, copper, iron, iodine, magnesium, phosphorus, potassium, and selenium, while at the same time being low in saturated fat, cholesterol, and calories. Wow; how swimming!

Selecting and Cooking Fish

If, as the expression goes, carpenters are only as good as their tools, then so too can your fish entrée be only as good as the fish you start with and the way you prepare it. For example, if you choose fish (good choice) but then deep-fry it and then smother it in a rich tartar sauce (ah, bad choices), you have taken a potentially healthy food choice and made it less healthy than a typical burger. In this section, we look at how you can keep your fish dinner healthy and appetizing at the same time.

Choosing fish

Fish are delicate creatures and begin to deteriorate as soon as they're lifted out of the water. Obtaining the freshest fish possible could be the difference between loving and hating fish. (As if anyone could hate fish, eh?)

Here are ways you can be sure to purchase high-quality, fresh fish:

- **Seek out a reputable retailer.** (This is rule number one.) You might start by asking your neighbours where they buy their fish. Also, don't feel shy about "interviewing" your local fish sellers and asking them about some of the points we note in this list.

- **Inspect the fish.** It should be blemish-free, and the flesh should be firm and spring back when touched. The fish should smell like the water it came from; if the fish smells fishy, it's not fresh. (Yeah, we know that sounds weird; wanting *fish* that doesn't smell *fishy*.)

- **Ask your retailer about the fish.** Ask how long ago it was caught; try to purchase fish that is no more than a day or two old. Ask where the fish was caught; the nearer it was caught, the more likely it is to be fresh. Ask if the fish has been previously frozen; if it has then you shouldn't refreeze it. (If the fish has been flash-frozen, its texture and taste will likely not have been compromised by the freezing process.)

- **Check out the bed of ice the fish are sitting on.** The ice should have no staining or grey areas.

The most economical way to purchase fish is whole. Look for clear, bulging eyes; shiny red gills; shiny, close-fitting scales; and a firm body. Avoid fish with cloudy, sunken eyes; blemishes; curled, brittle tails; or a fishy smell.

To make preparing and cooking fish easier and faster, consider purchasing fish in bone-free fillet or steak form. (If you are purchasing a whole, fresh fish, you can ask your fish vendor to cut it into fillets or steaks for you.) A fresh 4 oz. (120 g) fillet will cook to a 3-oz. (90 g) size.

Cooking fish

You can cook fish in an amazing number of ways: You can bake, steam, poach, sauté, boil, broil, barbecue, microwave, or plank it. Fish can even be dishwashered (Ian's mom's favourite way of preparing salmon), to coin a verb.

Regardless of which way you choose to cook your fish, the cardinal rule to follow is "Don't overcook it." Because fish is so delicate, it's easy to over-cook, leaving you with a dried-out product. In order to retain fish's moisture, cook it quickly over high heat or, alternatively, cook it with a liquid. A quick rule of thumb is to measure the fish at its thickest point and cook at high heat (425 degrees Fahrenheit or 220 degrees Celsius) for 10 minutes per inch (2.5 cm) of thickness.

Perfectly cooked fish should flake easily with a fork and be opaque with the faintest amount of translucency in the middle.

Oh, and if you're wondering how Ian's mom makes her dishwasher salmon, she wraps the fish in tin foil and puts it through the entire wash and dry cycle (without soap!). You can find other dishwasher salmon recipes on the Internet.

Baking fish

Here's a good way to bake fish:

1. Sprinkle both sides of a 1 lb. (450 g) fish fillet with a small amount of salt and pepper.

2. Melt 1½ tbsp (22 ml) soft margarine and mix together with 1 tbsp (15 ml) lemon juice and 1 tbsp (15 ml) diced onion.

3. Dip both sides of the fish into the margarine mixture and lay the fillet flat in an ungreased casserole dish or pan. Pour the remaining margarine mixture over the fillet.

4. Cook, uncovered, at 425 degrees Fahrenheit (220 degrees Celsius) for 10 minutes or until the fish flakes easily with a fork.

Broiling Fish

Try broiling fish using this technique:

1. Sprinkle both sides of a 1 lb. (450 g) fish fillet with a small amount of salt and pepper.

2. Melt 1½ tbsp (22 ml) soft margarine and mix in ¼ tsp (1 ml) dried dill, ⅛ tsp (0.5 ml) dried thyme, and 1 tbsp (15 ml) diced onion.

3. Line a broil pan with foil, place the fish on the foil, and brush with half the margarine mixture.

4. Set the oven to broil and with the pan 2 to 3 inches (5–7.5 cm) from the element, cook the fish until light brown, about 5 minutes.

5. Gently turn the fish over, brush with the remaining margarine mixture, and broil for about 5 minutes longer until the fish easily flakes with a fork.

Steaming Fish

This is a foolproof way of creating scrumptious steamed fish:

1. Rub the fillet with spices, chopped herbs, ginger, garlic, or chili peppers. Lay the seasoned fish flat in a bamboo steamer or folding steamer basket.

2. Pour about 1½ inches (3.75 cm) water into a pot, cover and bring the water to a boil. Place the steamer over the pot.

3. Check the fish for doneness after about 10 minutes. The fish should flake easily with a fork when done.

Tasty Fish Dinners

In the preceding section, we outline some easy ways to prepare fish. Here, we offer some great recipes if you need some inspiration.

Salmon Loaf

Salmon is an excellent source of protein and omega-3 fatty acids. To make this a truly special meal, serve it with our Cucumber Sauce (the recipe follows this one).

Preparation Time: *20 minutes*

Cooking Time: *40 minutes*

Yield: *4 servings*

2 - 7.5 oz/426 g cans salmon	*½ cup (125 ml) celery, chopped*
2 tbsp (30 ml) lemon juice	*½ tsp (2 ml) salt*
2 eggs, beaten	*¼ tsp (1 ml) pepper*
1 cup (250 ml) rolled oats	*½ tsp (2 ml) dried dill*
¼ cup (50 ml) ground flaxseed	*½ cup (125 ml) 1% milk*
½ cup (125 ml) onion, chopped	*½ tsp (2 ml) dry mustard*

1 Preheat oven to 350 degrees Fahrenheit (175 degrees Celsius). Lightly grease an 8-x-4-inch (20-x-10-cm) loaf pan with canola oil.

2 Mash the salmon, bones, and juice together in a food processor or blender at medium speed until well mixed. If you don't have a food processor or blender, use a hand blender, potato masher, or fork. Place the salmon in a medium-sized bowl.

3 Add the remaining ingredients to the bowl and blend well until thoroughly mixed.

4 Evenly spread the salmon mixture across the bottom of a loaf pan, making sure to fill the corners.

5 Fill a jelly roll pan or 9-x-13-inch (20-x-30-cm) pan with 1 inch (2.5 cm) of boiling water. Place the loaf pan inside the jelly pan of water and bake for about 40 minutes, until a knife inserted into the centre of the salmon loaf comes out clean.

6 Let the loaf cool for 7 minutes before slicing. Top with Cucumber Sauce, if desired (see following recipe).

Per Serving: (1 slice, 2⅖-inch cm wide, 150 g) Calories 316; Available carbohydrate 16 g; Carbohydrate 21 g; Fibre 5 g; Fat 14 g; Protein 27 g; Cholesterol 153 mg; Phosphorus 521 mg; Potassium 592 mg; Sodium 809 mg.

1 Serving = 1 Carbohydrate Choice

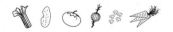

Pregnancy, children, fish, and mercury

Children, and women who may become pregnant, are pregnant, or are breastfeeding can eat fish as part of a healthy eating program, but because some fish are contaminated with mercury, these individuals need to limit the type and amount of fish they consume.

The fish that they need to limit are predatory fish like tuna, swordfish, marlin, orange roughy, and escolar. (Predatory fish accumulate mercury in their bodies by eating mercury-contaminated smaller fish.) Here is a list that shows safe levels of consumption of these fish:

✓ **General population:** 5 oz (150 g) per week

✓ **Women who may become pregnant, are pregnant, or are breastfeeding:** 5 oz (150 g) per month (For albacore/white tuna — 10 oz [300 g] per week)

✓ **Children 1–4 years old:** 2.5 oz (75 g) per month (For albacore/white tuna — 2.5 oz [75 g] per week)

✓ **Children 5–11 years old:** 4 oz (125 g) per month (For albacore/white tuna — 5 oz/150 g per week)

You can find out more about safe levels of fish consumption at `www.hc-sc.gc.ca/fn-an/securit/chem-chim/environ/mercur/cons-adv-etud-eng.php`.

☺ Cucumber Sauce

This light sauce makes a tasty addition to the Salmon Loaf.

Preparation Time: *10 minutes*

Yield: *4 servings*

½ cup (125 ml) low-fat mayonnaise

½ cup (125 ml) cucumber, grated (skin left on), drained

1½ tbsp (22 ml) lemon juice

¼ tsp (1 ml) dry mustard

¼ tsp (1 ml) salt

⅛ tsp (0.5 ml) pepper

1 green onion, chopped

1 In a small bowl, mix together all the ingredients, except the green onion, with a spoon or spatula.

2 Spoon ¼ cup (50 ml) of the sauce on top of each slice of Salmon Loaf, sprinkle with ¼ of the green onions, and serve.

Per Serving: *(¼ cup/50 ml, 4.5 g) Calories 77; Available carbohydrate 6 g; Carbohydrate 6 g; Fibre 0 g; Fat 6 g; Protein 0 g; Cholesterol 7.5 mg; Phosphorus 6 mg; Potassium 36 mg; Sodium 301 mg.*

1 Serving = 0 Carbohydrate Choices

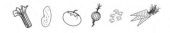

Greek Fish

Use either sole or tilapia for this recipe. Sole is a delicate, fine-textured fish with a mild flavour. Tilapia is also mild-flavoured but has a firm, flaky texture. Both are good sources of protein, vitamin B$_{12}$, and selenium.

Preparation Time: *15 minutes*

Cooking Time: *10 to 20 minutes (depending on the thickness of the fillet)*

Yield: *2 servings*

2 tbsp (15 ml) olive oil

2 cloves garlic, minced

½ cup (125 ml) onions, chopped

½ cup (125 ml) green pepper, thinly sliced

½ cup (125 ml) red pepper, thinly sliced

½ cup (125 ml) tomato, chopped

⅛ tsp (0.5 ml) salt

⅛ tsp (0.5 ml) pepper

½ lb (225 g) sole or tilapia

¼ cup (50 ml) low-fat feta cheese

2 tbsp (30 ml) kalamata olives, sliced

1 Preheat oven to 400 degrees Fahrenheit (200 degrees Celsius). Lightly grease a baking dish with canola oil.

2 Heat the oil in a medium-sized frying pan over medium heat. When it's warm, add the garlic, onions, and peppers, and sauté for 5 minutes, stirring occasionally with a spatula or egg lifter.

3 Add the tomatoes and sauté for another 2 minutes.

4 Sprinkle both sides of the fish with the salt and pepper.

5 Place the fish in the baking dish and top with the vegetable mixture, feta cheese, and olives.

6 Bake, uncovered, for 10 to 20 minutes, until the fish flakes easily when tested with a fork. Serve hot and enjoy.

Per Serving: *(1 fillet with ½ the topping, 145 g) Calories 314; Available carbohydrate 9 g; Carbohydrate 12 g; Fibre 3 g; Fat 19 g; Protein 30 g; Cholesterol 78 mg; Phosphorus 320 mg; Potassium 712 mg; Sodium 501 mg.*

1 Serving = ½ Carbohydrate Choice

Saffron Fish

In India, plain yogurt is used as a staple ingredient in many recipes, including this dish.

Preparation Time: *20 minutes*

Cooking Time: *13 minutes*

Yield: *2 servings*

½ lb (225 g) fish fillet (cod, sole, monkfish, or swordfish)

1 tsp (5 ml) fresh lemon juice

¼ cup (50 ml) warm water

2 saffron strands

1 tbsp (15 ml) canola oil

¼ cup (50 ml) onion, chopped

½ tsp (2 ml) ginger root, grated

½ tsp (2 ml) turmeric

¼ tsp (1 ml) ground cumin

1½ tsp (7 ml) parsley, chopped

Pinch of cinnamon

6 cherry tomatoes, halved

⅛ tsp (0.5 ml) salt

¼ cup (50 ml) low-fat plain yogurt

1 Remove any bones from the fish and cut into ½-inch (1.25-cm) cubes. Place the fish in a medium bowl with the lemon juice. Toss and set aside.

2 Add the warm water to a small bowl. Rub the saffron between your fingers to break it up. Add the saffron to the water and set aside.

3 Heat the oil in a wok or large frying pan (with a lid) over medium heat. Add the onion and ginger and sauté for about 3 minutes, until the onions are soft and translucent.

4 With a wooden spoon or spatula, stir in the turmeric, cumin, parsley, and cinnamon. Sauté for 1 minute.

5 Add the saffron water and tomatoes, and bring the mixture to a boil over high heat for 1 minute. Add the salt and fish, reduce the heat to low, cover, and let the fish cook for 5 to 6 minutes, until the fish can be flaked easily with a fork.

6 Add the yogurt to the wok and give it a quick stir (about 30 seconds) with a wooden spoon or spatula. Serve the fillets immediately.

Per Serving: *(1 cup/250 ml, 220 g) Calories 205; Available carbohydrate 6 g; Carbohydrate 7 g; Fibre 1 g; Fat 8 g; Protein 25 g; Cholesterol 57 mg; Phosphorus 324 mg; Potassium 776 mg; Sodium 240 mg.*

1 Serving = 0 Carbohydrate Choice

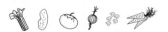

Japanese Fish Cakes

To add authentic Japanese flavour to these scrumptious fish cakes, serve them with grated daikon radish, pickled ginger, or reduced-sodium soy sauce.

Preparation Time: *15 to 20 minutes*

Cooking Time: *10 minutes*

Yield: *7 servings*

1 lb (45 g) fish fillets (cod, rockfish, tuna)	*2 tbsp (30 ml) miso*
2 tbsp (30 ml) sesame seeds	*1 egg, beaten*
1 leek, finely chopped	*1 tsp (5 ml) wasabi paste*
1½ tsp (7 ml) ginger, grated	*3 tbsp (45 ml) canola oil*

1 Rinse the fish under cool water and pat dry with paper towels. Remove any bones. Mince the fish using a food processor or blender. If you do not have a food processor or blender, use a sharp knife to finely chop the fish.

2 In a small, dry frying pan, toast the sesame seeds over medium-high heat for about 2 minutes, or until they are slightly brown. Remove from heat and let cool.

3 Combine all ingredients, except the oil, in a large bowl and mix well with a spatula, fork, or spoon.

4 With clean hands, shape the minced fish mixture into 7 equal-sized patties.

5 Heat the oil in a large frying pan over medium heat. Fry the patties for 4 to 5 minutes per side, until cooked through. Serve and enjoy.

Per Serving: (1 patty, 80 g) Calories 154; Available carbohydrate 3 g; Carbohydrate 4 g; Fibre 1 g; Fat 9 g; Protein 15 g; Cholesterol 61 mg; Phosphorus 194 mg; Potassium 356 mg; Sodium 236 mg.

1 Serving = 0 Carbohydrate Choices

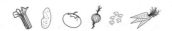

Mediterranean-Style Tuna Casserole

This is a gourmet-quality tuna casserole — everyone Cynthia has ever served this dish to has loved it!

Preparation Time: 22 minutes

Cooking Time: 20 minutes

Yield: 4 servings

7 oz/200 g dry, whole wheat spaghetti

½ cup (125 ml) oil-based commercial Caesar salad dressing

1 medium onion, chopped

3 cloves garlic, minced

2 6.5 oz/184 g cans water-packed chunk tuna, drained

⅓ cup (75 ml) black olives, sliced

1 tbsp (15 ml) dried basil

¼ tsp (1 ml) hot pepper flakes

1 cup (250 ml) tomato, chopped

⅔ cup (150 ml) low-fat feta cheese, cubed

1 In a medium-sized saucepan, bring 8 cups (2,000 ml) of water to a boil over high heat. Add the pasta and stir. Cook for 8 minutes, stirring occasionally. Drain the pasta in a strainer, then return the pasta back to the dry saucepan.

2 While the pasta is cooking, heat the salad dressing over medium heat for 1 minute in a large frying pan. Add the onions and garlic and sauté for about 3 minutes, stirring occasionally, until the onions are soft but not brown.

3 Add the tuna, olives, basil, and pepper flakes and sauté for 1 minute.

4 Add the tomato and feta and sauté for about 1 minute, until the tomatoes are warm throughout and the cheese cubes are just starting to melt at the edges. Remove from heat.

5 Mix all the ingredients together in the saucepan with a spatula or wooden spoon. Serve hot.

Per Serving: (1 cup/250 ml, 180 g) Calories 413; Available carbohydrate 45 g; Carbohydrate 47 g; Fibre 2 g; Fat 13 g; Protein 32 g; Cholesterol 30 mg; Phosphorus 302 mg; Potassium 496 mg; Sodium 964 mg.

1 Serving = 3 Carbohydrate Choices

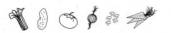

Crispy Coated Sole

This recipe is quick to make, and the fish and ground flaxseed are excellent sources of fibre and omega-3 fatty acids.

Preparation Time: *12 minutes*

Cooking Time: *6 minutes*

Yield: *2 servings*

½ lb (225 g) sole fillets	1 egg
2 tbsp (30 ml) cornmeal	1 tbsp (15 ml) 1% milk
2 tbsp (30 ml) ground flaxseed	1 tbsp (15 ml) canola oil
¼ tsp (1 ml) salt	1 tbsp (15 ml) soft margarine
⅛ tsp (0.5 ml) pepper	1 lemon, cut into wedges, if desired

1 Rinse the fish under cool water, pat dry with paper towel. Remove any bones.

2 In a small bowl, combine the cornmeal, flaxseed, salt, and pepper with a spatula or spoon.

3 In another small bowl, beat the egg and milk together with a whisk or fork.

4 Dip the fish in the egg mixture and then the cornmeal mixture.

5 In a large frying pan, heat the oil and margarine over medium heat. Fry the fish in the pan for 2 to 3 minutes on each side. The fish will be done when it turns golden brown and flakes easily when tested with a fork. Serve immediately, with lemon wedges if desired.

Per Serving: *(1 fillet, 125 g) Calories 335; Available carbohydrate 7 g; Carbohydrate 11 g; Fibre 4 g; Fat 20 g; Protein 28 g; Cholesterol 113 mg; Phosphorus 340 mg; Potassium 583 mg; Sodium 464 mg.*

1 Serving = ½ Carbohydrate Choice

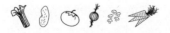

Seafood Suppers

Shellfish can be part of your balanced, healthy eating program. Clams, scallops, shrimp, lobster, mussels, oysters, and abalone are low in calories and saturated fat and are an excellent source of protein, omega-3 fatty acids, iron, zinc, copper, and vitamin B_{12}.

Although shellfish are an appropriate part of a healthy diet — whether or not you have diabetes — be careful not to undo the goodness of eating shellfish by loading it up with excessive amounts of butter or creamy sauces, as doing this will add significant amounts of calories and fat. Also, some types of shellfish (such as prawns, crab, and lobster) are high in cholesterol and thus should be consumed in limited quantities.

Seared Scallops

Scallops are a very good source of potassium, phosphorus, protein, and selenium, and are low in saturated fat.

Preparation Time: 10 minutes

Cooking Time: 5 minutes

Yield: 4 servings

1 lb (450 g) scallops	4 tbsp (60 ml) fine bread crumbs
¼ tsp (1 ml) salt	2 tbsp (30 ml) canola oil
¼ tsp (1 ml) pepper	1 lemon, cut into wedges, if desired

1 Place the scallops on a plate or cutting board and sprinkle them with the salt and pepper.

2 Place the bread crumbs in a clean plastic bag. Add a few scallops to the bag, twist the top so no crumbs escape, and shake until the scallops are coated. Remove the scallops from the bag, and repeat until all the scallops are breaded.

3 In a medium-sized frying pan, heat the oil over medium-high heat.

4 Place the scallops in the frying pan and sear them on one side for 1 to 2 minutes, until they are golden. Using an egg lifter, flip the scallops to sear them on the other side until they turn opaque in the centre, about another 1 to 2 minutes. Remove from heat and serve immediately. Garnish with lemon wedges, if desired.

Per Serving: (¼ lb, 108 g) Calories 291; Available carbohydrate 8 g; Carbohydrate 8 g; Fibre 0 g; Fat 21 g; Protein 16 g; Cholesterol 30 mg; Phosphorus 212 mg; Potassium 328 mg; Sodium 424 mg.

1 Serving = ½ Carbohydrate Choice

Chinese Jewelled Rice

With a wide variety of ingredients, this dish is a meal in itself! Crab, a main ingredient in this recipe, is low in fat — only 1 gram per ½ cup (125 ml) — and high in chromium, selenium, zinc, and protein.

Preparation Time: *10 minutes*

Cooking Time: *20 minutes*

Yield: *6 servings*

1 cup (250 ml) basmati rice	*1 cup (250 ml) shiitake mushrooms, sliced*
4 tsp (20 ml) canola oil	*½ cup (125 ml) frozen peas*
1 medium onion, chopped	*2 tbsp (30 ml) oyster sauce*
½ cup (125 ml) cooked ham, diced	*1 tsp (5 ml) sugar*
¾ cup (175 ml) canned crab meat	*⅛ tsp (0.5 ml) salt*
⅓ cup (75 ml) canned sliced water chestnuts	

1 Place the rice in a strainer and rinse under cool water for 1 minute.

2 In a large pot, bring 2 cups (500 ml) of water to a boil over high heat. Add the rice and stir. Cover the pot with a lid and simmer on low heat for 12 minutes. Remove the pot from the heat and let stand for 5 minutes. Fluff the rice with a fork.

3 Over medium heat, warm 2 tsp (10 ml) of the oil in a wok or large frying pan. Add the rice and stir-fry for 2 minutes. Remove from heat, transfer the rice back to the pot, and set aside.

4 Add 2 tsp (10 ml) oil to the wok or frying pan and place over medium-high heat. Add the onion and sauté for 2 minutes until the onions are soft but not brown.

5 Add the remaining ingredients (except the rice), to the wok or frying pan and stir-fry for 2 minutes.

6 Return the rice to the wok or frying pan and stir-fry for another 2 minutes. Serve hot.

Per Serving: *(1 cup/250 ml, 190 g) Calories 232; Available carbohydrate 34 g; Carbohydrate 36 g; Fibre 2 g; Fat 5 g; Protein 11 g; Cholesterol 29 mg; Phosphorus 149 mg; Potassium 256 mg; Sodium 267 mg.*

1 Serving = 2 Carbohydrate Choices

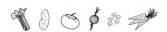

Sustainable seafood

Concern about the progressively worsening depletion of many types of fish and seafood stocks from the world's oceans is growing. You can support responsible stewardship of our marine resources by making a point of purchasing fish species that are not at risk: so-called sustainable fish species.

You can learn more about sustainable fish (and at-risk fish) — and how to go about selectively purchasing them — by visiting SeaChoice (www.seachoice.org). This site provides information, wallet cards you can take with you when shopping, and even an iPhone app that'll help keep you informed about the best fish to buy.

Chapter 14

Birds of a Feather: Poultry Dinners

Canadians love chicken . . . the taste, the value, the affordability, the versatility, the convenience, and, last but certainly not least, chicken's important role in a well-balanced, healthy eating program — especially if you have diabetes.

In this chapter, we look at a wide variety of ways you can prepare terrific, family-pleasing chicken recipes. But before we get cookin', we share some important chicken-handling tips.

Handling, Cooking, and Cleaning Up Poultry

All foods, including red meat, poultry, fruit, and vegetables, have the potential to cause foodborne illnesses due to contamination with bacteria. Infections (typically *gastroenteritis* — "gastro" for short) from eating "bad" chicken are very common. For this reason, you must properly handle food — especially chicken.

REMEMBER

The Canadian Partnership for Consumer Food Safety Education (www.canfightbac.org) sets out four steps to food safety:

1. **Clean:** Wash your hands with warm water and soap for at least 20 seconds before and after handling each food item. Wash utensils, countertops, and cutting boards with hot soapy water after preparing each food and before you go to the next food. Clean countertops using paper towels with hot soapy water or a bleach mixture of 1 tsp (5 ml) bleach to 3 cups (750 ml) water. If you use a cloth towel, wash it often on the hot cycle because it can harbour bacteria. Sponges are not recommended. Rinse fruits and vegetables under cool running water. Use a brush to scrub skins of potatoes, cantaloupes, lemons, and so on under cool running water.

2. **Separate:** Use one cutting board for fruits and vegetables and another for raw meat, poultry, and seafood. Separate raw meat, poultry, and seafood from other foods in the grocery cart, grocery bags, and in the refrigerator. Do not place cooked food on an unwashed plate that previously had raw meat, poultry, seafood, or eggs on it.

3. **Cook:** Use an instant-read food thermometer to check the internal temperatures of cooked meats. (Remember, you can't tell if a food is cooked by looking at it!) Place the food thermometer in the thickest part of the meat or, in the case of a whole chicken, into the thickest part of the thigh. (Bring soups, sauces, and gravy to the boil when reheating.)

4. **Chill:** Bacteria multiply the fastest at temperatures between 40 degrees Fahrenheit (4 degrees Celsius) and 140 degrees Fahrenheit (60 degrees Celsius), so chilling food properly is one of the best ways to reduce foodborne illnesses. Chill food within two hours in a refrigerator at 40 degrees Fahrenheit (4 degrees Celsius) or below. Refrigerate or freeze perishable foods as soon as you get home from the store. Never defrost food at room temperature; instead, thaw it in the refrigerator, in cold water, or in the microwave. Freeze uncooked poultry if you will not be using it within two days. Never refreeze previously frozen red meats, poultry, or seafood, unless you have cooked it and are then refreezing it.

Checking Out Chicken

Chicken is a good source of protein, niacin, phosphorus, selenium, and vitamin B_6. White meat has less fat than dark meat, but dark meat has more iron and zinc.

Two-thirds of the fat in chicken is in the skin. By way of illustration, a 4-ounce (130 g) chicken breast without the skin has 0.1 ounce (2.9 g) of fat whereas the same size breast with the skin has 0.3 ounces (8.3 g) of fat. Since it's important for people living with diabetes to avoid undue fat consumption, in this section we've specifically chosen recipes that don't contain poultry skin. Don't you worry though; the recipes in this section are scrumptious.

There are a variety of recipes here; some don't take long to prepare and others take a bit longer. If you don't have much time, save the longer preparation recipes for weekends. Some of the quicker recipes are Butter Chicken, Parmesan Chicken, Cinnamon Lime Chicken, Bok Choy with Chicken, Chicken with Cashews, Walnut Chicken, Curried Turkey in a Pita, and Turkey à la King.

Apricot Brie Chicken

Brie gives this dish a luxuriously creamy filling that also keeps the chicken moist.

Preparation Time: *25 minutes*

Cooking Time: *26 minutes*

Yield: *4 servings*

1 lb (450 g) skinless, boneless chicken (approximately 4 breasts)

2 oz (60 g) brie cheese, rind removed, sliced

4 dried apricots, finely chopped

½ cup (125 ml) sliced almonds

1 tsp (5 ml) rosemary

½ tsp (2 ml) salt

1 tsp (5 ml) fresh cracked pepper

⅓ cup (75 ml) bread crumbs

2 tbsp (30 ml) ground flaxseed

1 egg, beaten

2 tbsp (30 ml) soft margarine

1 Preheat oven to 375 degrees Fahrenheit (190 degrees Celsius). Lightly grease a baking dish with canola oil.

2 With a sharp knife, cut into the side of each chicken breast widthwise until it opens like a book.

3 In a small bowl, mix together the brie, the apricots, ¼ cup (50 ml) of the almonds, the rosemary, salt, and pepper. With a spoon, spread a quarter of the mixture over the inside of each chicken breast. Close the breast and secure with a toothpick.

4 In a shallow dish, combine the bread crumbs, flaxseed, and remaining almonds. Dip each piece of chicken in the egg and then evenly cover it with a thin layer of the crumb mixture.

5 In a large frying pan, melt the margarine over medium-high heat. Add the chicken breasts and brown for 3 minutes on each side.

6 Transfer the chicken to the baking dish and bake for 15 to 20 minutes, until cooked through. Remove the toothpicks and serve.

Per Serving: *(1 breast, 200 g) Calories 393; Available carbohydrate 10 g; Carbohydrate 14 g; Fibre 4 g; Fat 21 g; Protein 37 g; Cholesterol 136 mg; Phosphorus 393 mg; Potassium 526 mg; Sodium 592 mg.*

1 Serving = ½ Carbohydrate Choice

Butter Chicken

This favourite Indian dish is rich and tender. Serve it on its own, or with naan, basmati rice, or other traditional Indian fare. If you like it spicy, increase the cayenne pepper.

Preparation Time: *15 minutes*

Cooking Time: *30 minutes*

Yield: *4 servings*

2 tbsp (30 ml) canola oil	1 tsp (5 ml) garam masala
1 lb (450 g) skinless, boneless chicken breast, cut into cubes	1 tsp (5 ml) cumin
2 tbsp (30 ml) canola oil	¼ tsp (1 ml) salt
1 medium yellow onion, chopped	¼ tsp (1 ml) black pepper
2 cloves garlic, minced	¼ tsp (1 ml) cayenne pepper
1 tbsp (15 ml) ginger, grated	1 cup (250 ml) tomato sauce
2 tbsp (30 ml) butter	1 cup (250 ml) light evaporated milk
2 tsp (5 ml) lemon juice	¼ cup (50 ml) low-fat plain yogurt

1 Heat 2 tbsp (30 ml) of the oil in a large frying pan over medium-high heat. When the oil is warm, add the chicken pieces to the pan and stir with a spatula or wooden spoon until the chicken is lightly browned, about 10 minutes. Remove the chicken from the pan, place it in a bowl, and set it aside.

2 In the same frying pan, add the rest of the oil and sauté the onion, garlic, and ginger over medium-high heat until the onions are soft, about 3 to 5 minutes.

3 Add the butter, lemon juice, and spices, and continue to stir for 1 minute.

4 Add the tomato sauce and cook for 2 minutes. Add the milk and yogurt, reduce the heat to low, cover, and simmer for 10 minutes, stirring occasionally.

5 Add the chicken to the frying pan, increase the heat to high, and bring the sauce to a boil.

6 Reduce the heat to low, cover, and simmer for 15 minutes, until the sauce has thickened and the chicken is cooked through.

7 Serve hot with naan or rice. Enjoy.

Per Serving: *(1 cup/250 ml, 227 g) Calories 330; Available carbohydrate 13 g; Carbohydrate 15 g; Fibre 2 g; Fat 15 g; Protein 35 g; Cholesterol 90 mg; Phosphorus 399 mg; Potassium 802 mg; Sodium 664 mg.*

1 Serving = 1 Carbohydrate Choice

Chicken in Dijon Sauce

This chicken has a mustard flavour, so serve it with a simple side dish like mashed potatoes or plain brown rice.

Preparation Time: *25 minutes*

Cooking Time: *35 minutes*

Yield: *4 servings*

2 tbsp (30 ml) soft margarine

1 lb (450 g) skinless, boneless chicken breasts (approximately 4 breasts)

¾ cup (175 ml) yellow onion, chopped

1½ cup (375 ml) mushrooms, sliced

1½ tbsp (22 ml) flour

¾ cup (175 ml) reduced-sodium chicken broth

¾ cup (175 ml) 1% milk

¼ cup (50 ml) Dijon mustard

⅛ tsp (0.5 ml) salt

⅛ tsp (0.5 ml) pepper

2 tbsp (30 ml) sliced almonds

1 In a large frying pan, melt 1 tbsp (15 ml) of the margarine over medium-high heat. Add the chicken and cook until it is lightly browned, about 3 minutes per side. Remove the chicken from the pan, place on a plate, and set aside.

2 Add the rest of the margarine to the frying pan and place over medium-high heat. Add the onions and mushrooms, and sauté, stirring occasionally, for about 5 minutes, until the onions and mushrooms are tender. Add the flour and stir for 1 minute.

3 Slowly add the chicken broth and stir until the mixture thickens, about 3 minutes. Then stir in the milk, Dijon mustard, salt, and pepper and bring to a boil.

4 Add the chicken, cover the frying pan with a lid, and cook over medium-low heat for 15 minutes, until the chicken is cooked through.

5 In a small, dry frying pan, lightly toast the almonds over medium-high heat for 3 to 5 minutes, stirring often with a spatula or wooden spoon. When the almonds are lightly browned, remove the pan from the heat and allow the almonds to cool.

6 Sprinkle the chicken with the almonds and serve.

Per Serving: (1 breast, 280 g) Calories 320; Available carbohydrate 11 g; Carbohydrate 12 g; Fibre 1 g; Fat 16 g; Protein 32 g; Cholesterol 71 mg; Phosphorus 354 mg; Potassium 571 mg; Sodium 360 mg.

1 Serving = ½ Carbohydrate Choice

African Curry

This simple, spicy dish is a delicious way to enjoy international flavour with easily obtained ingredients. It can be served over rice or with naan bread if you wish. Of the many curry recipes Cynthia has sampled, this one is her favourite!

Preparation Time: *20 minutes (plus a minimum of 30 minutes for the chicken to marinate)*

Cooking Time: *22 minutes*

Yield: *4 servings*

1 lb (450 g) skinless, boneless chicken, cut into cubes	2 tbsp (30 ml) curry powder
½ cup (125 ml) low-fat plain yogurt	1 tbsp (15 ml) olive oil
2 tsp (10 ml) turmeric	1 large yellow onion, chopped
¼ tsp (2 ml) pepper	4 cloves garlic, minced
2 tsp (10 ml) ground coriander	1 bay leaf
2 tsp (10 ml) cumin	14 oz (398 ml) can diced tomatoes, drained
1 tsp (5 ml) chili powder	½ cup (125 ml) "lite" coconut milk
	2 tbsp (30 ml) lemon juice

1 In a large bowl, combine the yogurt, turmeric, pepper, coriander, cumin, chili, and curry powder with a spatula or spoon. Add the chicken, toss to coat it in the sauce, and place the bowl in the refrigerator to marinate for 30 minutes to 2 hours. Stir occasionally.

2 Add the oil to a large frying pan and set over medium-high heat. When the oil is warm, add the onions, garlic, and bay leaf. Sauté for 2 minutes, until the onions are soft. Reduce the heat to medium and add the tomatoes. Cook for 5 minutes, stirring occasionally with a spatula or wooden spoon.

3 Remove the chicken mixture from the fridge and add it to the frying pan. Cook over medium-high heat for 10 to 15 minutes, until the chicken is cooked through.

4 Reduce the heat to low and gradually blend in the coconut milk. Add the lemon juice. Remove the bay leaf. Stir well and serve.

Per Serving: *(1 cup/250 ml, 243 g) Calories 279; Available carbohydrate 15 g; Carbohydrate 19 g; Fibre 4 g; Fat 8 g; Protein 34 g; Cholesterol 74 mg; Phosphorus 385 mg; Potassium 939 mg; Sodium 253 mg.*

1 Serving = 1 Carbohydrate Choice

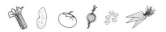

Tandoori Chicken

This is another tasty Indian dish. Traditionally, the chicken is brightly dyed with red food colouring. However, this step is optional and doesn't affect the flavour of the dish.

Preparation Time: *35 minutes (plus time for the chicken to marinate)*

Cooking Time: *35 minutes*

Yield: *4 servings*

1 lb (450 g) skinless, boneless chicken breasts (approximately 4 breasts)

Juice of 2 lemons

8 drops of red food colouring (optional)

⅛ tsp (0.5 ml) salt

2 tsp (10 ml) ginger, grated

3 cloves garlic, minced

1 tsp (5 ml) cumin

1 tsp (5 ml) paprika

1 tsp (5 ml) coriander

½ tsp (2 ml) nutmeg

1 tsp (5 ml) turmeric

½ tsp (2 ml) chili powder

½ tsp (2 ml) pepper

1¾ cups (375 ml) low-fat plain yogurt

1 With a sharp knife, make several ⅛-inch (0.3-cm) deep slits in the chicken breasts ¾ inch (1.8 cm) apart. Place the chicken in a medium-sized bowl.

2 If you are choosing to use red food colouring, mix it together with the lemon juice. Pour the lemon juice over the chicken. Add the salt and toss until the chicken is evenly coated.

3 To make the marinade, combine the remaining ingredients in a medium-sized bowl and stir well with a spatula or spoon. Pour this mixture over the chicken and stir well. Cover the bowl of chicken with plastic wrap and place in the refrigerator for several hours or overnight, if possible. Stir occasionally.

4 When you're ready to cook the chicken, preheat your oven to 350 degrees Fahrenheit (175 degrees Celsius). Cover a baking sheet with foil.

5 Remove the chicken from the marinade and place it on the baking sheet. Do not throw out the marinade; you will need it later.

6 Place the baking sheet on the middle rack of the oven and allow the chicken to cook for 10 minutes. Remove the sheet from the oven, spoon half of the marinade over the chicken, and put it back in the oven. Bake the chicken for another 10 minutes, then remove the sheet from the oven again. Flip the chicken and spoon on the rest of the marinade. Bake for another 15 minutes, until the chicken is cooked through. Serve and enjoy.

Per Serving: *(1 breast, 250 g) Calories 223; Available carbohydrate 11 g; Carbohydrate 12 g; Fibre 1 g; Fat 4 g; Protein 35 g; Cholesterol 78 mg; Phosphorus 411 mg; Potassium 662 mg; Sodium 234 mg.*

1 Serving = ½ Carbohydrate Choice

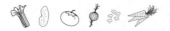

Parmesan Chicken

Parmesan chicken is a popular Italian dish that is usually paired with pasta. When preparing this dish, choose whole wheat pasta, and remember that ½ cup (125 ml) of cooked pasta is 1 Carbohydrate Choice. You can even splurge and add some low-fat mozzarella to the top of the chicken if you like.

Preparation Time: *10 minutes*

Cooking Time: *20 minutes*

Yield: *4 servings*

¼ cup (50 ml) whole wheat flour

1 lb (450 g) skinless, boneless chicken breasts (approximately 4 breasts)

1 egg, beaten

1 tbsp (15 ml) 1% milk

¼ cup (50 ml) bread crumbs

¼ tsp (1 ml) salt

¼ tsp (1 ml) pepper

1 tsp (5 ml) Italian seasoning

2 tbsp (30 ml) low-fat Parmesan cheese, grated

2 tbsp (30 ml) ground flaxseed

1 Preheat oven to 400 degrees Fahrenheit (200 degrees Celsius).

2 Sprinkle the flour onto a flat plate. Coat each chicken breast in the flour. Set aside.

3 In a small bowl, mix together the egg and milk with a whisk or fork. Set aside.

4 To make the coating, use a spoon to mix together the bread crumbs, salt, pepper, seasoning, Parmesan cheese, and flaxseed in a flat-bottomed dish.

5 With your fingers or a fork, dip each piece of flour-coated chicken first into the egg mixture and then into the coating, making sure each breast is evenly coated.

6 Place the chicken in a shallow baking dish and bake for about 20 minutes, until the chicken is cooked through and the juices run clear. Serve.

Per Serving: *(1 breast, 175 g) Calories 242; Available carbohydrate 9 g; Carbohydrate 12 g; Fibre 3 g; Fat 6 g; Protein 34 g; Cholesterol 128 mg; Phosphorus 360 mg; Potassium 432 mg; Sodium 344 mg.*

1 Serving = ½ Carbohydrate Choice

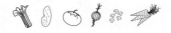

Bok Choy with Chicken

Bok choy is a vegetable commonly included in Asian cuisine. It can be found at most farmers' markets and large chain grocery stores.

Preparation Time: *12 minutes*

Cooking Time: *12 minutes*

Yield: *4 servings*

1 cup (250 ml) reduced-sodium chicken broth

2 tbsp (30 ml) reduced-sodium soy sauce

2 tsp (10 ml) fish sauce

½ tsp (2 ml) freshly ground black pepper

6 cups (1,500 ml) bok choy, chopped

1 lb (450 g) skinless, boneless chicken, cut into narrow strips

⅛ tsp (0.5 ml) salt

1½ tbsp (22 ml) cornstarch

3 tbsp (45 ml) cold water

¼ cup (50 ml) cilantro, chopped

1 In a large saucepan, bring the chicken broth, soy sauce, fish sauce, and pepper to a boil over high heat. Stir occasionally with a spoon.

2 Add the bok choy, chicken, and salt to the broth mixture and bring the mixture back to a boil. Reduce heat to medium, cover, and cook for about 4 minutes, until the bok choy is tender-crisp and the chicken is cooked through.

3 In a small bowl, add the cornstarch to the cold water. Stir with a fork until no lumps remain.

4 Add the cornstarch mixture to the saucepan and bring to a boil over high heat, stirring until the mixture thickens, about 4 minutes.

5 Spoon into bowls, sprinkle with cilantro, and serve.

Per Serving: *(1 cup/250 ml, 265 g) Calories 173; Available carbohydrate 5 g; Carbohydrate 6 g; Fibre 1 g; Fat 2 g; Protein 32 g; Cholesterol 72 mg; Phosphorus 305 mg; Potassium 674 mg; Sodium 875 mg.*

1 Serving = 0 Carbohydrate Choice

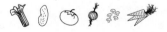

Cinnamon Lime Chicken

This Hispanic dish is a snap to make and has sensational flavour.

Preparation Time: *15 minutes*

Cooking Time: *25 minutes*

Yield: *2 servings*

½ lb (225 g) skinless, boneless chicken breasts (approximately 2 breasts)

¼ tsp (1 ml) salt

2 tsp (10 ml) cinnamon

1 tbsp (15 ml) olive oil

1 small yellow onion, chopped

1 clove garlic, minced

⅓ cup (75 ml) fresh lime juice

1 Preheat oven to 400 degrees Fahrenheit (200 degrees Celsius). Line a rimmed baking sheet with parchment paper and set aside.

2 In a small, flat-bottomed bowl, combine the salt and cinnamon. Rub this mixture onto each piece of chicken, evenly coating each breast.

3 Place the chicken on the baking sheet and cook for 15 to 20 minutes, until the juices run clear.

4 While the chicken is cooking, add the oil to a large frying pan and set over medium-heat. When the oil is warm, add the onion and garlic and sauté for about 3 minutes, until the onion is soft. Set aside.

5 When the chicken is done, add it to the frying pan with the onions and pour on the lime juice. Cover and simmer over low heat for 15 minutes. Serve and enjoy.

Per Serving: (1 breast, 140 g) Calories 213; Available carbohydrate 6 g; Carbohydrate 8 g; Fibre 2 g; Fat 14 g; Protein 16 g; Cholesterol 47 mg; Phosphorus 143 mg; Potassium 252 mg; Sodium 339 mg.

1 Serving = 0 Carbohydrate Choice

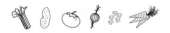

Chicken with Cashews

In Chinese culture, this dish can be prepared as an entrée or a side dish. Either way it's tasty and great when accompanied by rice.

Preparation Time: *25 minutes*

Cooking Time: *15 minutes*

Yield: *5 servings*

2 tbsp (30 ml) reduced-sodium soy sauce	*1 medium green pepper, chopped*
½ tsp (2 ml) ginger, grated	*1 tsp (5 ml) cornstarch*
1 clove garlic, minced	*4 tbsp (60 ml) cold water*
½ lb (225 g) skinless, boneless chicken (about 2 breasts), cut into bite-sized pieces	*1 tbsp (15 ml) Hoisin sauce*
2 tbsp (30 ml) canola oil	*1 tbsp (15 ml) water*
½ cup (125 ml) yellow onion, chopped	*1 tsp (5 ml) honey*
1 cup (250 ml) carrot, thinly sliced	*½ cup (125 ml) unsalted cashews*

1 To make the marinade, use a spoon to mix together the soy sauce, ginger, and garlic in a medium-sized bowl. Add the chicken and toss until the chicken is coated with the marinade. Set aside.

2 In a wok or large frying pan, warm 1 tbsp (15 ml) of the oil over medium-high heat. Add the onion, carrots, and green pepper and sauté, stirring occasionally with a wooden spoon, for 4 minutes. Remove the vegetables from the wok or pan and set them aside in a bowl.

3 Add the rest of the oil to the wok and warm over medium-high heat. Add the marinated chicken and cook for 7 minutes, until the chicken is almost cooked. Remove the wok from the heat.

4 In a small bowl, mix together the cornstarch and cold water, stirring with a whisk or fork until no lumps remain. Set the bowl aside.

5 In another small bowl, mix together the Hoisin sauce, water, and honey. Stir well with a spoon.

6 Place all the ingredients, except the cashews, into the wok and set over medium heat, stirring occasionally with a wooden spoon until the sauce thickens, about 3 minutes. Add the cashews, stir for 1 minute, and serve.

Per Serving: (1 cup/250 ml, 242 g) Calories 219; Available carbohydrate 11 g; Carbohydrate 13 g; Fibre 2 g; Fat 13 g; Protein 15 g; Cholesterol 29 mg; Phosphorus 195 mg; Potassium 377 mg; Sodium 392 mg.

1 Serving = ½ Carbohydrate Choice

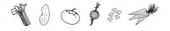

Walnut Chicken

This Chinese dish is delicious with rice. For a change, try wild or brown basmati rice — or even or a mixture of the two — with lots of veggies on the side.

Preparation Time: *20 minutes*

Cooking Time: *15 minutes*

Yield: *3 servings*

2 tsp (10 ml) cornstarch

4 tbsp (60 ml) rice wine (sake or mirin)

1 lb (450 g) skinless, boneless chicken, cut into bite-sized pieces

½ cup (125 ml) walnuts, coarsely chopped

3 tbsp (45 ml) canola oil

5 green onions, chopped into 1-inch (2.5 cm) pieces

1 tsp (5 ml) ginger, grated

3 tbsp (45 ml) low-sodium soy sauce

⅓ cup (75 ml) water

1 In a medium-sized bowl, mix together the cornstarch and 2 tbsp (30 ml) of the rice wine with a whisk or fork. Add the chicken and stir until it is coated. Set aside.

2 In a small, dry frying pan, lightly toast the walnuts over medium-high heat for 3 minutes, stirring often with an egg lifter or wooden spoon. Remove the pan from the heat and allow the walnuts to cool.

3 Heat the oil in a wok or large frying pan or large saucepan over medium-high heat. Add the chicken and stir-fry for 3 minutes, stirring occasionally with an egg lifter or spoon. Add the onion and ginger and stir-fry for another 3 minutes.

4 Add the remaining rice wine, soy sauce, water, and walnuts. Stir-fry for 5 minutes over medium-high heat, making sure the chicken is cooked through. Serve and enjoy.

*****Per Serving:*** *(1 cup/250 ml, 210 g) Calories 405; Available carbohydrate 6 g; Carbohydrate 7 g; Fibre 1 g; Fat 21 g; Protein 41 g; Cholesterol 96 mg; Phosphorus 382 mg; Potassium 566 mg; Sodium 718 mg.*

1 Serving = 0 Carbohydrate Choice

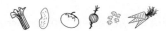

It's Okay to Have a Turkey

We're so proud of these delicious turkey recipes that we're sure you and your family will just gobble them up! (Do you have any idea how hard it is to not make puns about turkeys when writing a cookbook? Hmm, we bet you do now.)

You can buy turkey either as a whole bird or as turkey breasts. Without the skin, turkey has fewer calories and less fat than chicken. Turkey is a good source of protein, niacin, phosphorus, selenium, vitamin B_6, and zinc. Like chicken, white turkey meat has less fat than dark turkey meat.

Turkey can be easily substituted for chicken in most recipes.

Curried Turkey in a Pita

Stuff this curried turkey into a pita or wrap for a tasty lunch. Or, if you prefer, serve it as an appetizer with mini pitas. It even tastes great on its own! Making this dish is an excellent way to use up leftover turkey.

Preparation Time: *15 minutes*

Yield: *4 servings*

4 tbsp (60 ml) sliced almonds	*1½ tsp (7 ml) curry powder*
2 cups (500 ml) cooked turkey, cut into small cubes	*⅔ cup (150 ml) low-fat mayonnaise*
1 cup (250 ml) celery, chopped	*¼ tsp (1 ml) salt*
½ cup (125 ml) seedless grapes, cut in half	*¼ tsp (1 ml) pepper*
1 tbsp (15 ml) lemon juice	*⅛ cup (25 ml) ground flaxseed*
	2 whole wheat pitas

1 In a small, dry frying pan, lightly toast the almonds over medium-high heat for 3 to 5 minutes, stirring often with a spatula or wooden spoon. When the almonds are lightly browned, remove the pan from the heat and allow the almonds to cool.

2 In a medium-sized bowl, use a spoon to thoroughly mix together all the ingredients (except the pitas).

3 Cut each pita in half, across its diameter, to make 4 half circles. Fill each pita pocket with 1 cup (250 ml) of the chicken mixture. Serve and enjoy.

Per Serving: *(½ pita with 1 cup/250 ml filling, 265 g) Calories 452; Available carbohydrate 25 g; Carbohydrate 31 g; Fibre 6 g; Fat 25 g; Protein 28 g; Cholesterol 60 mg; Phosphorus 349 mg; Potassium 559 mg; Sodium 812 mg.*

1 Serving = 1½ Carbohydrate Choices

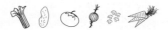

Cheesy Turkey Bake

This tasty casserole is a great addition to a buffet table.

Preparation Time: *25 minutes*

Cooking Time: *28 minutes*

Yield: *8 servings*

4 cups (1,000 ml) broad egg noodles	1 tsp (5 ml) garlic powder
1½ cup (375 ml) tomato sauce	2½ cups (625 ml) cooked turkey, cut into cubes
5 ½ oz (156 ml) can tomato paste	1½ cups (325 ml) low-fat cottage cheese
1 cup (250 ml) yellow onion, chopped	½ cup (125 ml) low-fat ricotta cheese
2 tbsp (30 ml) Italian seasoning	½ tsp (2 ml) nutmeg
1 tsp (5 ml) sugar	2 cups (500 ml) low-fat mozzarella cheese, grated

1 Preheat the oven to 350 degrees Fahrenheit (175 degrees Celsius).

2 Fill a large pot with water and bring to a boil over high heat. Add the pasta, stir with a spoon, and bring back to a boil. Cook, stirring occasionally, for 7 minutes. Drain the noodles in a strainer, rinse with cold water, and drain again. Set aside.

3 In a large bowl, mix together the tomato sauce, tomato paste, onion, spices, and sugar with a spatula or spoon.

4 Add the noodles and turkey to the large bowl and mix well.

5 In a medium-sized bowl, purée the cottage cheese, ricotta cheese, and nutmeg with a hand blender or potato masher.

6 Spoon half the noodle mixture into the bottom of a 2-quart (2.5-litre) glass baking dish. Spread the cheese mixture evenly over the noodles. Spoon on the rest of the noodles and top with the mozzarella cheese. Bake for 20 minutes or until bubbling and hot. Serve hot.

Per Serving: (1 cup/250 ml, 240 g) Calories 336; Available carbohydrate 27 g; Carbohydrate 30 g; Fibre 3 g; Fat 10 g; Protein 33 g; Cholesterol 81 mg; Phosphorus 434 mg; Potassium 678 mg; Sodium 600 mg.

1 Serving = 2 Carbohydrate Choices

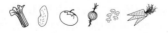

Turkey à la King

This dish is a tasty way to use up leftover turkey from the holidays.

Preparation Time: *15 minutes*

Cooking Time: *10 minutes*

Yield: *5 servings*

½ cup (125 ml) soft margarine	1½ tsp (7 ml) instant chicken bouillon
2½ cup (625 ml) mushrooms, sliced	1½ cups (375 ml) 1% milk
1 small green pepper, chopped	1¼ cups (300 ml) hot water
½ cup (125 ml) flour	2 cups (500 ml) cooked turkey, cut into cubes
¼ tsp (1 ml) pepper	

1 In a large frying pan or pot, melt the margarine over medium-high heat. Add the mushrooms and green pepper. Sauté for 5 minutes, stirring occasionally with a wooden spoon or spatula.

2 Add the flour and pepper, reduce heat to low, and stir for 1 minute.

3 Add the bouillon, milk, and water. Increase heat to high and bring to a boil, stirring constantly for 1 minute.

4 Reduce the heat to medium and add the turkey to the frying pan or pot. Stir occasionally until the turkey is warm, about 3 minutes. Serve over cooked rice or pasta — don't forget to count the extra Carbohydrate Choices!

Per Serving: (1 cup turkey/250 ml, 285 g) Calories 360; Available carbohydrate 15 g; Carbohydrate 16 g; Fibre 1 g; Fat 21 g; Protein 25 g; Cholesterol 50 mg; Phosphorus 265 mg; Potassium 486 mg; Sodium 458 mg.

1 Serving = 1 Carbohydrate Choice

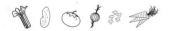

Chapter 15

Mighty Meat

*B*eef is chock-a-block full of nutrients, including protein, iron, magnesium, niacin, phosphorus, pantothenic acid, potassium, riboflavin, selenium, thiamin (vitamin B_1), vitamin B_6, vitamin B_{12}, vitamin D, and zinc. Also, your body absorbs the iron you get from eating meat more easily than the iron you get from plant sources.

In this chapter, we offer a whole host of recipes made with beef, pork, lamb, and venison. If meat's your thing, you've come to the right chapter.

Having diabetes makes avoiding excess amounts of fat especially important. Buy lean cuts of meat and trim any visible fat before cooking.

Beef It Up!

With the exception of short ribs, all trimmed cuts of beef are lean, containing no more than 7.5 to 10 percent fat. These are extra lean cuts:

✔ Blade steak

✔ Brisket

✔ Cross rib

✔ Extra lean ground beef

✔ Eye of round

✔ Flank

✔ Inside/outside round

✔ Porterhouse

✔ Rib-eye

✔ Rump roast

✔ Sirloin tip roast

✔ Stewing cubes

✔ Strip loin

✔ T-bone

✔ Tenderloin

✔ Top sirloin

The type of cooking method you choose will also influence the amount of fat remaining on the meat after it's been cooked. Baking, barbequing, broiling, microwaving, roasting, or stir-frying rather than deep-frying will help to lower the fat content.

Shepherd's Pie

Shepherd's Pie is a favourite comfort food, and combining white and sweet potatoes (a suggestion from Cynthia's friend, Patti Harvey) will make the dish even more flavourful. This recipe has a lot of steps, but don't be intimidated — they're all straightforward.

Preparation Time: *30 minutes*

Cooking Time: *20 to 25 minutes*

Yield: *6 servings*

2 medium-sized new white potatoes	*1 cup (250 ml) reduced-sodium beef broth*
1 medium-sized sweet potato	*1½ tbsp (22 ml) flour*
1 lb (450 g) extra lean ground beef	*3 tbsp (45 ml) cold water*
1 cup (250 ml) mushrooms, sliced	*½ cup (125 ml) frozen green peas*
¾ cup (175 ml) yellow onion, chopped	*½ cup (125 ml) frozen corn*
2 cloves garlic, minced	*1 tbsp (15 ml) soft margarine*
½ tsp (2 ml) Montreal steak spice	*½ cup (125 ml) 1% milk*
1 tsp (5 ml) Worcestershire sauce	*¼ tsp (1 ml) salt*
1–2 drops Tabasco sauce	

1 Preheat the oven to 375 degrees Fahrenheit (190 degrees Celsius) and lightly grease a 6-cup (1,500-ml) casserole dish.

2 Peel and rinse the potatoes.

3 Cut the potatoes into 2-inch (5-cm) pieces and place in a medium-sized saucepan. Add enough water to cover the potatoes. Place a lid on the saucepan and bring to a boil over high heat.

4 When the potatoes have started to boil, partially remove the lid to prevent the water from boiling over. Continue to cook for 15 minutes or until the potatoes are soft and can be easily pierced with a fork.

5 While the potatoes are cooking, place the beef, mushrooms, onion, and garlic in a large frying pan. Cook over medium-high heat, stirring, until the beef is cooked, about 4 minutes. Drain the fat.

6 Add the Montreal steak spice, Worcestershire sauce, Tabasco, and broth to the beef mixture and stir thoroughly.

7 Mix the flour into the cold water and stir with a fork until all the lumps have disappeared. Add this to the beef mixture and stir until it thickens.

8 Combine the frozen vegetables with the beef mixture and stir thoroughly. Evenly spread the mixture over the bottom of the casserole dish.

9 When the potatoes are done, drain them in a strainer. Return them to the saucepan with the margarine, milk, and salt. Mash with a potato masher until they are smooth. Use a spoon to evenly spread the potatoes over the beef mixture in the casserole dish.

10 Bake, uncovered, for 25 minutes or until the top is bubbly and lightly browned. Serve.

Per Serving: *(1 cup/250 ml, 230 g) Calories 269; Available carbohydrate 22 g; Carbohydrate 25 g; Fibre 3 g; Fat 10 g; Protein 29 g; Cholesterol 50 mg; Phosphorus 240 mg; Potassium 684 mg; Sodium 354 mg.*

1 Serving = 1½ Carbohydrate Choices

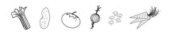

Hamburger Stroganoff

This dish is tastier than Hamburger Helper and much healthier. Cynthia's teenagers love it and it freezes well too — an ideal dish to send off with students living away from home at college or university!

Preparation Time: *20 minutes*

Cooking Time: *14 minutes*

Yield: *5 servings*

1 lb (450 kg) extra lean ground beef

¾ cup (175 ml) yellow onion, chopped

1½ cups (375 ml) mushrooms, sliced

2 tbsp (30 ml) whole wheat flour

1 clove garlic, minced

¼ tsp (1 ml) pepper

10 oz (284 ml) low-fat condensed cream of chicken soup

½ cup (125 ml) low-fat plain yogurt

2 tbsp (30 ml) ground flaxseed

2½ cups (625 ml) cooked egg noodles

1 In a large frying pan, brown the hamburger, onion, and mushrooms on medium-high heat for 4 minutes. Drain the fat.

2 Stir in the flour, garlic, and pepper. Cook for 3 minutes on medium-high heat.

3 Add the soup and bring to a boil, reduce heat, and simmer for 5 minutes over low heat. Stir in the yogurt and flaxseed and heat through, about 2 minutes.

4 Remove from heat and serve over a ½-cup (125-ml) portion of hot egg noodles.

*****Per Serving:*** *(¾ cup/175 ml, 204 g on ½ cup/125 ml noodles) Calories 365; Available carbohydrate 30 g; Carbohydrate 33 g; Fibre 3 g; Fat 14 g; Protein 26 g; Cholesterol 89 mg; Phosphorus 323 mg; Potassium 569 mg; Sodium 379 mg.*

1 Serving = 2 Carbohydrate Choices

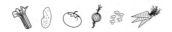

Stir-Fried Beef with Rice Noodles

This Thai recipe is very easy to make. The rice noodles used in this recipe are the same variety that is used to make Pad Thai.

Preparation Time: *30 minutes*

Cooking Time: *10 minutes*

Yield: *7 servings*

8 oz (225 g) dry wide rice noodles	*¼ cup (50 ml) canola oil*
1 lb (450 g) beef tenderloin or rib-eye	*2 tbsp (30 ml) oyster sauce*
7 cups (1,750 ml) bok choy	*1 tbsp (15 ml) fish sauce*
1 large onion, chopped	*2 tsp (10 ml) sugar*
3 cloves garlic, minced	*⅔ cup (150 ml) roasted peanuts, chopped*

1 Cook the rice noodles according to directions on the package. When they are cooked, drain the water and set them aside.

2 Slice the beef, against the grain, into thin strips.

3 Wash the bok choy under running water. Cut the bok choy into wide strips by cutting it in half lengthwise and then crosswise.

4 In a wok or large frying pan, heat the oil over medium-high heat until it's warm. Add the beef and sauté with the onion and garlic for 5 minutes. Add the bok choy and continue to sauté for another 3 minutes.

5 Add the remaining ingredients and the noodles. Heat thoroughly while stirring for 2 minutes. Serve hot.

Per Serving: (1 cup/250 ml, 210 g) Calories 448; Available carbohydrate 32 g; Carbohydrate 35 g; Fibre 3 g; Fat 26 g; Protein 19 g; Cholesterol 43 mg; Phosphorus 267 mg; Potassium 518 mg; Sodium 419 mg.

1 Serving = 2 Carbohydrate Choices

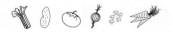

Groundnut Stew

In Africa, peanuts are commonly referred to as groundnuts. This recipe, which includes a peanut butter–based sauce, is one of Cynthia's favourites — you won't believe how well it turns out!

Preparation Time: *40 minutes*

Cooking Time: *30 minutes*

Yield: *8 servings*

1 large sweet potato	*2 medium tomatoes, chopped*
1 tbsp (15 ml) canola oil	*1 large green pepper, chopped*
2 lbs (900 g) beef tenderloin or rib-eye (or equal parts of beef and chicken), cut into cubes	*1 cup (250 ml) yellow onion, chopped*
¼ tsp (1 ml) salt	*1 clove garlic, minced*
¼ tsp (1 ml) black pepper	*1 tsp (5 ml) chili pepper paste*
½ cup (125 ml) reduced-sodium beef broth	*3 cups (750 ml) eggplant, cut into cubes*
1 tbsp (15 ml) canola oil	*½ cup (125 ml) peanut butter*

1 Use a fork to pierce the sweet potato in a few places. Wrap the potato in a paper towel and place in the microwave for 2 minutes to partially cook. (If you don't have a microwave, place the pierced potato in a steamer over a pot of boiling water for 5 minutes.)

2 When the potato is cool to touch, peel the skin, and use a sharp knife to cut it into cubes. Set aside.

3 In a large saucepan, warm the oil over medium-high heat and add the beef. With a wooden spoon, stir the beef until it is browned, about 3 minutes. Add the salt, pepper, and broth, and simmer, covered, over low heat for 10 minutes.

4 While the beef is cooking, warm the oil over medium-high heat in a large frying pan. Add the cubed sweet potato, tomatoes, green pepper, onions, garlic, and chili pepper paste, and sauté for 2 minutes, stirring occasionally.

5 Reduce the heat under the frying pan, with the vegetables, to medium-low, add the eggplant and peanut butter, and stir well. Cover and simmer for 8 minutes.

6 Add the vegetable mixture to the meat mixture, mix thoroughly, and continue to simmer until the meat is cooked and the vegetables are tender, about 2 minutes.

7 Serve hot over ⅔ cup (150 ml) of rice or 1 cup (250 ml) of couscous (but don't forget to count the extra two Carbohydrate Choices). Serve and enjoy.

Per Serving: *(1 cup/250 ml, 230 g) Calories 484; Available carbohydrate 10 g; Carbohydrate 14 g; Fibre 4 g; Fat 36 g; Protein 28 g; Cholesterol 75 mg; Phosphorus 304 mg; Potassium 780 mg; Sodium 229 mg.*

1 Serving = ½ Carbohydrate Choice (without rice or couscous)

Meatloaf with Mushroom Sauce

Here's another great comfort food. Leftovers can be used in sandwiches or frozen for later.

Preparation Time: *15 minutes*

Cooking Time: *45 minutes*

Yield: *6 servings*

1 lb (450 g) extra lean ground beef

1 cup (250 ml) mushrooms, sliced

2 tbsp (30 ml) dry, low fat, onion soup mix

2 tbsp (30 ml) whole wheat bread crumbs

2 tbsp (30 ml) ground flaxseed

¼ cup (50 ml) 1% milk

1 egg, beaten

⅛ tsp (0.5 ml) salt

⅛ tsp (0.5 ml) pepper

Sauce:

2 tbsp (30 ml) 1% milk

1 tbsp (15 ml) cornstarch

1 tbsp (15 ml) soft margarine

1½ cups (375 ml) mushrooms, sliced

3 tbsp (45 ml) onion, chopped

1 cup (250 ml) reduced-sodium beef broth

1 Preheat the oven to 350 degrees Fahrenheit (175 degrees Celsius).

2 Combine the meatloaf ingredients in a large bowl. Use a large spoon or clean hands to combine the ingredients until they are evenly mixed.

3 Evenly distribute the meatloaf mixture in a loaf pan and bake for 45 minutes.

4 To prepare the sauce, combine the milk and cornstarch in a small bowl. Using a fork, stir until the mixture is smooth and no lumps appear.

5 Melt the margarine in a medium-sized frying pan over medium-high heat. Add the mushrooms and onions. Stir until the onions are soft and light golden, about 5 minutes.

6 Mix in the beef broth, bring to a boil, and add the cornstarch mixture. Cook, stirring constantly, for about 1 minute, until the sauce is slightly thickened. Remove from heat. (If necessary, the sauce can be reheated prior to serving.)

7 When the meatloaf is cooked (the meat should be slightly pulling away from the sides of the pan), let it cool slightly, about 4 minutes. While the meatloaf is in the pan, use a knife to cut it into 1¼-inch (3.2-cm) slices. Top with 2½ tbsp (37 ml) of warm sauce, if desired, and serve.

Per Serving: *(1¼ inch/3.2 cm slice, 112 g) Calories 186; Available carbohydrate 5 g; Carbohydrate 6 g; Fibre 1 g; Fat 10 g; Protein 18 g; Cholesterol 85 mg; Phosphorus 205 mg; Potassium 359 mg; Sodium 393 mg.*

1 Serving = 0 Carbohydrate Choice

Per Serving: *(2½ tbsp/37 ml sauce) Calories 37; Available carbohydrate 3 g; Carbohydrate 3 g; Fibre 0 g; Fat 2 g; Protein 2 g; Cholesterol 0 mg; Phosphorus 34 mg; Potassium 105 mg; Sodium 32 mg.*

1 Serving = 0 Carbohydrate Choice

Aboriginal Tacos with Fried Bannock

Don't be afraid to try this recipe — it is so good. But the bannock and beans have a lot of carbohydrate, so watch how much you eat. This low-fat version is healthier than the traditional bannock because it's not deep-fried.

Preparation Time: *30 minutes*

Cooking Time: *16 minutes*

Yield: *6 servings*

1 lb (450 g) extra lean ground beef	**Toppings:**
28 oz (796 ml) can diced tomatoes	*1½ cups (375 ml) low-fat cheddar cheese, shredded*
1 large green pepper, chopped	*2 cups (500 ml) lettuce, shredded*
1 large yellow onion, chopped	*1½ cups (375 ml) tomato, diced*
1 cup (250 ml) mushrooms, sliced	**Fried Bannock:**
19 oz (540 ml) can kidney beans	*2 cups (500 ml) flour*
14 oz (398 ml) can refried beans	*2 tsp (10 ml) baking powder*
1 tsp (5 ml) chili powder	*½ tsp (2 ml) salt*
2 drops Tabasco sauce	*1 cup warm water*
	Canola oil for hands and frying

1 Place the hamburger in large frying pan and set over medium-high heat. Stir frequently with a spatula until no pink appears, about 4 minutes. Drain the fat.

2 Add the tomatoes, pepper, onion, and mushrooms to the frying pan with the hamburger and cook for another 4 minutes.

3 Place the kidney beans in a strainer and rinse under cool water for 2 minutes.

4 Add the beans, chili powder, and Tabasco sauce to the frying pan. Stir until the ingredients are heated through.

5 While the meat and vegetables are cooking, prepare the toppings.

6 To make the bannock, mix together the flour, baking powder, and salt in a medium-sized bowl. Slowly add the warm water and stir with a spoon until the ingredients form a sticky ball. Sprinkle some flour on a clean, dry surface. Rub some oil on your hands (make sure they're clean first!) and knead the dough 6 times.

7 Divide the dough into 6 equal parts. Heat a thin layer of oil in a large frying pan over medium-high heat. On a floured surface, use your greased hands to flatten the dough balls into thin pancakes about ¼ inch (0.6 cm) thick. Place the bannock in the frying pan. Cook until the bannock is golden brown, about 2 minutes on each side.

8 To serve, place each hot bannock on a plate and cover with ⅔ cup (150 ml) of the meat mixture. Top each bannock with ¼ cup (50 ml) cheese, ⅓ cup (75 ml) of lettuce, and ¼ cup (50 ml) of tomatoes. Enjoy.

Per Serving: (83 g bannock with ⅔ cup/150 ml meat and toppings, 315 g) Calories 578; Available carbohydrate 61 g; Carbohydrate 74 g; Fibre 13 g; Fat 15 g; Protein 37 g; Cholesterol 54 mg; Phosphorus 553 mg; Potassium 1,295 mg; Sodium 1,265 mg.

1 Serving = 4 Carbohydrate Choices

Pork on Your Fork

Many cuts of pork are lean and can be part of a healthy diet. Pork provides protein (which, as we discuss in detail in Chapter 2, plays an invaluable role in growing and maintaining healthy body tissues), and the fat in pork is the better, monounsaturated and polyunsaturated variety. Fat-trimmed pork is suitable for a low-cholesterol, heart-friendly diet.

Listed from leanest to least lean, these are the cuts of pork with the least fat:

- Tenderloin
- Chops
- Pork leg (ham)
- Steaks
- Roast
- Cutlets

Spanish Pork Chops

In Spanish, these marinated pork chops from Madrid are called "Chuletas de Cerdo." Now you can impress your family!

Preparation Time: *10 minutes (plus 2 hours to marinate)*

Cooking Time: *30 to 40 minutes*

Yield: *2 servings*

2 lean boneless pork chops, about ½ lb (225 g)	*1 tsp (5 ml) sun-dried tomatoes, finely chopped*
2 cloves garlic, minced	*⅛ tsp (0.5 ml) salt*
1 bay leaf, torn into small pieces	*⅛ tsp (0.5 ml) ground pepper*
1 tbsp (15 ml) parsley, chopped	*¼ cup (50 ml) red wine*
½ tsp (2 ml) fresh thyme	*2 tbsp (30 ml) canola oil*

1 Place the trimmed pork chops in a small casserole dish.

2 Cover the pork chops with the garlic, bay leaf, parsley, thyme, tomatoes, salt, and pepper.

3 In a small bowl mix together the wine and oil with a fork. Gently pour the mixture over the pork chops. Cover the dish and refrigerate for 2 hours, flipping after 1 hour.

4 After 2 hours, preheat the oven to 350 degrees Fahrenheit (175 degrees Celsius). Remove the cover from the dish and bake the pork chops for 30 to 40 minutes, basting about halfway through with the marinade. When the pork chops are cooked, the internal temperature should be 160 degrees Fahrenheit (70 degrees Celsius). Serve and enjoy.

Per Serving: *(1 pork chop, 103 g) Calories 200; Available carbohydrate 2 g; Carbohydrate 2 g; Fibre 0 g; Fat 9 g; Protein 24 g; Cholesterol 71 mg; Phosphorus 257 mg; Potassium 475 mg; Sodium 227 mg.*

1 Serving = 0 Carbohydrate Choice

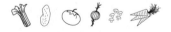

Pork Chow Mein

This speedy meal is a family favourite, and using sesame oil gives it an authentic Chinese taste. You should be able to find the chow mein noodles in vacuum-sealed packages in the produce department of the grocery store.

Preparation Time: *20 minutes*

Cooking Time: *15 minutes*

Yield: *6 servings*

8 oz (250 g) package chow mein noodles, uncooked

2 tbsp (30 ml) sesame seeds

1 tbsp (15 ml) canola oil

2 cups (500 ml) pork tenderloin, bite-sized pieces

1 tbsp (15 ml) sesame oil

2 cloves garlic, minced

1 large red pepper, chopped

1 large green pepper, chopped

3 tbsp (45 ml) reduced-sodium soy sauce

3 tbsp (45 ml) Chinese rice wine

6 green onions, chopped

2 cups (500 ml) bean sprouts

⅓ cup (75 ml) parsley, chopped

1 Place the noodles in a large pot. Add enough boiling water to cover the noodles by 1 inch (2.5 cm). Stir gently, cover, and let sit for approximately 5 minutes, until the noodles are tender.

2 Drain the noodles in a strainer, then rinse with cold water. Drain the noodles again.

3 Add the sesame seeds to a small, dry frying pan and stir continuously over medium-high heat until they are lightly toasted, about 3 minutes. Remove from heat and let cool.

4 Add the canola oil to a wok or large frying pan and warm over medium-high heat. Add the pork and stir with a wooden spoon or spatula until the pork is golden brown. Continue to let the pork cook for 6 minutes.

5 Add the sesame oil to the wok or frying pan with the garlic and peppers. Stir over medium-high heat for 4 minutes.

6 Reduce the heat to medium and add the noodles, soy sauce, and rice wine. Toss the noodles and stir-fry for 2 minutes.

7 Add the green onions and bean sprouts to the wok and stir-fry for another 2 minutes. Stir in the parsley and sesame seeds. Serve.

Per Serving: *(1⅓ cups/325 ml, 93 g) Calories 385; Available carbohydrate 28 g; Carbohydrate 32 g; Fibre 4 g; Fat 20 g; Protein 19 g; Cholesterol 29 mg; Phosphorus 315 mg; Potassium 617 mg; Sodium 636 mg.*

1 Serving = 2 Carbohydrate Choices

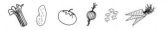

Mary Had a Little Lamb — So Can You

Lamb is a good source of protein, iron, niacin, vitamin B$_{12}$, and zinc.

One-third of the fat in lamb is saturated (the bad type of fat), but it can be easily removed before cooking and doing so won't take away from lamb's unique taste.

Lamb is tastiest when served slightly pink; the internal temperature should be 155 degrees Fahrenheit (68 degrees Celsius). Lamb tastes best when served hot and on a heated plate.

Glazed Asian Lamb

The lemon and honey make this glazed lamb recipe a savoury dish. Lamb has little marbled fat, and most of it is on the edges so it's easy to trim.

Preparation Time: *25 minutes*

Cooking Time: *10 minutes*

Yield: *3 servings*

⅔ lb (300 g) boneless lean lamb, cut into strips

1 tbsp (15 ml) sesame oil

2 cups (500 ml) pea pods, topped and tailed

1 tbsp (15 ml) honey

2 tbsp (30 ml) lemon juice

1 tbsp (15 ml) sesame seeds

2 tbsp (30 ml) coriander, chopped

2 green onions, chopped

⅛ tsp (0.5 ml) salt

⅛ tsp (0.5 ml) pepper

1 Warm the oil in a wok or large frying pan over medium heat. Add the lamb and stir until it's browned, about 4 minutes. Remove the lamb from the wok.

2 Place the pea pods, honey, lemon juice, and sesame seeds in the wok, bring to a boil over medium-high heat, and stir-fry for 1 minute.

3 Return the lamb to the wok and stir-fry for 3 minutes. Add the coriander, onions, salt, and pepper and stir-fry for 1 minute.

4 Serve and enjoy.

Per Serving: *(1 cup/250 ml, 140 g) Calories 196; Available carbohydrate 9 g; Carbohydrate 11 g; Fibre 2 g; Fat 7 g; Protein 22 g; Cholesterol 66 mg; Phosphorus 240 mg; Potassium 428 mg; Sodium 166 mg.*

1 Serving = ½ Carbohydrate Choice

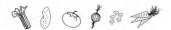

Lamb with Chinese Oyster Sauce

Modern oyster sauce doesn't contain actual oysters, but an oyster essence or extract. Not that you'd know it from this scrumptious oyster sauce recipe!

Preparation Time: *25 minutes*

Cooking Time: *8 minutes*

Yield: *4 servings*

1¼ lb (565 g) leg of lamb

2 tsp (10 ml) cornstarch

1 tbsp (15 ml) rice wine (mirin, sake)

1 tbsp (15 ml) water

Dash of salt

2 tbsp (30 ml) reduced-sodium soy sauce

3 tbsp (45 ml) oyster sauce

1 tsp (5 ml) sugar

1 tsp (5 ml) sesame oil

¼ cup (50 ml) canola oil

1 leek, cut in ½-inch (1.25-cm) rings

2 cups (500 ml) shiitake mushrooms, stems discarded and caps sliced

½-inch (1.25 cm) ginger, peeled and grated

2 cloves garlic, minced

1 Remove any fat from the lamb and slice into thin strips, ¼ inch (0.6 cm) thick.

2 In a medium-sized bowl, mix together the cornstarch, rice wine, water, and salt. Add the meat to the bowl and stir until the meat is coated. Set aside.

3 For the sauce, mix together the soy sauce, oyster sauce, sugar, and sesame oil in a small bowl. Stir with a spoon until the sugar is dissolved. Set aside.

4 In a wok or large frying pan, warm the canola oil over medium-high heat. Add the lamb to the wok and stir for 6 minutes using a wooden spoon or spatula. Remove the lamb from the wok and set aside.

5 Add the leek and mushrooms to the wok and stir-fry for 3 minutes. Add the ginger and garlic and stir-fry for another minute.

6 Return the lamb to the wok and add the sauce. Stir well to heat thoroughly. Serve.

Per Serving: *(1 cup/250 ml, 197 g) Calories 373; Available carbohydrate 9 g; Carbohydrate 10 g; Fibre 1 g; Fat 22 g; Protein 31 g; Cholesterol 91 mg; Phosphorus 336 mg; Potassium 695 mg; Sodium 705 mg.*

1 Serving = ½ Carbohydrate Choice

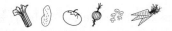

Going Wild

Game meat is usually very lean so it's often helpful to cook it in a sauce or to marinate it. Marinating game will add flavour and help keep the meat moist and tender. Watch game meat closely while cooking and never overcook, as it will quickly become dry. Cook game to medium-rare.

Venison, the meat in the recipe that follows, is lower in fat than beef and is a source of iron, protein, selenium, and zinc.

Venison Steak in Cranberry Sauce

Many Aboriginal groups believe that the hunter who kills a deer must thank it. To do this, a hunter will sometimes return to the place where a deer was felled to bury its heart. While there, it is also common for a hunter to pinch his sides to show the deer spirit how fat and grateful he is for having eaten the meat.

Preparation Time: *25 minutes*

Cooking Time: *18 to 20 minutes*

Yield: *4 servings*

8 allspice, whole	*¼ tsp (1 ml) thyme*
8 juniper berries (optional)	*½ cup (125 ml) reduced-sodium beef broth*
⅛ tsp (0.5 ml) salt	*1½ tbsp (25 ml) soft margarine*
⅛ tsp (0.5 ml) pepper	*¼ cup (50 ml) shallots, chopped*
1 1b (450 g) venison steak, sliced into 1½-inch (4 cm) thick strips	*1 clove garlic, minced*
	⅛ tsp (0.5 ml) salt
¼ cup (50 ml) red wine or cranberry juice	*1 tsp (5 ml) cold water*
¼ cup (50 ml) frozen cranberries	*½ tsp (2 ml) cornstarch*

1 Use a coffee grinder to process the allspice and juniper berries until they are finely ground.

2 In a small bowl, combine half of the allspice and juniper berries with the salt and pepper. Set the venison on a cutting board and sprinkle with the allspice mixture. Set aside.

3 To prepare the sauce, combine the red wine or cranberry juice, frozen cranberries, thyme, and beef broth in a small saucepan. Bring the mixture to the boil over high heat, remove from heat, cover, and set aside.

4 In a large frying pan, melt 2 teaspoons (10 ml) of the margarine over medium-high heat and sauté the shallots and garlic for 2 minutes. Add the sauce, the rest of the ground allspice (and juniper berries), and the salt. Bring to a boil over high heat. Reduce heat to simmer and cook uncovered for 3 minutes.

5 In a small bowl, combine the cold water and cornstarch. Stir well with a fork. When the mixture is smooth and no lumps appear, add it to the sauce, bring to a boil over high heat, and cook for 1 minute, stirring constantly. Remove from heat and cover to keep warm.

6 Melt the rest of the margarine in a medium-large frying pan over medium heat. Add the venison and cook for 5 minutes on each side until browned.

7 Pour the sauce over the venison and cook for about 5 more minutes until cooked through. Serve.

Per Serving: *(¾ cup/175 ml, 227 g) Calories 223; Available carbohydrate 6 g; Carbohydrate 7 g; Fibre 1 g; Fat 7 g; Protein 27 g; Cholesterol 96 mg; Phosphorus 262 mg; Potassium 509 mg; Sodium 254 mg.*

1 Serving = 0 Carbohydrate Choice

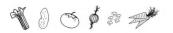

Chapter 16

Vegetarian Variety

· ·

In This Chapter

▶ Looking at the benefits of a vegetarian diet

▶ Cooking filling and flavourful vegetarian mains

· ·

More and more people are choosing to eat some, most, or even all their meals without meat. Fortunately, wherever you fall on the spectrum from meat lover to meat abstainer, you can enjoy great vegetarian recipes.

If you are a longstanding vegetarian, you have likely discovered that following a vegetarian diet is much easier than it was years ago because stores now carry numerous vegetarian products — even convenience foods — including soymilk, juices, breakfast cereals, veggie burgers, veggie dogs, and frozen entrées. In this chapter, we share a wide variety of vegetarian recipes that are rich not only in nutrition, but in taste, too.

Benefits to Eating the Vegetarian Way

The health benefits of vegetarian meals are numerous. Vegetarian meals are typically low in saturated fat and cholesterol. They are also high in fibre, magnesium, folate, and antioxidants. The main sources of protein for most vegetarians are legumes (beans, peas, and lentils), nuts, and seeds. *Eating Well with Canada's Food Guide* suggests that everyone should frequently consume these and other meat alternatives.

The different types of vegetarianism

A vegetarian diet is one that is free of meat, fish, seafood, and poultry. There are, however, different types or classifications of vegetarians:

✔ A lacto-ovo-vegetarian avoids meat, fish, seafood, and poultry.

✔ A lacto-vegetarian avoids meat, fish, seafood, poultry, and eggs.

✔ An ovo-vegetarian avoids meat, fish, seafood, poultry, and milk.

✔ A vegan avoids meat, fish, seafood, poultry, eggs, milk, and honey.

Several different types of vegetarianism exist (see the sidebar "The different types of vegetarianism"), but one unofficial category applies to most people (including us): the *flexitarian;* that is, the occasional vegetarian.

Compared with non-vegetarians, vegetarians have a lower risk of the following:

✔ Certain types of cancer, including colon cancer

✔ Heart disease

✔ Hypertension (high blood pressure)

✔ Lipid abnormalities (including elevated LDL cholesterol)

✔ Obesity

Vegetarian diets may not provide sufficient quantities of all necessary nutrients. As a result, vegetarians are prone to iron deficiency, and vegans are at additional risk for deficiency of vitamin B_{12}, vitamin D, calcium, zinc, and, occasionally, riboflavin (vitamin B_2). For this reason, if you are a vegetarian (and especially if you are vegan) you should speak to a registered dietitian to find out how to ensure you get all the nutrients you need. You may need to take supplements of certain nutrients.

Paying a vegetarian "complement" . . . or not

Amino acids are the building blocks of proteins. There are over 20 different amino acids. In the past, scientists believed that different food sources of amino acids had to be balanced or matched ("complemented") at each meal in order to obtain the maximum protein benefit from a vegetarian meal. However, new research has shown otherwise. As long as you eat an assortment of plant foods *over the course of a day,* all your amino acid requirements will be met.

Meatless Marvels

Meat-free meals can be every bit as tasty as meat-containing meals and are often more nutritious. It is no coincidence that more and more Canadians — including newcomers from countries where meat is not routinely available — are making most of their meals without meat.

A serving in the Meat and Alternate group of *Eating Well with Canada's Food Guide* for meatless options includes

- ✓ ¾ cup (175 ml) legumes or tofu
- ✓ 2 eggs
- ✓ ¼ cup (50 ml) of nuts or seeds
- ✓ 2 tbsp (30 ml) peanut butter or nut butter
- ✓ ½ cup (125 ml) soy-based meat substitutes

Because legumes are a source of protein and carbohydrate, ½ cup (125 ml) contains one protein and one carbohydrate choice on average, a person with diabetes needs to be mindful of portion sizes.

☺ Curry Tofu with Noodles

On its own, tofu (soybean curd) tastes bland, but when added to curry, the tofu takes on a wonderful flavour.

Preparation Time: *20 minutes*

Cooking Time: *15 minutes*

Yield: *6 servings*

7 oz (200 g) rice vermicelli noodles	*1 large red pepper, cut into thin, lengthwise strips*
Warm water	
3 tbsp (45 ml) canola oil	*1 tbsp (15 ml) reduced-sodium soy sauce*
1½–2½ tbsp (22–37 ml) curry paste (to taste)	*⅛ tsp (0.5 ml) salt*
8 oz (225 g) firm tofu, cut into 1-inch (2.5 cm) cubes	*⅛ tsp (0.5 ml) pepper*
	2 green onions, finely chopped
1 cup (250 ml) green beans, cut into 1-inch (2.5 cm) pieces	*1 lime, cut into wedges, for garnish*

1 Place the vermicelli noodles in a medium-sized bowl and cover with warm water. Let the noodles soak for about 10 minutes. Drain the water from the noodles using a strainer.

2 Add 1½ tbsp (22 ml) of the oil to a wok or large frying pan and set over medium heat. Add the curry paste and stir-fry for 1 minute. Add the tofu to the wok and continue to stir-fry until the tofu is lightly browned, about 3 minutes. Remove the tofu from the wok and set aside.

3 Add the remaining oil to the wok and stir-fry the green beans and red pepper over medium heat for about 5 minutes, until the vegetables are tender.

4 Add the vermicelli, tofu, soy sauce, salt, and pepper to the wok and stir-fry until heated through, about 5 minutes.

5 Transfer to a serving dish, sprinkle with green onions, and serve with a lime wedge on the side.

Per Serving: *(1 cup/250 ml, 132 g) Calories 226; Available carbohydrate 30 g; Carbohydrate 32 g; Fibre 2 g; Fat 9 g; Protein 4 g; Cholesterol 0 mg; Phosphorus 106 mg; Potassium 175 mg; Sodium 239 mg.*

1 Serving = 2 Carbohydrate Choices

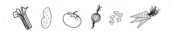

♨ *Barbecued Eggplant*

This dish is quick and easy to prepare and tastes great done on the barbecue. If it's not barbecue season, this dish can be easily cooked in the oven.

Preparation Time: *15 minutes*

Cooking Time: *10 minutes*

Yield: *4 servings (as an entrée)*

1 large eggplant, cut into 1-inch (2.5 cm) slices	*3 firm, ripe tomatoes, cut into ½-inch (1.25 cm) slices*
2 tbsp (30 ml) olive oil	
1 tbsp (15 ml) Italian seasoning	*1½ cups (375 ml) Asiago cheese, grated*
¼ tsp (2 ml) salt	*½ cup (125 ml) fresh basil, chopped*
¼ tsp (2 ml) pepper	

1 Set the barbecue to medium heat. (If you're using an oven, turn on the broiler element.)

2 Brush both sides of the eggplant with oil.

3 Sprinkle the seasonings, salt, and pepper on the eggplant. Place the eggplant on the grill or under the broiler of the oven. Cover the eggplant and cook until grill marks form on one side, about 5 minutes. Flip the eggplant and grill the other side for 5 minutes until the eggplant is tender.

4 Brush both sides of each tomato slice with oil. Grill the tomatoes for 5 minutes, flipping often, until the tomatoes are warmed through.

5 Remove the eggplant and tomato from the barbecue or oven. Place the eggplant on a dinner plate, add the tomato, and sprinkle with the cheese and basil. Serve hot.

Per Serving: (2 slices, 240 g) Calories 273; Available carbohydrate 7 g; Carbohydrate 13 g; Fibre 6 g; Fat 18 g; Protein 17 g; Cholesterol 33 mg; Phosphorus 334 mg; Potassium 603 mg; Sodium 726 mg.

1 Serving = ½ Carbohydrate Choice

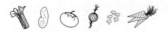

⏲ Nutty Rice and Mushroom Stir-Fry

Basmati is a type of long, thin rice with a nutty aroma. It is very popular in many Asian diets.

Preparation Time: *20 minutes*

Cooking Time: *25 minutes*

Yield: *3 servings*

½ cup (125 ml) basmati rice	¼ cup (50 ml) pecans, chopped
1 cup (250 ml) water	¼ cup (50 ml) almonds, chopped
1½ tbsp (22 ml) canola oil	¼ cup (50 ml) parsley, chopped
1 shallot, chopped	⅛ tsp (0.5 ml) salt
1 cup (250 ml) white mushrooms, sliced	⅛ tsp (0.5 ml) pepper
¼ cup (50 ml) hazelnuts, chopped	

1 Place the rice in a strainer and rinse with cool running water until it runs clear.

2 Place the rice and water in a medium-sized saucepan with a tight-fitting lid. Bring to a boil over high heat. Stir and reduce heat to low, cover with the lid, and simmer for 12 minutes. Do not remove the lid while the rice is simmering.

3 Remove the saucepan from the heat and let sit for 5 minutes. Fluff the rice with a fork, then rinse the rice in a strainer under cold running water. Let drain.

4 Add half the oil to a wok or large frying pan and stir-fry the rice for 2 minutes over medium-high heat. Remove from heat and set aside.

5 Add the remaining oil to the wok and stir-fry the shallot for 2 minutes until it is soft. Add the mushrooms and stir-fry for another 2 minutes. Add the nuts and stir-fry for 1 minute. Return the rice to the wok and stir-fry for another 3 minutes. Add the salt, pepper, and parsley. Stir well and serve.

Per Serving: (¾ cup/175 ml, 156 g) Calories 357; Available carbohydrate 27 g; Carbohydrate 31 g; Fibre 4 g; Fat 24 g; Protein 7 g; Cholesterol 0 mg; Phosphorus 156 mg; Potassium 314 mg; Sodium 105 mg.

1 Serving = 2 Carbohydrate Choices

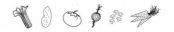

☺ Three-Bean Chili

When Cynthia first made this recipe several years ago, her father turned up his nose and asked where the meat was. Later, he asked to take home the leftovers!

Preparation Time: *18 minutes*

Cooking Time: *40 minutes*

Yield: *6 servings*

19 oz (540 ml) can of kidney beans	*2–3 tbsp (30–45 ml) chili powder*
19 oz (540 ml) can of romano beans	*1 tsp (5 ml) dried oregano*
19 oz (540 ml) can of black beans	*28 oz (796 ml) canned diced tomatoes*
1 tbsp (15 ml) canola oil	*Water*
2 onions, coarsely chopped	*½ tsp (2 ml) pepper*
4 cloves garlic, minced	*⅓ cup (75 ml) cilantro, chopped*

1 Place the beans in a strainer and rinse under cool running water for 2 minutes. Drain.

2 Heat the oil in a large pot over medium heat. Add the onion. Stir-fry for 2 minutes, until the onion is tender.

3 Add the garlic, chili powder, and oregano. Stir until well mixed.

4 Stir in the canned tomatoes and cook for 5 minutes. Add the beans to the pot along with water, if necessary, so the beans are covered by 1 inch (2.5 cm) of liquid. Cover the pot and simmer on low heat for 30 to 35 minutes.

5 Add the pepper and cilantro. Stir until the ingredients are thoroughly mixed. Serve.

Per Serving: (1⅓ cups/325 ml, 339 g) Calories 381; Available carbohydrate 49 g; Carbohydrate 69 g; Fibre 20 g; Fat 4 g; Protein 21 g; Cholesterol 0 mg; Phosphorus 336 mg; Potassium 1413 mg; Sodium 631 mg.

1 Serving = 3 Carbohydrate Choices

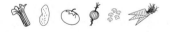

○ Tofu Mushroom Caps

Tofu is high in protein and very low in fat — a versatile and healthy source of protein for a vegetarian.

Preparation Time: *15 minutes*

Cooking Time: *10 minutes*

Yield: *4 servings*

8 large open mushrooms	*⅓ cup (75 ml) corn*
2 green onions, sliced	*2 tsp (10 ml) ground flaxseed*
1 clove garlic, minced	*⅛ tsp (0.5 ml) salt*
2 tbsp (30 ml) oyster sauce	*⅛ tsp (0.5 ml) pepper*
5 oz (135 g) firm tofu, cut into cubes	*4 tsp (20 ml) sesame oil*
½ cup (125 ml) low-fat mozzarella cheese, grated	

1 Preheat the oven to 400 degrees Fahrenheit (200 degrees Celsius).

2 Carefully remove the stems from the mushroom caps. To make the filling, finely chop the mushroom stems and add them to a medium-sized bowl with the onions, garlic, and oyster sauce.

3 Stir in the tofu, cheese, corn, flaxseed, salt, and pepper.

4 Brush the edges of the mushrooms with the sesame oil. Spoon the filling equally into the mushroom caps and place on a baking dish or jelly roll sheet.

5 Bake for 10 to 12 minutes until the mushrooms are tender. Serve.

Per Serving: (2 mushroom caps, 150 g) Calories 142; Available carbohydrate 7 g; Carbohydrate 8 g; Fibre 1 g; Fat 9 g; Protein 8 g; Cholesterol 8 mg; Phosphorus 168 mg; Potassium 296 mg; Sodium 371 mg.

1 Serving = ½ Carbohydrate Choice

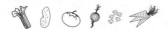

☺ Quesadillas

Quesadillas are quick and effortless to make for a quick Mexican meal. They're also a great way to use up leftovers!

Preparation Time: *8 minutes*

Cooking Time: *8 minutes*

Yield: *1 serving*

8-inch (20 cm) whole wheat tortilla

1½ tbsp (22 ml) salsa

¼ cup (50 ml) low-fat mozzarella cheese, grated

1½ tbsp (22 ml) red pepper, diced

2 tsp (10 ml) green onion, chopped

2 tbsp (30 ml) black beans, rinsed and drained

2 tbsp (30 ml) tomato, chopped

1 In a small bowl, mix together all the ingredients except the tortilla.

2 Place the tortilla in a dry medium-sized frying pan. Place the contents of the bowl onto half of the tortilla. Fold the tortilla in half.

3 Warm the tortilla in the frying pan over medium heat, about 4 minutes per side until the sides become golden brown and the cheese has melted.

4 Serve warm with light sour cream for dipping, if desired.

Per Serving: *(1 quesadilla, 135 g) Calories 288; Available carbohydrate 31 g; Carbohydrate 36 g; Fibre 5 g; Fat 10 g; Protein 14 g; Cholesterol 15 mg; Phosphorus 257 mg; Potassium 321 mg; Sodium 590 mg.*

1 Serving = 2 Carbohydrate Choices

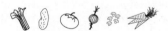

☺ White Pizza

Using prepared pizza dough makes this recipe simple. To save even more time, the mushroom mixture can even be made a day in advance and stored in the refrigerator until needed.

Preparation Time: 35 minutes

Cooking Time: 15 minutes

Yield: 3 servings

1 tbsp (15 ml) canola oil

1½ cups (375 ml) shiitake mushrooms, stems removed and sliced

1 cup (250 ml) cremini mushrooms, sliced

3 cloves garlic, minced

1 tbsp (15 ml) cooking sherry

1 tsp (5 ml) lemon juice

¼ tsp (1 ml) salt

⅛ tsp (0.5 ml) pepper

2 tbsp (30 ml) cornmeal

½ lb (225 g) whole wheat pizza dough

¼ cup (50 ml) fresh chopped herbs (mixture of parsley, thyme, and rosemary)

3 oz (85 g) brie, sliced

1 Preheat the oven to 450 degrees Fahrenheit (230 degrees Celsius).

2 In a medium-sized frying pan, heat the oil over medium-high heat. Add the mushrooms and cook for 5 minutes, stirring with a spatula or wooden spoon.

3 Add the garlic, sherry, lemon juice, salt, and pepper to the mushrooms and continue to cook for 3 more minutes, stirring occasionally. Remove from heat and set aside.

4 Sprinkle the cornmeal onto a large, rimmed baking sheet or pizza pan and set aside.

5 Divide the pizza dough into 3 equal pieces so it's easier to handle. Lightly coat the inside of a clean plastic bag with canola oil. Place a ball of dough ball into the plastic bag. (The dough is easier to roll this way.) Flatten the dough with a rolling pin or your hands to form a flat oval. Remove the dough from the bag and place it on a baking sheet. Repeat with the remaining two balls of dough.

6 Evenly spread a third of the mushroom mixture over each of the 3 pizzas. Cover each pizza with a third of the herbs and brie.

7 Bake on the middle rack of the oven for 7 to 8 minutes, until the crusts are golden brown. Serve warm.

Per Serving: (1 pizza, 147 g) Calories 459; Available carbohydrate 56 g; Carbohydrate 64 g; Fibre 8 g; Fat 14 g; Protein 19 g; Cholesterol 28 mg; Phosphorus 146 mg; Potassium 358 mg; Sodium 960 mg.

1 Serving = 4 Carbohydrate Choices

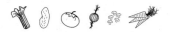

☙ Chapati

A chapati (pronounced chuh-paa-teeh) is a flatbread and a staple at most traditional Indian meals. There are numerous versions of chapati — this one comes from Cynthia's friend, Dr. Nita Rajesh.

Preparation Time: *10 minutes (plus 15 minutes stand time)*

Cooking Time: *20 minutes*

Yield: *10 chapatis*

2 cups (500 ml) whole wheat flour

1 tsp (5 ml) salt

Water, (approximately ¾ cup/175 ml), depending on the fineness of the flour)

1 tbsp (15 ml) olive oil

1 Mix the flour and salt in a medium-sized bowl. Make a well in the middle of the flour and slowly add the water. Continue mixing with clean hands until a dough ball forms.

2 Add the oil and mix well using your hands.

3 Place the dough on a lightly floured surface and knead the dough into a smooth ball. Add more flour or water as required to make the dough workable and elastic. The dough should not stick to your fingers, nor should it be too dry.

4 Cover the dough with a clean tea towel and let sit for 15 minutes.

5 Divide the dough into ten golf-ball-sized pieces.

6 Lightly coat each ball in flour. On a lightly floured surface, flatten each ball using a rolling pin and roll into a thin round circle about 6 inches (15 cm) wide. Roll from the middle out.

7 Heat a dry frying pan or tawah (a special Indian frying pan) over medium heat and add the chapati. When it has lightly browned, about 1 to 2 minutes, flip the chapati over with a spatula or egg lifter. Cook the second side until it turns light brown.

8 Using a clean tea towel, gently press the chapati into the pan around the edges and turn the chapati in circles so it puffs up. The chapati is done when it turns golden brown.

9 Place the chapati on a plate while you cook the others. Place a sheet of paper towel between the chapatis to prevent them from sticking together.

10 Serve warm with dal, curry, soup, stew, cheese, or diet jam.

Per Serving: (1 chapati, 40 g) Calories 117; Available carbohydrate 18 g; Carbohydrate 22 g; Fibre 4 g; Fat 2 g; Protein 4 g; Cholesterol 0 mg; Phosphorus 104 mg; Potassium 122 mg; Sodium 293 mg.

1 Serving = 1 Carbohydrate Choice

Chapter 17

Delectable Endings

For many people, a meal is simply not complete without dessert. (Indeed, for many people, dessert is the highlight of a meal!)

Having diabetes doesn't magically make your appetite for dessert go away, nor should it. If you're living with diabetes you can eat anything you want — including dessert. As you might expect, some "buts" go along with this open invitation. As we look at in the next section, however, the overriding point is that having diabetes is not a punishment and nothing is forbidden!

Diabetes, Desserts, and You

If you have diabetes, you're likely well aware of how important eating nutritiously is to your health. You may, however, be less aware that "sweets" are an acceptable part of your diet. Indeed, the Canadian Diabetes Association notes that up to 10 percent of your daily calories can come from sweets (in the form of sucrose-based foods) as "there is no evidence that sucrose intake up to this level has any deleterious effect on (blood glucose) control or lipid(s)" if you have diabetes. Nice!

Please keep in mind the 10 percent limit, however, because consumption of greater quantities of sucrose-based foods may increase blood glucose levels and adversely affect lipids. So yes, you can have dessert, but no, not in unlimited quantities (not that *anyone* should — whether or not living with diabetes).

Using Sugar Substitutes

Using a sugar substitute is one way of including desserts in your diabetes meal plan without also incorporating excess sugar in your diet. (We discuss sugar substitutes in Chapter 3.) Sucralose and aspartame, two popular sugar substitutes, are heat stable and so can be used for baking.

These are the acceptable daily limits for sugar substitutes, based on body weight:

- The acceptable daily limit for sucralose (as is found in Splenda) is 9 mg per kg body weight per day. One cup (250 ml) of Splenda has 250 mg sucralose. Sucralose is 400 to 800 times sweeter than sugar.

- The acceptable daily limit for aspartame (which goes by the trade names NutraSweet or Equal) is 40 mg per kg body weight per day. One can (355 ml) of diet pop has 200 mg of aspartame. Aspartame is 200 times sweeter than sugar.

To help baked goods rise when using Splenda Granulated Sweetener, the manufacturer suggests adding ½ cup (125 ml) of dry skim milk powder and ½ tsp (2 ml) of baking soda for every 1 cup (250 ml) of Splenda Granulated Sweetener (not Splenda Brown Sugar Blend). Following this suggestion increases the carbohydrate content and the number of calories (from the skim milk powder) and the amount of sodium (from the baking soda).

As you read the recipes in this chapter (or, even better, make them!), you may notice that some of the recipes call for sugar, whereas other recipes call for either sugar or a sugar substitute. When only sugar is listed, it is because the recipe tastes significantly better — or was significantly healthier — when made this way, or that the carbohydrate and sodium content was too high when the skim milk powder, baking soda, and Splenda were added.

Baking Up a Storm: Pies and Cakes

These pie and cake recipes are easy to prepare without sacrificing taste. The recipes call for frozen pie shells (to save you time), but you are, of course, welcome to make your own pie shell if you wish. (You can also use prepared pie crusts, which you can find in the refrigerator section of your grocery store. These need to be unrolled into a pie plate following the manufacturer's directions.)

☺ Rhubarb Cake

We commonly refer to rhubarb as a fruit, but it is actually a vegetable. One cup (250 ml) of rhubarb has only 26 calories! Rhubarb has a unique type of fibre that may confer health benefits; indeed, researchers are looking into its cholesterol-lowering properties.

Preparation Time: *30 minutes*

Cooking Time: *30 to 35 minutes*

Yield: *12 servings*

1 cup (250 ml) sugar or Splenda

2 tbsp (30 ml) cornstarch

5 cups (1,250 ml) rhubarb, chopped into ½-inch (1.25 cm) pieces

½ cup (125 ml) 1% milk

1 tbsp (15 ml) vinegar

1½ cups (375 ml) flour

½ cup (125 ml) soft margarine

½ tsp (2 ml) baking soda

½ tsp (2 ml) baking powder

1 egg, beaten

1 Preheat the oven to 350 degrees Fahrenheit (175 degrees Celsius). Lightly oil an 8-x-8-inch (20-x-20-cm) baking pan.

2 In a medium-sized saucepan, combine ½ cup (125 ml) of the sugar (or Splenda) and the cornstarch. Add the rhubarb and cook over medium-high heat for about 5 minutes, stirring constantly. The mixture is done when the rhubarb softens and the mixture thickens slightly. Remove from heat and set aside.

3 In a measuring cup, combine the milk and vinegar. Set aside to sour for 5 minutes.

4 In a large bowl, combine the flour, margarine, and remaining sugar or Splenda with a spatula. Stir until the mixture becomes crumbly. Set aside ⅓ cup (75 ml) to use as the topping later.

5 Add the baking soda and baking powder to the flour mixture and stir well.

6 Add the egg to the milk and vinegar and mix well. To finish the batter, add the egg and milk mixture to the flour and stir until thoroughly blended.

7 Spread half the batter over the bottom of the baking pan. Spoon the rhubarb mixture evenly over the batter, then cover with the remaining batter. Sprinkle the topping over the cake.

8 Bake for 30 to 35 minutes until the cake turns light golden and a toothpick inserted in the centre comes out dry. Serve warm or cold.

Per Serving *(with sugar): (2 x 2½ inches/5 x 6.25 cm, 108 g) Calories 216; Available carbohydrate 32 g; Carbohydrate 33 g; Fibre 1 g; Fat 8 g; Protein 3 g; Cholesterol 18 mg; Phosphorus 46 mg; Potassium 186 mg; Sodium 152 mg.*

1 Serving = 2 Carbohydrate Choices

Per Serving *(with Splenda): (2 x 2½ inches/5 x 6.25 cm, 85 g) Calories 158; Available carbohydrate 17 g; Carbohydrate 18 g; Fibre 1 g; Fat 8 g; Protein 3 g; Cholesterol 18 mg; Phosphorus 46 mg; Potassium 186 mg; Sodium 152 mg.*

1 Serving = 1 Carbohydrate Choice

♨ Pumpkin Pie

There is no reason for a person with diabetes not to enjoy pumpkin pie. When Cynthia's mother, Bonnie Payne, makes this recipe, everyone runs to grab a slice before there is none left!

Preparation Time: *10 minutes*

Cooking Time: *75 to 85 minutes with sugar/65 to 85 minutes with Splenda*

Yield: *8 servings*

2 eggs, beaten

14 oz (398 ml) can of pure pumpkin

¾ cup (175 ml) brown sugar or 6 tbsp (90 ml) Brown Sugar Splenda

1½ tsp (7 ml) pumpkin pie spice

¼ tsp (1 ml) salt

⅔ cup (150 ml) 1% milk

9-inch (22.5 cm) deep-dish frozen pie shell

1 Preheat the oven to 400 degrees Fahrenheit (200 degrees Celsius).

2 In a medium-sized bowl, use an electric beater, whisk, or spoon to thoroughly blend together the eggs, pumpkin, brown sugar (or Brown Sugar Splenda), spice, and salt.

3 Add the milk and mix well. Pour the mixture into the pie shell.

4 Bake for 15 minutes at 400 degrees Fahrenheit (200 degrees Celsius), then reduce heat to 350 degrees Fahrenheit (175 degrees Celsius) and continue baking for 60 to 70 minutes if using sugar or 50 to 60 minutes if using Brown Sugar Splenda. The pie is done when a knife inserted in the centre comes out clean.

5 Serve warm or cold.

Per Serving *(with sugar): (⅛ pie, 96 g) Calories 232; Available carbohydrate 34 g; Carbohydrate 36 g; Fibre 2 g; Fat 9 g; Protein 4 g; Cholesterol 54 mg; Phosphorus 73 mg; Potassium 196 mg; Sodium 355 mg.*

1 Serving = 2 Carbohydrate Choices

Per Serving *(with Splenda): (⅛ pie, 100 g) Calories 175; Available carbohydrate 19 g; Carbohydrate 21 g; Fibre 2 g; Fat 9 g; Protein 4 g; Cholesterol 54 mg; Phosphorus 72 mg; Potassium 174 mg; Sodium 350 mg.*

1 Serving = 1 Carbohydrate Choice

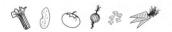

☞ Blueberry Pie

Small, wild, or low-bush blueberries are better for baking than the large, high-bush varieties. Search for blueberries that are uniformly blue in colour. If they have a reddish tinge, pass them up — they're not ripe and won't ripen any further.

Preparation Time: *15 to 20 minutes*

Cooking Time: *30 to 35 minutes*

Yield: *8 servings*

¼ cup (50 ml) sugar or Splenda

3 tbsp (45 ml) flour

9-inch (22.5 cm) frozen prepared regular pie crust (thaw on counter for 10 minutes)

3 cups (750 ml) blueberries

1 tbsp (15 ml) lemon juice

Topping:

6 tbsp (90 ml) rolled oats

3 tbsp (45 ml) flour

3 tbsp (45 ml) brown sugar or 1½ tbsp (22 ml) Brown Sugar Splenda

3 tbsp (45 ml) soft margarine

1 Preheat oven to 400 degrees Fahrenheit (200 degrees Celsius).

2 In a medium-sized bowl, mix together the sugar (or Splenda) and flour. Sprinkle the bottom of the pie crust evenly with 3 tablespoons (45 ml) of the flour mixture.

3 Add the blueberries and lemon juice to the flour mixture and stir gently until evenly mixed. Pour the blueberry mixture into the pie shell.

4 To make the topping, use a fork to mix together the rolled oats, flour, brown sugar (or Brown Sugar Splenda), and margarine until crumbly. Evenly coat the blueberries with the topping.

5 Bake for 10 minutes. Reduce the heat to 350 degrees Fahrenheit (175 degrees Celsius) and bake for another 20 to 25 minutes if using sugar or 15 to 20 minutes if using Splenda. The crumb mixture should be golden. Serve and enjoy!

Per Serving (with sugar): (⅛ pie, 103 g) Calories 260; Available carbohydrate 35 g; Carbohydrate 37 g; Fibre 2 g; Fat 12 g; Protein 2 g; Cholesterol 0 mg; Phosphorus 42 mg; Potassium 96 mg; Sodium 179 mg.

1 Serving = 2 ½ Carbohydrate Choices

Per Serving (with Splenda): (⅛ pie, 98 g) Calories 227; Available carbohydrate 27 g; Carbohydrate 29 g; Fibre 2 g; Fat 12 g; Protein 2 g; Cholesterol 0 mg; Phosphorus 41 mg; Potassium 90 mg; Sodium 179 mg.

1 Serving = 2 Carbohydrate Choices

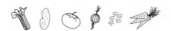

☞ Chocolate Zucchini Muffins

Nobody will think these chocolaty muffins have a healthy zucchini base. Cynthia's daughter, Kristen, made these and loved them.

Preparation Time: *14 minutes*

Cooking Time: *18 minutes*

Yield: *17 muffins*

2 cups (500 ml) flour	*½ cup (125 ml) chocolate chips*
¼ cup (50 ml) cocoa powder	*¾ cup (175 ml) canola oil*
1 tsp (5 ml) baking soda	*¾ cup (175 ml) sugar*
1½ tsp (7 ml) baking powder	*2 eggs, beaten*
1 tsp (5 ml) cinnamon	*½ cup (125 ml) 1% milk*
1 tsp (5 ml) ground cloves	*2 cups (500 ml) zucchini, grated*
½ tsp (2 ml) salt	

1 Preheat the oven to 350 degrees Fahrenheit (175 degrees Celsius). Lightly oil the muffin pan.

2 In a large bowl, mix together the flour, cocoa, baking soda, baking powder, cinnamon, cloves, and salt with a spatula or spoon. Stir in the chocolate chips.

3 In another medium-sized bowl, mix together the remaining ingredients.

4 Add the contents of the medium-sized bowl to the larger one and mix well.

5 Spoon ⅓ cup (75 ml) of batter into each muffin cup and bake for 18 minutes or until a toothpick inserted into the centre of the muffin comes out dry.

6 Cool on wire racks for at least 10 minutes. Serve.

Per Serving: *(1 muffin, 62 g) Calories 214; Available carbohydrate 24 g; Carbohydrate 25 g; Fibre 1 g; Fat 12 g; Protein 3 g; Cholesterol 25 mg; Phosphorus 64 mg; Potassium 112 mg; Sodium 200 mg.*

1 Serving = 1½ Carbohydrate Choices

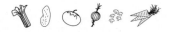

Sour Cream Chocolate Chip Cake

This recipe has been passed down through the Payne family and is always a crowd pleaser.

Preparation Time: *25 minutes*

Cooking Time: *20 to 25 minutes*

Yield: *15 servings*

6 tbsp (90 ml) soft margarine	*1 tsp (5 ml) baking soda*
¾ cup (175 ml) sugar	*1 tsp (5 ml) cinnamon*
2 eggs	*1 cup (250 ml) low-fat sour cream*
1½ cups (375 ml) flour	*¾ cup (175 ml) semi-sweet chocolate chips*
1½ tsp (7 ml) baking powder	

1 Preheat the oven to 350 degrees Fahrenheit (175 degrees Celsius). Lightly oil and flour a 9-x-13-inch (22.5-x-32.5-cm) baking pan.

2 In a medium-sized bowl, mix together the margarine, sugar, and eggs with a hand mixer or spatula until creamy.

3 In another medium-sized bowl, mix together the flour, baking powder, baking soda, and cinnamon using a spatula or spoon. Add this mixture to the bowl with the eggs and mix well.

4 Mix in the sour cream and chocolate chips. When the batter is well blended, pour it into the baking pan.

5 Bake for 20 to 25 minutes until a toothpick inserted into the centre of the cake comes out dry. Serve warm or cold.

Per Serving: (3 x 2½ inches/7.5 x 6.25 cm, 59 g) Calories 198; Available carbohydrate 25 g; Carbohydrate 26 g; Fibre 1 g; Fat 10 g; Protein 3 g; Cholesterol 34 mg; Phosphorus 59 mg; Potassium 89 mg; Sodium 195 mg.

1 Serving = 2 Carbohydrate Choices

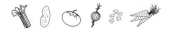

✎ Mini Cheesecakes

People with diabetes can have their mini cheesecakes and eat them too — in moderation!

Preparation Time: *30 minutes*

Cooking Time: *25 to 35 minutes*

Yield: *12 servings*

12 vanilla wafer cookies	*6 tbsp (90 ml) sugar or Splenda*
1 tbsp (15 ml) soft margarine	*8 oz (250 g) light cream cheese, softened*
1 cup (250 ml) apples, peeled, and finely chopped	*1 egg*
½ tsp (2 ml) cinnamon	*⅓ cup (75 ml) low-fat sour cream*
	1 tsp (5 ml) vanilla

1 Preheat the oven to 325 degrees Fahrenheit (165 degrees Celsius). Place paper liners in the cups of a 12-muffin pan.

2 Place a cookie in the bottom of each paper-lined cup and set the pan aside.

3 Melt the margarine in a small frying pan over medium heat and add the apples. Cook for 5 minutes, stirring often with a spatula or wooden spoon, until the apples are tender.

4 Stir in the cinnamon and 1 tablespoon (15 ml) of sugar or Splenda and cook for 1 minute. Spoon the apple mixture evenly over the cookies.

5 In a medium-sized bowl, beat the cream cheese, egg, sour cream, vanilla, and the remaining sugar or Splenda until smooth. Spoon evenly over the apples.

6 Bake 35 minutes for the sugar version and 25 minutes for the Splenda version, or until the cheesecake is set.

7 Cool the cheesecakes in the pan on a wire rack. Serve warm or cold.

Per Serving *(with sugar): (1 cheesecake, 40 g) Calories 123; Available carbohydrate 14 g; Carbohydrate 14 g; Fibre 0 g; Fat 6 g; Protein 3 g; Cholesterol 31 mg; Phosphorus 48 mg; Potassium 88 mg; Sodium 132 mg.*

1 Serving = 1 Carbohydrate Choice

Per Serving *(with Splenda): (1 cheesecake, 35 g) Calories 102; Available carbohydrate 9 g; Carbohydrate 9 g; Fibre 0 g; Fat 6 g; Protein 3 g; Cholesterol 31 mg; Phosphorus 48 mg; Potassium 88 mg; Sodium 132 mg.*

1 Serving = ½ Carbohydrate Choice

↺ Carrot Cake

This cake has been adapted from a recipe from Cynthia's friend, Debbie Smith, and is always moist and tasty — the cream cheese icing adds a special touch.

Preparation Time: *25 minutes*

Cooking Time: *20 to 30 minutes with sugar/15 to 25 minutes with Splenda*

Yield: *15 servings*

¾ cup (175 ml) sugar or Splenda

¾ cup (175 ml) canola oil

3 eggs, beaten

½ tsp (2 ml) salt

1 tsp (5 ml) baking soda

1 tsp (5 ml) baking powder

1½ tsp (7 ml) cinnamon

1⅓ cups (325 ml) flour

2 cups (500 ml) carrots, grated

For the Icing:

8 oz (250 g) light cream cheese, softened

½ cup (125 ml) icing sugar

4 tbsp (60 ml) orange juice

½ tsp (2 ml) vanilla

½ tsp (2 ml) orange rind

1 Preheat the oven to 350 degrees Fahrenheit (175 degrees Celsius). Lightly grease a 9-x-13-inch (22.5-x-32.5-cm) baking pan.

2 Mix together the sugar or Splenda, oil, and eggs in a medium-sized bowl with an electric mixer, whisk, or spatula.

3 Combine the remaining ingredients, except the carrots, in another medium-sized bowl with a spatula or wooden spoon. Add this mixture to the first bowl and blend well. Add the carrots and mix thoroughly.

4 Pour the batter into the baking pan and bake for 20 to 30 minutes if using sugar or 15 to 25 minutes if using Splenda. When the cake is ready, a toothpick inserted in the centre of the cake will come out dry.

5 To prepare the icing, mix together the ingredients in a medium-sized bowl using an electric beater or spatula until smooth. After the cake has cooled, evenly spread the icing over the cake. Serve and enjoy.

Per Serving *(with sugar): (3 x 2½ inches/7.5 x 6.25 cm, 66 g) Calories 250; Available carbohydrate 25 g; Carbohydrate 26 g; Fibre 1 g; Fat 15 g; Protein 4 g; Cholesterol 51 mg; Phosphorus 67 mg; Potassium 108 mg; Sodium 265 mg.*

1 Serving = 1½ Carbohydrate Choices

Per Serving *(with Splenda): (3 x 2½ inches/7.5 x 6.25 cm, 55 g) Calories 221; Available carbohydrate 17 g; Carbohydrate 18 g; Fibre 1 g, Fat 15 g; Protein 5 g; Cholesterol 51 mg; Phosphorus 81 mg; Potassium 134 mg; Sodium 301 mg.*

1 Serving = 1 Carbohydrate Choice

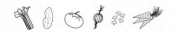

○ Fruit Trifle

This recipe is so simple, but the end result is elegant and delicious.

Preparation Time: *15 minutes*

Yield: *4 servings*

2 cups (500 ml) angel food cake, cut into cubes

2 cups (500 ml) fresh fruit, chopped

1 cup (250 ml) sugar-free, fat-free vanilla yogurt

In the first of four parfait glasses or bowls, layer 2 tbsp (30 ml) of cubed cake, 2 tbsp (30 ml) of fresh fruit, and 2 tablespoons (30 ml) of yogurt. Repeat twice per glass. Serve and enjoy.

Per Serving: (176 g) Calories 100; Available carbohydrate 19 g; Carbohydrate 21 g; Fibre 2 g; Fat 0 g; Protein 4 g; Cholesterol 1 mg; Phosphorus 116 mg; Potassium 223 mg; Sodium 116 mg. (The phosphorus and potassium will vary depending on the type of fruit used.)

1 Serving = 1 Carbohydrate Choice

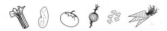

Fruit counts as dessert!

Cynthia is always surprised when people tell her they never eat dessert only to then acknowledge, when asked, that they regularly eat fruit after a meal. Many people simply don't think of fruit as a dessert. As it turns out, however, fruit has all the traits of any good dessert: It is both sweet and satisfying. Fruit contains sugar and can, therefore, raise your blood glucose, but eaten in moderation it's a perfectly acceptable component of a healthy diabetes eating plan and is also an integral part of *Eating Well with Canada's Food Guide.* (Other benefits of fruit are its abundance of vitamins, minerals, and, especially when the skin is consumed, fibre.)

If you're eating canned fruit, be sure to choose canned fruit that has no added sugar or that is packed in its own juice.

Pudding on the Ritz

In the U.K., they call just about every dessert "pudding." In this book, however, when we refer to pudding, we're talking about the delicious, sweet treat in a bowl that you know and love. With a few exceptions, pudding is a great choice when you're looking for a quick weekday dessert.

ᗝ Orange Frost

This dessert is very light — a good choice after a big meal.

Preparation Time: 15 minutes (plus 2 hours in the freezer)

Yield: 6 servings

1 egg, separated

⅓ cup (75 ml) water

⅓ cup (75 ml) skim milk powder

4 tbsp (60 ml) sugar

1½ tsp (7 ml) orange rind

4 tbsp (60 ml) orange juice

Dash of salt

4 tbsp (60 ml) graham cracker crumbs, plus 1 tbsp (15 ml) for dusting

1 In a small bowl, combine the egg white, water, and milk powder with an electric beater or whisk. Beat until stiff peaks form, about 3 minutes.

2 In a medium-sized bowl, lightly beat the egg yolk then add the sugar, orange rind, orange juice, and salt. Fold this mixture into the egg white mixture with a spatula.

3 Place 2 teaspoons (10 ml) of the graham crumbs into the bottom of a small dessert dish. Repeat with the other 5 dishes. Divide the orange mixture evenly between the 6 bowls and dust each bowl with ½ teaspoon (2 ml) graham crumbs.

4 Freeze until firm, about 2 hours. Serve chilled.

Per Serving: (½ cup/125 ml, 46 g) Calories 85; Available carbohydrate 17 g; Carbohydrate 17 g; Fibre 0 g; Fat 1 g; Protein 1 g; Cholesterol 35 mg; Phosphorus 22 mg; Potassium 38 mg; Sodium 66 mg.

1 Serving = 1 Carbohydrate Choice

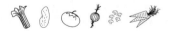

Strawberry Dream

This easy mousselike dessert is light and low in calories, too!

Preparation Time: *15 minutes (plus 1 hour to refrigerate)*

Yield: *6 servings*

½ cup (125 ml) package light strawberry Jell-O

½ cup (125 ml) boiling water

½ cup (125 ml) very cold water

8 oz (250 g) light cream cheese, softened

1 tsp (5 ml) vanilla

2 cups (500 ml) fat-free whipped topping, thawed

1 cup (250 ml) strawberries, sliced

1 cup (250 ml) blueberries

1 Add the Jell-O powder to a small bowl and add the boiling water. Stir with a fork or whisk for 2 minutes until the powder is completely dissolved.

2 Add the cold water to the Jell-O and stir until well mixed.

3 In a large bowl, use an electric mixer or a spatula to beat the cream cheese and vanilla until smooth.

4 Slowly add the Jell-O to the cream cheese mixture. Beat with an electric mixer, fork, or whisk until well blended. Gently stir in the whipped topping and fruit, reserving 12 slices of strawberries to place on top of the mousse.

5 Divide ⅔ cup (150 ml) of the mixture between 6 small dessert dishes or parfait glasses. Top each dish with 2 sliced strawberries. Refrigerate for 1 hour, until the mixture is firm. Serve.

Per Serving: *(⅔ cup/150 ml, 164 g) Calories 148; Available carbohydrate 14 g; Carbohydrate 15 g; Fibre 1 g; Fat 1 g; Protein 5 g; Cholesterol 26 mg; Phosphorus 110 mg; Potassium 188 mg; Sodium 245 mg.*

1 Serving = 1 Carbohydrate Choice

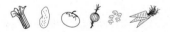

⌒ *Aboriginal Wild Rice Pudding*

This Aboriginal recipe was adapted from Audrey Smoke, an elder at the Alderville First Nations Reserve where Cynthia works. Every time there is a community function, you can be sure everyone will be there if Audrey brings her rice pudding!

Preparation Time: *12 minutes*

Cooking Time: *90 minutes*

Yield: *6 servings*

½ cup (125 ml) wild rice	*½ cup (125 ml) low-fat evaporated milk*
Dash salt	*½ tsp (2 ml) vanilla*
1 cup (250 ml) water	*¼ cup (50 ml) sugar or Splenda*
2 eggs, beaten	*¼ cup (50 ml) raisins*
1½ cups (375 ml) 1% milk	

1 Place the wild rice in a strainer and rinse with cool water until the water runs clear. Drain.

2 Add the rice, salt, and water to a medium-sized saucepan with a tight-fitting lid. Bring to a boil over high heat. Reduce the heat to low and let the rice simmer with the lid on for 1 hour.

3 When the rice is done, preheat the oven to 400 degrees Fahrenheit (200 degrees Celsius).

4 In a large bowl, thoroughly mix together the remaining ingredients using a spatula or spoon. Add the rice and stir. Place the entire mixture into a 2-quart (2.5-litre) glass casserole dish. Cover and bake at 400 degrees (200 degrees Celsius) for 15 minutes.

5 Reduce the heat to 300 degrees Fahrenheit (150 degrees Celsius) and bake for another 15 minutes. Serve warm.

Per Serving *(with sugar): (½ cup/125 ml, 145 g) Calories 167; Available carbohydrate 28 g; Carbohydrate 29 g; Fibre 1 g; Fat 2 g; Protein 8 g; Cholesterol 74 mg; Phosphorus 196 mg; Potassium 294 mg; Sodium 103 mg.*

1 Serving = 2 Carbohydrate Choices

Per Serving *(with Splenda): (½ cup/125 ml, 106 g) Calories 139; Available carbohydrate 21 g; Carbohydrate 22 g; Fibre 1 g; Fat 2 g; Protein 8 g; Cholesterol 74 mg; Phosphorus 196 mg; Potassium 294 mg; Sodium 103 mg.*

1 Serving = 1 Carbohydrate Choice

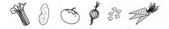

✿ Luscious Lemon Pudding Cake

The lemon flavour in this dish makes it a refreshing end to a meal or a lovely snack with afternoon tea.

Preparation Time: *30 minutes*

Cooking Time: *25 to 30 minutes with sugar/20 to 25 minutes with Splenda*

Yield: *9 servings*

4 eggs, separated

Dash of salt

½ cup (125 ml) sugar or Splenda

¼ cup (50 ml) soft margarine

2 tbsp (30 ml) lemon rind

⅓ cup (75 ml) flour

1 cup (250 ml) 1% milk

½ cup (125 ml) lemon juice

¼ cup (50 ml) skim milk powder, if using Splenda

¼ tsp (1 ml) baking soda, if using Splenda

1 tsp (5 ml) icing sugar, for dusting

1 Preheat the oven to 350 degrees Fahrenheit (175 degrees Celsius). Lightly grease an 8-x-8-inch (20-x-20-cm) baking dish.

2 In a small bowl, beat the egg whites and salt with an electric beater or whisk until they become light. Gradually add 2 tablespoons (30 ml) of sugar or Splenda and continue beating until firm peaks form. Set aside.

3 In a medium-sized bowl, using clean beaters, cream the margarine with the rest of the sugar or Splenda. Add the egg yolks and lemon rind. Gently stir in the flour (and skim milk powder and baking soda, if using Splenda) until mixed. Add the milk and lemon juice to the batter.

4 Gently fold the egg whites into the batter. Spoon the batter evenly into the baking dish.

5 Place the baking dish in a larger baking dish — for example, a 9-x-13-inch (22.5-x-32.5-cm) dish. Fill the larger baking dish with enough water to come halfway up the sides of the smaller baking dish. Place the dishes in the oven and bake for 20 to 30 minutes, until the cake is lightly brown on top. The bottom layer of the cake will resemble a saucelike mixture.

6 Remove the pudding cake from the oven and let it cool. Dust the cake with 1 teaspoon (5 ml) of icing sugar just before serving. Serve warm or cold.

Per Serving: *(with sugar) (2½-x-2½ inch/6.25-x-6.25 cm slice, 92 g) Calories 153; Available carbohydrate 18 g; Carbohydrate 18 g; Fibre 0 g; Fat 8 g; Protein 4 g; Cholesterol 95 mg; Phosphorus 74 mg; Potassium 92 mg; Sodium 105 mg.*

1 Serving = 1 Carbohydrate Choice

Per Serving: (with Splenda) (2½-x-2½-inch/6.25-x-6.25 cm slice, 67 g) Calories 121; Available carbohydrate 9 g; Carbohydrate 9 g; Fibre 0 g; Fat 8 g; Protein 5 g; Cholesterol 96 mg; Phosphorus 93 mg; Potassium 124 mg; Sodium 150 mg.

1 Serving = ½ Carbohydrate Choice

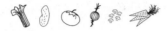

⟲ Baked Custard

This is an old favourite comfort food, great as a dessert or a snack when you're not feeling well.

Preparation Time: *10 minutes*

Cooking Time: *25 to 35 minutes*

Yield: *2 servings*

1 egg, lightly beaten	¾ cup (175 ml) 1% milk
½ tsp (2 ml) vanilla	Pinch of nutmeg
1 tsp (5 ml) sugar	Hot water

1 Preheat the oven to 350 degrees Fahrenheit (175 degrees Celsius).

2 In a small bowl, mix together all the ingredients except the nutmeg and hot water. Divide the mixture equally between two 6-ounce (175-ml) oven-safe custard cups. Sprinkle each with nutmeg.

3 Place the custard cups in a larger baking dish and fill the larger baking dish with enough hot water to come halfway up the sides of the custard cups. Bake for 25 to 35 minutes, until a knife inserted in the centre of the custard comes out clean.

4 Serve warm or cold.

Per Serving: (½ cup/125 ml, 99 g) Calories 86; Available carbohydrate 7 g; Carbohydrate 7 g; Fibre 0 g; Fat 3 g; Protein 6 g; Cholesterol 110 mg; Phosphorus 135 mg; Potassium 173 mg; Sodium 75 mg.

1 Serving = ½ Carbohydrate Choice

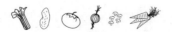

Bite-Sized Fun: Cookies

Cookies are a great, portable dessert, and small cookies can offer a perfectly sized tiny treat when you're not looking for anything more. They're also a great addition to a child's lunch.

☙ Jam Jewel Cookies

These cookie are like shortbread thumbprint cookies with a delightful jam jewel on top. They are lovely even without the diet jam.

Preparation Time: *20 minutes*

Cooking Time: *9 to 10 minutes*

Yield: *28 cookies*

½ cup (125 ml) soft margarine	2 tsp (10 ml) lemon juice
¼ cup (50 ml) sugar	1 cup (250 ml) flour
1 egg yolk, beaten	⅓ cup (75 ml) diet jam

1 Preheat the oven to 350 degrees Fahrenheit (175 degrees Celsius).

2 In a medium-sized bowl, cream the margarine and sugar with an electric beater or spatula until the mixture becomes light and fluffy. Add the egg yolk and lemon juice and continue to mix. Add the flour and stir until well blended.

3 Shape the dough into 1-inch (2.5-cm) balls and place them on a baking sheet. Using your thumb, press a small indent in the centre of each ball to hold the diet jam.

4 Bake for 9 to 10 minutes until the cookies are lightly brown at the edges.

5 Remove the cookies from the oven and allow them to cool. Add ½ teaspoon (2 ml) of diet jam to the top of each cookie. Serve.

Per Serving: *(2 cookies, 20 g) Calories 116; Available carbohydrate 13 g; Carbohydrate 13 g; Fibre 0 g; Fat 7 g; Protein 1 g; Cholesterol 15 mg; Phosphorus 15 mg; Potassium 16 mg; Sodium 58 mg.*

1 Serving = 1 Carbohydrate Choice

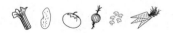

♻ Chocolate Chip Cookies

Everyone needs a chocolate chip cookie once in a while. These will hit the spot despite the low sugar content.

Preparation Time: *30 minutes*

Cooking Time: *7 to 8 minutes*

Yield: *36 cookies*

½ cup (125 ml) soft margarine	½ tsp (2 ml) baking soda
½ cup (125 ml) brown sugar, lightly packed	¼ tsp (1 ml) salt
1 egg, beaten	1 cup (250 ml) rolled oats
1 tsp (5 ml) vanilla	½ cup (125 ml) semi-sweet chocolate chips
1 cup (250 ml) flour	

1 In a medium-sized bowl, cream the margarine and sugar using an electric beater or spatula until the mixture becomes light and fluffy.

2 Add the egg and vanilla to the bowl and mix well.

3 In another bowl, combine the flour, baking soda, and salt. Add this mixture to the first bowl and stir thoroughly.

4 Fold in the oats and chocolate chips with a spatula.

5 Take 1 tablespoon (15 ml) of dough, roll into a ball, and place onto a baking sheet. Flatten each ball with a fork.

6 Bake for 7 to 8 minutes, until the cookies begin to brown around the edges.

7 Allow the cookies to cool on a wire rack. Serve.

Per Serving: *(2 cookies, 28 g) Calories 130; Available carbohydrate 14 g; Carbohydrate 15 g; Fibre 1 g; Fat 7 g; Protein 2 g; Cholesterol 12 mg; Phosphorus 38 mg; Potassium 50 mg; Sodium 118 mg.*

1 Serving = 1 Carbohydrate Choice

⌀ Rocky Road Balls

This is a no-bake dessert that's fun for kids!

Preparation Time: *30 minutes (plus 60 minutes to chill)*

Cooking Time: *3 minutes (plus 60 minutes to harden)*

Yield: *36 balls*

¾ cup (175 ml) semi-sweet chocolate chips	1½ cups (375 ml) puffed wheat cereal
¾ cup (175 ml) milk chocolate chips	½ cup (125 ml) mini coloured marshmallows
½ package (125 g) light cream cheese, softened	¾ cup (175 ml) shredded sweetened coconut

1 Place the chocolate chips and cream cheese in a small saucepan and set over low heat. Stir constantly for about 3 minutes or until the ingredients have melted. Remove from heat.

2 Add the cereal and marshmallows to the saucepan and stir until they are evenly mixed. Place the saucepan in the refrigerator to chill for about 1 hour.

3 Wash your hands and lightly coat them in canola oil. Using your hands, roll 1 tablespoon (15 ml) of dough into a ball. Continue until no dough is left.

4 Cover the bottom of a flat plate with the shredded coconut. Roll each ball in the coconut until it is lightly coated.

5 Place the balls in a sealed container lined with waxed paper and let them harden in the refrigerator for an hour. Serve and enjoy.

Per Serving: (3 balls, 39 g) Calories 164; Available carbohydrate 17 g; Carbohydrate 19 g; Fibre 2 g; Fat 10 g; Protein 2 g; Cholesterol 6 mg; Phosphorus 54 mg; Potassium 118 mg; Sodium 49 mg.

1 Serving = 1 Carbohydrate Choice

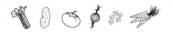

✎ Flax Cookies

These cookies taste so good you'd never know they're healthy for you! Ground flaxseed is a great source of omega-3 fatty acids.

Preparation Time: *25 minutes*

Cooking Time: *5 to 7 minutes*

Yield: *36 cookies*

½ cup (125 ml) soft margarine

½ cup (125 ml) brown sugar

1 egg

1 tsp (5 ml) vanilla

1¼ cups (300 ml) flour

1 tsp (5 ml) baking soda

⅛ tsp (0.5 ml) salt

¾ cup (175 ml) ground flaxseed

1 cup (250 ml) rolled oats

½ cup (125 ml) lightly crushed flaxseed (for appearance)

1 Preheat the oven to 350 degrees Fahrenheit (175 degrees Celsius). Line a cookie sheet with parchment paper.

2 In a large bowl, cream the margarine and sugar with an electric beater or spatula until it becomes light in consistency. Add the egg, then the vanilla. Mix well.

3 In a medium-sized bowl, combine the flour, baking soda, salt, and ground flaxseed. Add this mixture to the large bowl.

4 Stir in the rolled oats and the lightly crushed flaxseed. Mix well.

5 Roll 1 tbsp (15 ml) of the dough into a ball. Continue until no dough is left. Place the balls on the parchment-lined baking sheet. Flatten the cookies with a fork, so they are only ¼ inch (0.6 cm) thick.

6 Bake for 5 to 7 minutes, until the cookies are lightly golden. Remove the cookies from the oven and allow them to cool on a wire rack. Serve.

Per Serving: *(2 cookies, 26 g) Calories 176; Available carbohydrate 16 g; Carbohydrate 19 g; Fibre 3 g; Fat 10 g; Protein 4 g; Cholesterol 12 mg; Phosphorus 98 mg; Potassium 120 mg; Sodium 140 mg.*

1 Serving = 1 Carbohydrate Choice

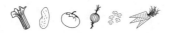

♻ Cocoa Oatmeal Cookies

The batter for these cookies may seem too runny at first, but the oats and cocoa will absorb the extra moisture.

Preparation Time: *25 minutes*

Cooking Time: *9 to 11 minutes with sugar/7 minutes with Splenda*

Yield: *75 cookies with sugar/80 cookies with Splenda*

1½ cups (375 ml) sugar or Splenda

½ cup (125 ml) soft margarine

½ cup (125 ml) low-fat plain yogurt

¼ cup (50 ml) water

1 tsp (5 ml) vanilla

1 egg, beaten

3 cups (750 ml) rolled oats

1¼ cups (300 ml) flour

⅓ cup (75 ml) cocoa powder

½ tsp (2 ml) baking soda or 1¼ tsp (6 ml), if using Splenda

¼ tsp (1 ml) salt

¾ cup (175 ml) skim milk powder, if using Splenda

1 Preheat the oven to 350 degrees Fahrenheit (175 degrees Celsius).

2 In a large bowl, mix together the sugar or Splenda, margarine, yogurt, water, vanilla, and egg with an electric beater or spatula. Stir in the remaining ingredients and mix well.

3 With clean hands, roll the batter into 1-inch (2.5-cm) balls. Place the balls on the baking sheet 2 inches (5 cm) apart.

4 Bake the cookies for 9 to 11 minutes if you made them with sugar, 7 minutes if you used Splenda, or until they feel firm. Remove the cookies from the baking sheet and allow them to cool on a wire rack. Serve.

Per Serving (with sugar): (2 cookies, 28 g) Calories 100; Available carbohydrate 16 g; Carbohydrate 17 g; Fibre 1 g; Fat 3 g; Protein 2 g; Cholesterol 6 mg; Phosphorus 44 mg; Potassium 50 mg; Sodium 59 mg.

1 Serving = 1 Carbohydrate Choice

Per Serving (with Splenda): (4 cookies, 44 g) Calories: 139; Available carbohydrate 16 g; Carbohydrate 18 g; Fibre 2 g; Fat 6 g; Protein 4 g; Cholesterol 11 mg; Phosphorus 107 mg; Potassium 135 mg; Sodium 171 mg.

1 Serving = 1 Carbohydrate Choice

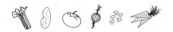

Snickers

These cookies are soft and chewy, and no, they aren't made with Snickers bars!

Preparation Time: *20 minutes*

Cooking Time: *6 to 7 minutes*

Yield: *42 cookies*

½ cup (125 ml) sugar or Splenda	1 tsp (5 ml) cinnamon
½ cup (125 ml) soft margarine	⅛ tsp (0.5 ml) salt
1 egg	½ cup (125 ml) raisins
1 tsp (5 ml) vanilla	½ cup (125 ml) dried cranberries
¾ cup (175 ml) all-purpose flour	**Topping:**
¾ cup (175 ml) whole wheat flour	2 tsp (10 ml) sugar or Splenda
¾ tsp (4 ml) baking soda	¼ tsp (1 ml) cinnamon

1 Preheat the oven to 400 degrees Fahrenheit (200 degrees Celsius).

2 In a large bowl, cream the sugar or Splenda and margarine with a spatula or an electric beater on medium speed. Add the egg and vanilla and beat until combined.

3 In a medium bowl, stir together the flours, baking soda, cinnamon, and salt with a spatula. Add this to the creamed mixture and mix well. Stir in the raisins and cranberries.

4 Roll the dough into 1-inch (2.5-cm) balls and place them on a baking sheet. Flatten the balls with a fork until each is about ½ inch (1.25 cm) thick.

5 In a small bowl, mix together the sugar or Splenda and cinnamon to make the topping. Sprinkle over the cookies and bake for 6 to 7 minutes or until the cookies are lightly browned at the edges.

6 Transfer the cookies to a wire rack to cool. Serve.

Per Serving *(with sugar): (2 cookies, 31 g) Calories 112; Available carbohydrate 16 g; Carbohydrate 17 g; Fibre 1 g; Fat 5 g; Protein 1 g; Cholesterol 10 mg; Phosphorus 28 mg; Potassium 53 mg; Sodium 101 mg.*

1 Serving = 1 Carbohydrate Choice

Per Serving *(with Splenda): (2 cookies, 25 g) Calories: 95; Available carbohydrate 11 g; Carbohydrate 12 g; Fibre 1 g; Fat 5 g; Protein 1 g; Cholesterol 10 mg; Phosphorus 28 mg; Potassium 53 mg; Sodium 101 mg.*

1 Serving = ½ Carbohydrate Choice

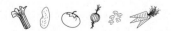

Chapter 18

Kooking for Kids

In This Chapter

▶ Bringing kids into the kitchen

▶ Cooking kid-friendly dinners

▶ Making desserts they'll love

Having a child with diabetes makes establishing and maintaining healthy eating practices especially important. Healthy nutrition is a mainstay of managing diabetes in all people, especially youngsters because their bodies are constantly growing and developing (as are your food bills!). Fortunately, healthy eating for children doesn't require any sacrifice in taste, food appeal, or simple food fun.

In this chapter, we present recipes that kids will love. Kids can also be involved in many aspects of preparing these recipes.

Kids in the Kitchen

If you or your child has diabetes, involve your age-appropriate child in the kitchen activities. It will be a great opportunity for you to teach your child about healthy eating, it'll provide him or her invaluable life skills, and it'll also be fun for the two of you.

Getting kids excited about healthy eating, food selection, and meal preparation will give them a sense of pride and ownership in the food they prepare and can lead to lifelong healthy eating habits.

Kids need to be encouraged to find variety in foods. Developing a wide repertoire of preferred foods to choose from creates a more interesting diet — a diet that supports growth and development and maintains optimal nutritional status.

You can foster your child's interest in kitchen activities in a number of ways:

✔ Ask your child to choose a favourite food from each of the four food groups of *Eating Well with Canada's Food Guide* (www.hc-sc.gc.ca/ fn-an/food-guide-aliment/index-eng.php). Using his or her picks, work as a team to create fun and interesting meals or snacks.

✔ Prepare foods that will foster your child's interest in helping out. Work together in making kid-friendly foods such as sandwiches, fajitas, pizza, and fruit kabobs.

✔ Ask your child to set the table using special child-friendly themed plates, cups, and even personalized cutlery.

✔ Have your child sweep the floor after a meal.

✔ Have your young child

• Decide what cereal to place on the table for breakfast and which vegetable to eat for dinner

• Gather recipe ingredients from the refrigerator and pantry

✔ Have your older child

• Measure ingredients

• Do some chopping

• Help plan a lunch or dinner and make up a shopping list

Always give age-appropriate tasks. Supervise children in the kitchen, especially around the stove, food processors, knives, and hot water. Teach food safety rules from an early age, including proper hand washing, cleaning fruits and vegetables, and post-meal cleanup.

Super Suppers

This is a selection of time-tested diabetes-friendly, supper favourites for kids, tweaked to ensure they are suitably nutritious. Kids don't need to know that, though . . .

Pizza Faces

This is a quick and easy dinner to make with kids in the kitchen. Kids can top their pizzas to their own tastes *and* show off their artistic abilities! This recipe makes one child-sized serving.

Preparation Time: *10 minutes*

Cooking Time: *2 to 3 minutes*

Yield: *1 serving*

½ whole wheat English muffin

2 tsp (10 ml) pizza sauce

2 tbsp (30 ml) low-fat mozzarella, shredded

1 tbsp (15 ml) low-fat ham, diced

1 tbsp (15 ml) vegetables of your choice

1 Move the oven rack to the highest setting. Turn on the broiler element.

2 Place half of the English muffin on a baking sheet. Use a spoon to evenly spread pizza sauce over the English muffin. Top with the mozzarella, ham, and mixed vegetables (in that order).

3 Place the baking sheet under the broiler for 2 to 3 minutes, until the cheese has melted and the muffin is warm. Serve.

Per Serving: *(½ English muffin, 79 g) Calories 127; Available carbohydrate 11 g; Carbohydrate 14 g; Fibre 3 g; Fat 4 g; Protein 9 g; Cholesterol 13 mg; Phosphorus 176 mg; Potassium 175 mg; Sodium 248 mg.*

1 Serving = ½ Carbohydrate Choice

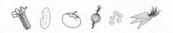

Sloppy Joes

Sloppy Joes are a family-friendly dish, but make sure to have napkins handy.

Preparation Time: *15 minutes*

Cooking Time: *15 minutes*

Yield: *7 servings*

1 lb (450 g) extra lean hamburger	*⅔ cup (150 ml) ketchup*
½ cup (125 ml) yellow onion, chopped	*¼ cup (50 ml) water*
⅔ cup (150 ml) mushrooms, sliced	*1 tbsp (15 ml) Worcestershire sauce*
⅓ cup (75 ml) celery, chopped	*½ tsp (2 ml) salt*
⅓ cup (75 ml) green pepper, chopped	*7 whole wheat hamburger buns*

1 In a large frying pan, brown the hamburger and onion over medium-high heat for 5 minutes, stirring frequently with a spatula or wooden spoon. Drain the fat from the meat.

2 Stir in the remaining ingredients, except the buns. Cover and simmer over low heat until the vegetables are tender, about 10 minutes.

3 Spoon ½ cup (125 ml) of the mixture over each bun. Serve and enjoy.

Per Serving: *(½ cup/125 ml meat, 115 g) Calories 146; Available carbohydrate 8 g; Carbohydrate 8 g; Fibre 0 g; Fat 7 g; Protein 14 g; Cholesterol 42 mg; Phosphorus 140 mg; Potassium 379 mg; Sodium 491 mg.*

1 Serving = ½ Carbohydrate Choice + 2 Carbohydrate Choices for the hamburger bun

Breaded Chicken Fingers

These baked chicken fingers are a healthy alternative to the fried version, and easy to clean up too. The breading is made with whole wheat bread crumbs, ground flaxseed, and wheat germ, so it's a source of fibre. The chicken fingers can be frozen for up to 2 weeks.

Preparation Time: *15 minutes*

Cooking Time: *16 to 20 minutes*

Yield: *4 servings*

Sauce (see the following recipe)

1 lb (450 g) skinless, boneless chicken breasts

4 tbsp (60 ml) low-fat plain yogurt

¼ cup (50 ml) whole wheat bread crumbs

⅛ cup (25 ml) ground flaxseed

⅛ cup (25 ml) wheat germ

½ tsp (2 ml) thyme

½ tsp (2 ml) marjoram

¼ tsp (1 ml) garlic powder

⅛ tsp (0.5 ml) salt

1 Preheat the oven to 400 degrees Fahrenheit (200 degrees Celsius). Line a baking sheet with parchment paper. (Lining the baking sheet with parchment paper makes for fast cleanup).

2 Trim the visible fat from the chicken and slice it into even strips, each about ¾ to 1 inch (2 to 2.5 cm) wide.

3 Place the yogurt in a small flat-bottomed bowl. Set aside.

4 In another flat-bottomed small bowl combine the rest of the chicken strip ingredients and mix well with a spoon.

5 Dip each strip of chicken into the yogurt to coat it, then dip the chicken in the bread crumb mixture until all sides are coated evenly. Place the strips on the baking sheet.

6 Bake for 8 to 10 minutes per side until the chicken is golden brown and no pink appears.

7 While the chicken is cooking, prepare the sauce.

8 Serve the chicken strips plain or with the dipping sauce.

Per Serving: *(3 chicken strips, 140 g) Calories 196; Available Carbohydrate 7 g; Carbohydrate 9 g; Fibre 2 g; Fat 4 g; Protein 29 g; Cholesterol 65 mg; Phosphorus 305 mg; Potassium 381 mg; Sodium 210 mg.*

1 Serving = ½ Carbohydrate Choice

Sauce

½ cup (125 ml) low-fat plain yogurt

2 tbsp (30 ml) ketchup

1 tsp (5 ml) celery seed

2 tsp (10 ml) reduced-sodium soy sauce

½ tsp (2 ml) garlic powder

¼ tsp (1 ml) pepper

Mix all the ingredients together in a small bowl.

Per Serving: *(2 tbsp/30 ml sauce) Calories 31; Available carbohydrate 5 g; Carbohydrate 5 g; Fibre 0 g; Fat 1 g; Protein 2 g; Cholesterol 2 mg; Phosphorus 54 mg; Potassium 118 mg; Sodium 194 mg.*

1 Serving = 0 Carbohydrate Choice

🍅 Macaroni and Cheese

It's difficult to find tasty low-fat mac and cheese, but here's one Cynthia invented that she hopes you'll enjoy.

Preparation Time: *25 minutes*

Cooking Time: *30 minutes*

Yield: *6 servings*

6 cups (1,500 ml) water

2½ cups (625 ml) dry, whole wheat macaroni noodles

¼ cup (50 ml) soft margarine

½ cup (125 ml) yellow onion, finely chopped

½ tsp (2 ml) salt

¾ tsp (4 ml) paprika

¾ tsp (4 ml) dry mustard

⅛ tsp (0.5 ml) pepper

¼ cup (50 ml) whole wheat flour

1 cup (250 ml) 1% milk

2 cups (500 ml) low-fat old cheddar cheese, grated

¼ cup (50 ml) low-fat parmesan cheese

1 Preheat the oven to 350 degrees Fahrenheit (175 degrees Celsius).

2 Place the water in a large pot and bring to a boil over high heat. Add the macaroni to the boiling water and cook until the noodles are tender, about 8 minutes. Drain the water from the macaroni using a strainer.

3 In a large frying pan, melt the margarine over medium-high heat. Add the onion, salt, paprika, mustard, pepper, and flour. Stir-fry with a spatula or wooden spoon for 3 minutes.

4 Reduce heat to medium and slowly add the milk, while continuing to stir. The ingredients should start to thicken. While continuing to stir, gradually add the cheeses. When all the cheese has been added and the sauce has thickened, combine it with the macaroni and mix well.

5 Pour the macaroni mixture into a large casserole dish. Bake for 20 minutes until the sauce starts to bubble. Serve.

Per Serving: *(¾ cup/175 ml, 161g) Calories 338; Available Carbohydrate 36 g; Carbohydrate 41g; Fibre 5g; Fat 12 g; Protein 19 g; Cholesterol 14 mg; Phosphorus 389 mg; Potassium 236 mg; Sodium 584 mg.*

1 Serving = 2 Carbohydrate Choices

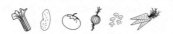

Desserts Kids Dig

Kids love dessert. (Hmm, so do most adults now that we think about it.) Although no food — including dessert foods — is forbidden just because you have diabetes, certain desserts do fit better into overall diabetes nutrition plans than others. In this section, we offer some diabetes-friendly dessert recipes for kids.

The more you restrict sweets from a child, the more powerfully the child may crave them. (You know, forbidden fruit and all that.) Although you may be able to control your children's eating when they are very young and under your constant supervision, eventually they will become more autonomous and will be spending time away from you at school, at camp, at a friend's house, and so forth. Providing occasional desserts and sweets as a treat at home will make your children more likely to be careful about how many sweets they eat in other settings.

☞ Baked Apple with Raspberries

This is a snap to prepare, but it can take a long time to cook in an oven. Using a microwave is much faster. This recipe tastes so great you won't believe it has no added sugar!

Preparation Time: 5 minutes

Cooking Time: 4 to 5 minutes (depending on size of apple)

Yield: 2 servings

2 large apples (Granny Smith, Cortland, Golden   ¼ cup (50 ml) raspberries, fresh or frozen
Delicious, or Empire)

1 Using a sharp knife, cut off the top ½ inch (1.25 cm) of each apple and remove the core.

2 Firmly press the raspberries into the hole where the core was.

3 Place the apples into a microwave/oven safe dish. Add 2 tablespoons (30 ml) of water to the bottom of dish.

4 Microwave on high for 4 to 5 minutes or until the pulp of the apples is soft. If you don't have a microwave, preheat your oven to 375 degrees Fahrenheit (190 degrees Celsius). Place the dish in the oven and bake for 30 to 40 minutes, until the pulp of the apples is soft.

5 Spoon the raspberries and sauce back into the apples. (Some of the fruit and juices may have escaped when heated.) Let the apples cool slightly and serve warm.

Per Serving: (1 apple, 176 g) Calories 118; Available carbohydrate 25 g; Carbohydrate 31 g; Fibre 6 g; Fat 0 g; Protein 1 g; Cholesterol 0 mg; Phosphorus 28 mg; Potassium 250 mg; Sodium 2 mg.

1 Serving = 1½ Carbohydrate Choices

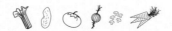

🍎 Apple Crisp

Here's an all-time favourite. The best baking apples are both sweet and tart. Cynthia suggests using Cortland, Empire, Golden Delicious, or Granny Smith apples.

Preparation Time: *30 minutes*

Cooking Time: *30 to 35 minutes*

Yield: *9 servings*

5 cups (1,250 ml) baking apples, peeled and sliced

1 tsp (5 ml) lemon juice

1 tsp (5 ml) cinnamon

1 tbsp (15 ml) white sugar or Splenda

Topping:

⅔ cup (150 ml) whole wheat flour

¼ cup (50 ml) ground flaxseed

⅓ cup (75 ml) rolled oats

⅓ cup (75 ml) brown sugar or 2½ tbsp (37 ml) Brown Sugar Splenda

⅓ cup (75 ml) soft margarine

1 Preheat the oven to 375 degrees Fahrenheit (190 degrees Celsius). Lightly grease an 8-x-8-inch (20-x-20-cm) baking dish with canola oil.

2 In a large bowl, combine the apples with the lemon juice, cinnamon, and white sugar or Splenda. Spread the apples evenly over the bottom of the baking pan.

3 Combine the topping ingredients in a medium-sized bowl. Mix well with a spatula, wooden spoon, or fork.

4 Gently spoon the topping evenly over the apples.

5 Bake in the oven for 30 to 35 minutes or until the topping is golden brown and the apples are tender. Serve warm or cold.

Per Serving *(with sugar): (2½-x-2½-inch/6.25-x-6.25 cm piece, 95 g) Calories 181; Available Carbohydrate 24 g; Carbohydrate 27g; Fibre 3 g; Fat 2 g; Protein 2 g; Cholesterol 0 mg; Phosphorus 70 mg; Potassium 140 mg; Sodium 4 mg.*

1 Serving = 1½ Carbohydrate Choices

Per Serving *(with Splenda): (2½-x-2½-inch/6.25-x-6.25 cm piece, 98 g) Calories 162; Available carbohydrate 19 g; Carbohydrate 22 g; Fibre 3 g; Fat 8 g; Protein 2 g; Cholesterol 0 mg; Phosphorus 70 mg; Potassium 134 mg; Sodium 58 mg.*

1 Serving = 1 Carbohydrate Choice

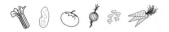

☺ *Brownies*

These brownies contain sour cream to make them extra moist. For the best results, bake them the day before they're needed. The brownies can also be frozen for up to 6 weeks.

Preparation Time: *12 minutes*

Cooking Time: *20 minutes*

Yield: *9 servings*

⅔ cup (150 ml) sugar

⅓ cup (75 ml) soft margarine

1 egg

1 tsp (5 ml) vanilla

⅓ cup (75 ml) cocoa powder

⅓ cup (75 ml) flour

1 tsp (5 ml) baking powder

¼ cup (50 ml) low-fat sour cream

3 tbsp (45 ml) walnuts, chopped

1 Preheat the oven to 350 degrees Fahrenheit (175 degrees Celsius). Lightly grease an 8-x-8-inch (20-x-20-cm) baking dish with canola oil.

2 In a medium-sized bowl, cream the sugar and margarine using an electric beater or spatula until light and fluffy, about 1 minute. Add the egg and vanilla to the bowl and mix well.

3 In another medium-sized bowl, use a spatula or wooden spoon to stir together the cocoa, flour, and baking powder. Blend in the sour cream and walnuts.

4 Add the ingredients of the second bowl to the first bowl, and mix well.

5 Pour the batter into the baking pan. Bake the brownies for 20 minutes or until a toothpick inserted into the centre comes out dry.

6 Cool the brownie on a wire rack, cut into squares, and serve.

Per Serving: *(2½-x-2½-inch/6.25-x-6.25 cm piece, 47 g) Calories 172; Available carbohydrate 20 g; Carbohydrate 21 g; Fibre 1 g; Fat 10 g; Protein 2 g; Cholesterol 26 mg; Phosphorus 63 mg; Potassium 86 mg; Sodium 123 mg.*

1 Serving = 1 Carbohydrate Choice

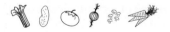

⏱ Happy Birthday Cake

This cake is nice and moist, perfect for party time. People with diabetes can have their cake and eat it too, in moderation!

Preparation Time: *12 minutes*

Cooking Time: *30 minutes with sugar/22 minutes with Splenda*

Yield: *15 servings for a 9-x-13-inch (22.5 x 32.5 cm) pan*

1½ cups (375 ml) sugar or Splenda

⅔ cup (150 ml) soft margarine

2 eggs

1½ tsp (7 ml) vanilla

2¾ cups (675 ml) flour

2½ tsp (12 ml) baking powder

1 tsp (5 ml) salt

1¼ cup (300 ml) 1% milk

¾ cup (175 ml) skim milk powder, if using Splenda

¾ tsp (4 ml) baking soda, if using Splenda

Frosting:

¾ cup (175 ml) whipping cream

1½ tbsp (22 ml) sugar or Splenda

¾ tsp (4 ml) vanilla

¾ cup (175 ml) low-fat yogurt, plain or flavoured

1 Preheat the oven to 350 degrees Fahrenheit (175 degrees Celsius). Grease and flour a 9-x-13-inch (22.5-x-32.5-centimetre) baking pan or two 8-x-8-inch (20-x-20-centimetre) pans, if you prefer to make a layer cake.

2 In a large bowl, mix together the sugar or Splenda, margarine, eggs, and vanilla with an electric mixer or whisk, until the ingredients become fluffy. Scrape the sides of the bowl often.

3 In a medium-sized bowl, mix together the flour, baking powder, and salt (if using Splenda, also add the skim milk powder and baking soda). On low speed, beat a third of the flour into the egg mixture. Mix in a third of the milk. Repeat until all the flour and milk has been added. Continue mixing until the batter is smooth.

4 Pour the batter into the cake pan(s). Bake for 30 minutes if using sugar or 22 minutes if using Splenda, or until a toothpick inserted in the centre comes out dry. Allow the cake(s) to cool, then remove from the baking pan(s) and place on a platter.

5 While the cake is cooking, prepare the frosting. Beat the whipping cream, sugar or Splenda, and vanilla together using an electric beater or whisk until peaks form in the frosting.

6 Gently fold the yogurt into the whipped cream mixture and blend until thoroughly combined.

7 If you are making a single-layer cake, evenly cover it with frosting. If you are making a layer cake, evenly spread diet jam over the top of one of the two cakes. Place the second cake on top and evenly cover the top and sides with frosting. Serve with candles. Make a wish!

Per Serving: *(with sugar-one layer cake) (3-x-2½-inch/7.5-x-6.25 cm piece, plus frosting, 68 g) Calories 300; Available carbohydrate 42 g; Carbohydrate 43 g; Fibre 1 g; Fat 12 g; Protein 5 g; Cholesterol 43 mg; Phosphorus 96 mg; Potassium 100 mg; Sodium 333 mg.*

1 Serving = 3 Carbohydrate Choices

Per Serving: *(with Splenda-one layer cake) (3-x-2½-inch/7.5-x-6.25 cm piece, plus frosting, 70 g) Calories 238; Available carbohydrate 25 g; Carbohydrate 26 g; Fibre 1 g; Fat 12 g; Protein 6 g; Cholesterol 44 mg; Phosphorus 129 mg; Potassium 158 mg; Sodium 415 mg.*

1 Serving = 1½ Carbohydrate Choices

✪ Chocolate Mud Cakes

This recipe is a great way to get kids involved in the kitchen — even the name sounds fun!

Preparation Time: *15 to 20 minutes*

Cooking Time: *20 to 25 minutes*

Yield: *9 servings*

3 tbsp (45 ml) soft margarine

⅓ cup (75 ml) sugar or Splenda

1 cup (250 ml) flour

1 tsp (5 ml) baking powder

¼ tsp (1 ml) salt

½ cup (125 ml) 1% milk

2½ tbsp (37 ml) skim milk powder, if using Splenda

⅛ tsp (0.5 ml) baking soda, if using Splenda

Topping:

½ cup (125 ml) sugar or Splenda

¼ tsp (1 ml) salt

¼ cup (50 ml) cocoa powder

1 cup (250 ml) plus 1 tbsp (15 ml) boiling water

1 Preheat the oven to 350 degrees Fahrenheit (175 degrees Celsius). Lightly grease an 8-x-8-inch (20-x-20-cm) cake pan with canola oil.

2 Using an electric beater or spatula, cream the margarine and sugar or Splenda together in a medium-sized bowl.

3 In another medium-sized bowl, mix together the flour, baking powder, and salt with a spatula or fork. Add the skim milk powder and baking soda as well if using Splenda.

4 Add a third of the flour mixture and a third of the milk to the creamed margarine and sugar. Stir well and repeat until all the flour mixture and milk have been mixed into the margarine and sugar.

5 Using a spatula, evenly spread the batter over the bottom of the cake pan and set aside.

6 To make the topping, combine the ingredients in a bowl, stir well, and gently pour over the cake batter.

7 Bake for 20 to 25 minutes, until a toothpick inserted into the centre of the cake comes out clean and dry.

8 Serve warm or cold.

Per Serving (with sugar): (2½-x-2½-inch/6.25-x-6.25 cm piece, 67 g) Calories 167; Available carbohydrate 30 g; Carbohydrate 31 g; Fibre 1 g; Fat 4 g; Protein 2 g; Cholesterol 1 mg; Phosphorus 57 mg; Potassium 72 mg; Sodium 224 mg.

1 Serving = 2 Carbohydrate Choices

Per Serving (with Splenda): (2 ½-x-2½-inch/6.25-x-6.25 cm piece, 55 g) Calories 146; Available carbohydrate 25 g; Carbohydrate 26 g; Fibre 1 g; Fat 4 g; Protein 2 g; Cholesterol 1 mg; Phosphorus 58 mg; Potassium 72 mg; Sodium 231 mg.

1 Serving = 1 ½ Carbohydrate Choices

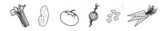

🍎 Banana Chocolate Chip Muffins

Here's a muffin the kids can still take to school — this recipe doesn't call for nuts!

Preparation Time: *12 minutes*

Cooking Time: *20 minutes with sugar/15 minutes with Splenda*

Yield: *12 muffins*

¼ cup (50 ml) 1% milk	*1 tbsp (15 ml) baking powder*
1 egg, beaten	*½ cup (125 ml) chocolate chips*
¼ cup (50 ml) canola oil	*2 tbsp (30 ml) ground flaxseed*
1 cup (250 ml) bananas, mashed	*½ tsp (2 ml) salt*
1¾ cups (425 ml) flour	*¼ cup (50 ml) skim milk powder, if using Splenda*
½ cup (125 ml) sugar or Splenda	*¼ tsp (1 ml) baking soda, if using Splenda*

1 Preheat the oven to 400 degrees Fahrenheit (200 degrees Celsius). Use canola oil to lightly grease a muffin pan or place paper liners in the cups.

2 In a medium-sized bowl, mix together the milk, egg, oil, and bananas using a spatula or wooden spoon.

3 In another medium-sized bowl, mix together the remaining ingredients.

4 Combine the contents of the two bowls and stir well. Spoon equal amounts of batter into the muffin cups.

5 Bake for 20 minutes if made with sugar and 15 minutes if made with Splenda. Remove from the oven and allow the muffins to cool on a wire rack. Serve.

Per Serving (with sugar): (1 muffin, 60 g) Calories 204; Available carbohydrate 30 g; Carbohydrate 32 g; Fibre 2 g; Fat 8 g; Protein 3 g; Cholesterol 18 mg; Phosphorus 78 mg; Potassium 135 mg; Sodium 228 mg.

1 Serving = 2 Carbohydrate Choices

Per Serving: (with Splenda) (1 muffin, 60 g) Calories 180; Available carbohydrate 23 g; Carbohydrate 25 g; Fibre 2 g; Fat 8 g; Protein 4 g; Cholesterol 18 mg; Phosphorus 92 mg; Potassium 159 mg; Sodium 262 mg.

1 Serving = 1½ Carbohydrate Choices

⏣ Little Jam Cupcakes

This cupcake recipe has been in Cynthia's family for as long as she can remember. The great thing about these cupcakes is that they don't need icing! Less fuss and mess and they taste fabulous.

Preparation Time: *20 minutes*

Cooking Time: *15 to 20 minutes with sugar/11 to 13 minutes with Splenda*

Yield: *10 cupcakes with sugar/8 cupcakes with Splenda*

2 eggs (egg whites separated from the yolks)

½ cup (125 ml) sugar or Splenda

½ tsp (2 ml) vanilla

½ tsp (2 ml) lemon juice

¾ cup (175 ml) flour

⅛ tsp (0.5 ml) salt

½ cup (125 ml) soft margarine, melted

½ cup (125 ml) diet jam

¼ cup (50 ml) skim milk powder, if using Splenda

¼ tsp (1 ml) baking soda, if using Splenda

1 Preheat the oven to 350 degrees Fahrenheit (175 degrees Celsius). Place paper liners in 10 muffin cups. (Using paper liners will reduce mess caused by the jam.)

2 In a small bowl, beat the egg whites with an electric beater or whisk until stiff peaks form, about 2 minutes. Set aside.

3 In a second small bowl, use clean beaters or a whisk to beat the egg yolks until they are thick.

4 Add the sugar or Splenda, vanilla, and lemon juice to the egg yolks. Mix well.

5 Fold the flour and salt, (and the skim milk powder and baking soda, if using Splenda) alternately with the melted margarine into the bowl with the egg yolk mixture. When the batter is smooth, fold in the egg whites as well.

6 Spoon 1 tablespoon (15 ml) of batter into each muffin cup. Add 1 teaspoon (5 ml) of diet jam and top with another 2 tablespoons (30 ml) of batter.

7 Bake for 15 to 20 minutes if using sugar or 11 to 13 minutes if using Splenda or until a toothpick inserted in the centre of the muffin comes out clean.

8 Cool on a wire rack. Serve.

Per Serving (with sugar): (1 cupcake, 44 g) Calories 184; Available carbohydrate 22 g; Carbohydrate 23 g; Fibre 1 g; Fat 10 g; Protein 2 g; Cholesterol 42 mg; Phosphorus 30 mg; Potassium 32 mg; Sodium 123 mg.

1 Serving = 1½ Carbohydrate Choices

Per Serving (with Splenda): (1 cupcake, 49 g) Calories 194; Available carbohydrate 18 g; Carbohydrate 19 g; Fibre 1 g; Fat 13 g; Protein 4 g; Cholesterol 53 mg; Phosphorus 59 mg; Potassium 76 mg; Sodium 205 mg.

1 Serving = 1 Carbohydrate Choice

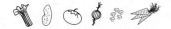

Part IV
The Part of Tens

In this part . . .

Here we offer three lists that provide you with some helpful information. We answer ten frequently asked questions about living with diabetes and set the record straight on ten diabetes nutrition myths.

Chapter 19

Ten Frequently Asked Questions

In This Chapter

▶ Finding out how diabetes affects how you eat

▶ Understanding the essentials of successful diabetes management

*O*ver the years we've been in practice, we've been asked many, many, different diabetes food-related questions. A few, however, come up much more often than others. In this chapter, we've collected the ten most frequently asked questions and provide our answers. One thing you will notice as you read our answers is that we use terms like "it depends" or "sometimes" or other such qualifiers. The reason for this isn't that we want to be evasive but, well, the answers do depend; they depend on a person's eating preferences, work, activities, medications, and so on.

Why Can't I Skip Meals to Lose Weight?

Most Canadians living with type 2 diabetes — and a significant number of Canadians living with type 1 diabetes — are overweight and are facing the challenge of how to shed extra pounds.

In Chapter 4, we discuss helpful strategies you can use to lose weight. Skipping meals isn't one of them! (Indeed we include it in our list of "Ways to sabotage your attempts at losing weight.")

In theory, skipping meals *could* help you lose weight. Since pretty well all foods and liquids (water, diet soft drinks, and the like aside) contain calories, if you skipped meals you would avoid the calories the meals would have contained and you would eventually lose weight. Well, as we say, that's the theory.

The reality is that if you skip meals you're going to feel that much hungrier as the day progresses and, if you're like most people in this situation, when your next meal comes around you'll eat more than enough to compensate for the food (and hence, calories) you deprived yourself of earlier in the day. Alternatively, as evening approaches (most often it is breakfast or lunch that is skipped) you'll repeatedly beat a path to the fridge or pantry in search of snacks until suppertime. Either way you'll end up consuming as many or possibly even more calories than if you hadn't skipped a meal in the first place.

If I Don't Eat Carbs, My Sugars Will Be Low, Right?

The term "carbs" is the short form for the word "carbohydrates." Carbohydrates, as we discuss in Chapter 2, can be loosely thought of as the wide variety of sugars you consume in your diet. Carbohydrates range from bread, rice, and pasta, to fruit and milk, to regular (non-diet) soft drinks, to sugar-rich desserts and snack foods like cakes and chocolate bars. Because carbohydrates are forms of sugar, they are the nutrients that will raise your blood glucose (your "blood sugar"). Given the preceding facts, it's probably not surprising that we are often asked "if carbs raise your blood sugar then wouldn't avoiding carbs cause low blood sugar?" To which we answer, well, yes . . . and no.

First the "no." Diabetes in and of itself does not cause low blood glucose. And if you have diabetes treated with lifestyle alone then avoiding carbohydrates will not cause you to have low blood glucose. Pure and simple.

And now the "yes." As we discuss in Chapter 1, some medications like insulin and sulfonylureas (especially glyburide) that are *used to treat diabetes* can lead to low blood glucose. Let's say, for example, its dinner time and you check your blood glucose and you find it to be 4.5 mmol/L (which is perfectly normal). You take your usual dose of rapid-acting meal-time insulin, but you then decide to deviate from your usual pattern of ingesting 100 grams of carbs as part of your dinner and on this occasion consume no carbs at all. Since your blood glucose was normal to start with and you didn't consume any carbs to raise your blood glucose yet you took insulin to reduce your blood glucose, the odds are good you'll end up developing low blood glucose (hypoglycemia).

If you take rapid-acting meal time insulin and your blood glucose levels after your meals are overly variable, this may be due to inconsistent intake of carbohydrates. An effective strategy to address this is to carbohydrate count. We discuss this strategy in detail in Chapter 1.

I'm Not Hungry for Breakfast — Do I Need It?

Most people have a pretty hectic time from the moment first thing in the morning that the alarm (be it the one that sits on the bedside table or the more mobile one with two little feet that comes running into your room) goes off until they're out the door (or have the rest of the family out the door). Given this fast pace, finding time for breakfast can be a challenge. Also, many people don't feel particularly hungry first thing in the morning.

If you find yourself with little time to eat breakfast or not much interest in eating breakfast, you might be wondering if it's okay to skip this meal altogether. Well, despite these challenges, we recommend you do indeed make a point of eating breakfast. Eating breakfast will

- Help provide you with the energy you will need to function in the morning
- Make you less hungry as the morning progresses and therefore less likely to snack excessively
- Allow you to distribute your carbohydrates over three meals (with or without snacks) per day, which will make it easier to prevent high blood glucose
- Reduce your likelihood of low blood glucose if you are taking medicines that can lead to hypoglycemia (see the FAQ that precedes this one)

Having said all this, we do recognize the realities of modern-day existence and appreciate that you may not always be able to eat breakfast. For most people, skipping the occasional breakfast will do no harm.

If you are taking insulin or sulfonylurea medication, be sure to ask your doctor what you are to do with these medicines when you are not going to be eating breakfast.

For some quick and easy breakfast ideas — which hopefully will make it less likely that you will skip breakfast — check out the Rise and Shine breakfast recipes in Chapter 7.

Do I Really Need Snacks?

For quite some time it has been considered gospel that everyone living with diabetes needs to eat snacks; typically midway between breakfast and lunch, again midway between lunch and dinner, and also at bedtime. However, many people living with diabetes simply don't desire a snack and therefore ask if it's really necessary to have one (or more).

The current Canadian Diabetes Association (CDA) Clinical Practice Guidelines have revisited the issues surrounding snacking and now advise that including snacks in a person's meal plan should be "individualized based on meal spacing, metabolic control, treatment regimen, and risk of hypoglycemia."

We are pleased with the CDA's recommendation because it recognizes that each person living with diabetes has his or her own needs and wants, and this applies to snacking also.

Factors that will influence whether or not you need to have snacks as part of your nutrition program include your

- Blood glucose control
- Meal spacing
- Diabetes medications
- Calorie requirements (and whether or not you are trying to lose weight)
- Exercise routine (including the type of exercise you do and the time you do it, as well as its duration and intensity)
- Being pregnant. If you are pregnant, because of your additional nutritional needs, snacking becomes more important.

- Risk of hypoglycemia. If you are prone to low blood glucose overnight, take a bedtime snack to reduce your risk of having hypoglycemia during the night. Also, speak to your doctor to see if your medications can be changed to help you avoid having low blood glucose overnight.

Should I Use Sugar Substitutes?

There are many different types of sugars *(carbohydrates)*, but in general when people talk about "sugar" in their diet they are not referring to the broad range of carbohydrates one consumes, but rather are specifically referring to consuming table sugar *(sucrose)*.

Because sucrose contains calories and can raise blood glucose whereas sugar substitutes (sugar alcohols, artificial sweeteners, and the natural sweetener stevia), when used in typical amounts, do not contain calories or raise blood glucose, a frequently asked question is whether a sugar substitute should be used instead of sucrose.

In general, using sugar substitutes in lieu of sucrose is reasonable when it comes to adding something sweet to coffee, tea, or cereal, choosing a soft drink, and so forth. You should, however be aware of a few caveats:

- ✔ Artificial sweeteners containing cyclamates or saccharin should not be consumed by pregnant women.

- ✔ Aspartame shouldn't be consumed if you have a medical condition called PKU.

- ✔ Artificial sweeteners are not always a suitable substitute for sugar in some baked goods.

- ✔ Sugar alcohols can cause diarrhea.

- ✔ Sugar-free foods can have just as many calories as their sugar-containing equivalent products.

Should I Check My Blood Sugar after Meals?

Most people with diabetes who test their blood glucose do so pretty well only before they eat. Before-meal testing is certainly very important, but testing one's blood glucose after meals can often provide very helpful, additional information to help you manage your diabetes.

Testing your blood glucose after meals will provide you with this additional information:

- ✔ If certain types of carbohydrates — or the way you've cooked them — are more likely than others to raise your blood glucose. (This often relates to the glycemic index of a food; see Chapter 4.)

- ✔ If a given serving size pushes your blood glucose level above target.

- ✔ For those people being treated with oral hypoglycemic agents: whether the doses or types of drugs should be changed. (Certain oral hypoglycemic agents are better than others at keeping after-meal blood glucose levels controlled.)

- ✔ For those people being treated with meal-time rapid-acting or regular insulin: whether the insulin doses need to be changed.

- ✔ For those people performing carbohydrate counting using an insulin to carbohydrate ratio (ICR) and using an insulin sensitivity factor (ISF; also called a correction factor): if these parameters need adjusting.

If your before-meal blood glucose readings are within target yet your A1C is above target, it is likely that your after-meal blood glucose readings are elevated.

Does It Matter When I Take My Meal-time Insulin?

Virtually all people with type 1 diabetes and many people with type 2 diabetes take meal-time, rapid-acting or regular insulin (see Chapter 1) in order to prevent the blood glucose levels from going up excessively after eating. A frequently asked question is when, relative to a meal, the insulin should be given.

In almost all situations (we discuss two exceptions in a moment), meal-time, rapid-acting or regular insulin should be taken *before you eat*. This way, the insulin has time to get absorbed from the injection site and make its way into your blood so it can be there at the ready to deal with the glucose molecules as they too reach the blood after being absorbed into your body from the food you eat.

Regular insulin should be injected about 30 minutes before you start to eat. The reason for this is that regular insulin takes about 30 minutes before it starts to work.

Because rapid-acting insulin acts, as the name suggests, rapidly, it can be given closer to the start of a meal than regular insulin. Taking it immediately before eating works sufficiently well for many people, but in general it is best to take rapid-acting insulin 10 to 15 minutes before eating as doing so will usually better control after-meal blood glucose levels.

In some special circumstances, rapid-acting insulin can be given *after* a meal. Here are two situations where this is sometimes done:

- ✔ **The young child whose eating is unpredictable.** As most parents of a young child know, there is no guarantee children are going to eat all the food they are given. Therefore it can be difficult to know how much meal-time insulin (the amount of which is based on the amount of carbohydrate being eaten) to give. In this situation, rapid-acting insulin is *sometimes* (that is, not routinely) administered after the child eats; this way the parent can give the dose based on what the child *actually* ate, not on what it was *anticipated* he would eat.

- ✔ **Diabetic Gastroparesis.** Gastroparesis is a condition in which the stomach is damaged from longstanding diabetes and as a result doesn't properly empty its contents into the small intestine. This delayed delivery of nutrients into the small intestine (from where nutrients are then absorbed into the body) results in a delayed — and often unpredictable — rise in blood glucose. This makes it very difficult to properly estimate how much insulin to give before a meal. One way of dealing with this is to delay giving insulin until an hour or so after eating, at which time you check your blood glucose and then give an insulin dose based on your blood glucose level.

Will I Always Need to Take Pills for My (Type 2) Diabetes?

Most people with type 2 diabetes are prescribed medication (oral hypoglycemic agents; see Chapter 1) to control their blood glucose levels. We are often asked by our patients if there is the possibility these medications can eventually be discontinued.

The quick answer to this question is, ah, well, there is no quick answer. Here's the less quick answer . . .

Not everyone with type 2 diabetes who takes oral hypoglycemic agents will need to stay on them indefinitely. You are most likely to be able to successfully have your oral hypoglycemic agents discontinued if the following statements apply to you:

✔ You've had your diabetes for a relatively short period of time.

✔ You are very attentive to healthy eating and regular exercise.

✔ You were overweight when you were diagnosed with diabetes and you then lost significant weight.

✔ On treatment, your blood glucose levels are now excellently controlled.

If these listed features apply to you, then your doctor may recommend to you that, *under his or her careful guidance and supervision,* you try weaning off your oral hypoglycemic agents. If an attempt is made to wean you off your medications, it would be prudent for you to keep a close eye on your blood glucose readings and for you to notify your doctor if they climb above target. (Alternatively, your doctor may possibly advise you in advance of your stopping your drugs to simply restart them if your readings climb.)

The preceding comments apply only to your oral hypoglycemic agents, not to blood pressure medicines, cholesterol drugs, and so forth. Whether or not these can be safely discontinued is an entirely different issue.

Is Fruit Juice Good or Bad?

Is fruit juice good or bad? Yes. And no.

Yes, fruit juice is good for you. Consuming fruit is part of a healthy diet (whether or not you have diabetes) and if that fruit comes in its natural state (be it a banana, orange, apple, and so on) or in the form of juice, you will be getting similar nutritional value so, yes, fruit juice is good for you.

No, fruit juice is bad for you. Well, not really bad. Just less good than consuming fruit in its natural state. Here are some reasons why fruit juice may be less healthful than eating whole fruit:

- ✔ If you get your fruit in the form of juice, unless you made it yourself there will have been processing involved, during which some nutrients may have been lost.
- ✔ Fruit juice may contain less fibre than fruit in its natural state.
- ✔ Fruit juice is typically less filling than whole fruit so you may find yourself consuming more juice than is necessary or healthy. (Fruit juice raises your blood glucose and contributes calories to your diet.)

If you're okay with eating whole fruit, we recommend you eat whole fruit. On the other hand, if you're unlikely to eat fruit unless it's in the form of juice, then have your juice, but just make sure you don't consume too much of it.

One place where fruit juice is definitely better than eating whole fruit is in the treatment of hypoglycemia since fruit juice will bring your blood glucose level up faster than whole fruit.

Can I Eat Birthday Cake?

Yes, you can eat birthday cake. Or wedding cake, apple cake, cheese cake, or any other type of cake you desire. Indeed, in Chapter 17, we present a whole bunch of recipes for cakes (and pies) and in Chapter 18, you'll find a recipe for Happy Birthday Cake. One of the dictums to which we most closely adhere is that no food — *no food!* — including cakes, pies, and other treats is forbidden if you have diabetes.

There is, of course, a flip side to this. Although you can indeed eat cake, you should only eat a limited quantity of this or other sweets.

When eating cake or other sweets, be mindful of portion sizes (which should be small) and the total amounts per day. No more than 10 percent of your daily calories should come from sweets. If you're on a 2,000 calorie per day diet, 10 percent works out to 200 calories per day, which is a small-sized piece of cake or pie.

There is one other, terribly important thing to bear in mind as you eat your piece of cake. Whatever you do, do NOT feel guilty as you eat your treat and do not let others make you feel guilty. Enjoy your birthday cake. And if people, however well intentioned, tell you that you can't eat birthday cake, show them this section of this book so that they will know you are indeed very much allowed.

Chapter 20

Ten Diabetes Nutrition Myths

In This Chapter

▶ Debunking misconceptions about diet and diabetes

*O*ne of our kids' (and our) favourite television shows is *MythBusters*. As the name indicates, this show is all about dispelling commonly held myths. Well, we aren't likely to appear on that show any time soon so, instead, in this chapter we do our own version of MythBusters and dispel ten commonly believed myths about diabetes nutrition.

I Know What to Eat; No Point Seeing a Dietitian

Perhaps you've done a fair bit of reading about diabetes nutrition, or perhaps you're using common sense to help you determine what foods are good choices and what foods are best left alone. In either case, it's terrific and we extend our congratulations. We also invite you to further enrich your knowledge about healthy eating strategies by availing yourself of the expertise of a registered dietitian.

A registered dietitian is the consummate pro when it comes to helping people optimize their health through nutrition. Also, many dietitians working in the diabetes field have done additional training and have become Certified Diabetes Educators.

See Chapter 1 for a discussion of some of the many ways that a dietitian can help you in your quest for good health.

If you have diabetes and you haven't yet met with a dietitian, you're missing out. If you're in this situation, be sure to ask your doctor to refer you to a dietitian or, instead, call your local diabetes education centre and see if you can refer yourself.

Omega-3 Fatty Acid Supplements Are of Proven Benefit if You Have Diabetes

As we discuss in Chapter 2, omega-3 fatty acids are a good type of fat. Consuming a diet that is rich in omega-3 fatty acids helps reduce your risk of developing hardening of the arteries *(atherosclerosis)* and, as a result, lowers the risk of heart attack and stroke.

Salmon, herring, sardines, mackerel, and trout are all excellent sources of omega-3 fatty acids. Other good dietary sources are ground flaxseed, omega-3 eggs, and canola oil.

Although it is known that consuming a *diet* rich in omega-3 fatty acids is a healthy thing to do, it is not as yet proven that people will derive the same health benefits if they get their omega-3 fatty acid in the form of *supplements.* Hopefully, future research will provide this answer.

If My Blood Sugar Goes Up Overnight It's Because of What I Ate

If you check your blood sugar before bed and it is very good — say 6.4 mmol/L, for example — yet you wake up in the morning and it's elevated — say 8.7 mmol/L, despite what many people think, this is not likely due to having eaten "something wrong" the night before.

The explanation, in fact, lies not in an overly large dinner or bedtime snack, or to a sleepwalking trip to the fridge at 3 in the morning. Rather, it lies in your liver and something called the *dawn phenomenon.*

Beginning in the middle of the night the amount of certain hormones (including growth hormone, cortisol, glucagon, and epinephrine) in the body normally goes up. These hormones, in turn, promote the release of glucose from the liver into the bloodstream. A person without diabetes can counteract the liver's tendency to release glucose into the bloodstream overnight by making more insulin, and as a result blood glucose levels remain normal. People with diabetes, however, may not be able to make enough insulin and as a result their blood glucose level goes up overnight (that is, their blood glucose level goes up as the dawn approaches, hence the name *dawn phenomenon*).

If you think you're experiencing the dawn phenomenon, speak to your doctor because a change in your medication may be required to keep your blood glucose levels in check overnight.

Soaking Rice or Lentils Will Help Prevent These Foods from Raising My Sugar Level

Eating rice and dal (which is a legume-based dish) is a perfectly acceptable part of a healthy diabetes diet. One myth is that soaking rice and lentils will make these foods less likely to raise your blood glucose levels.

In reality, soaking rice and lentils doesn't have any impact on their capability to affect your blood glucose levels. All that soaking does is lead to loss of certain vitamins from these foods.

Although you shouldn't soak rice, *rinsing* rice is okay. Rinsing rice will increase its quality, making it more flavourful and less sticky when prepared.

I Can't Eat My Homeland Food Now That I Have Diabetes

If you, like so many millions of other Canadians, have moved here from some other country, you may have heard that having diabetes means you can no longer eat foods from your homeland. This is definitely a myth.

Eating a healthy diabetes diet does *not* mean giving up your traditional foods. It may, however, require you to make some modifications. Under the expert guidance of a dietitian, you need to discover which of your traditional foods contain carbohydrate, salt, fat, and so forth and then to determine, with the dietitian's help, how often and how much of your favourite foods you can eat.

Sometimes new Canadians say they have concerns that a Canadian dietitian won't be familiar with their traditional foods and, as a result, they believe that it won't be worth their while to meet with a dietitian. If this applies to you, we are ever so glad that you're reading this section.

Registered dietitians are both highly trained and highly skilled. And their training includes being familiar not just with "Western" foods, but with foods from everywhere on the planet. Canada is, after all, a nation of immigrants, and therefore, dietitians must know all about food types, customs, and preferences from every corner of the world . . . including your corner. (You may find yourself surprised when you visit your dietitian for the first time — there's a darn good chance your dietitian may even come from the same country as you do!)

The Canadian Diabetes Association (CDA) has handouts and teaching tools on how to incorporate traditional foods from various regions of the world into a healthy diabetes eating program. The CDA also has local chapters for Chinese, Caribbean, Polish, Ukrainian, Pilipino, Jewish, South Asian, and other groups. To learn more about these resources visit the CDA website (www.diabetes.ca) or call the CDA at 1-800-BANTING.

Spices Make Blood Sugar Levels Go Up

You may have heard that eating spices makes blood glucose levels go up. Well, truth be told, this is not so. The reality is that the spices you love (and even those you hate) don't have any influence on your blood glucose levels.

Even better, since people love spices (and since they won't worsen your blood glucose or your blood pressure), they can be safely used as an alternative to salt.

A few years ago a report came out suggesting that cinnamon could actually *improve* blood glucose levels. Alas, further scientific research determined that this isn't the case. Like the taste of cinnamon? Then keep using it, but for its taste value, not its medicinal value.

All White Food Is Bad and Should Be Avoided

When it comes to the question of whether all white food is bad, we've got to say that this isn't, ahem, a black-and-white issue. Indeed, as we note a number of times in this book, *no* food is forbidden just because you have diabetes, and that includes any and all white foods — even white marshmallows! Of course, just because a food isn't forbidden doesn't automatically make that food a nutritious choice that should be consumed routinely or in unlimited quantities.

A main reason why white foods sometime have a bad reputation is because certain white foods have a high glycemic index, meaning that they have a greater tendency to raise blood glucose than do some other foods of equal carbohydrate content. (We discuss the glycemic index in Chapter 4.) There are, however, so many exceptions to this rule that it's not much of a rule at all.

For example, new potatoes have a lower glycemic index than some other types of potato, basmati rice (which is white) has a similar glycemic index to brown rice, white sugar's affect on blood glucose is no better or worse than brown sugar's, and, of course, milk and yogurt are excellent food choices.

Remember the old rule about not judging a book by its cover? We suggest adding a parallel phrase: Don't judge a food by its colour.

Eating Too Much Sugar Causes Type 2 Diabetes

Likely the most common diabetes myth of all is the notion that eating excess amounts of sugar causes type 2 diabetes. In a word (or two), it doesn't.

Type 2 diabetes develops due to a complex and incompletely understood interplay of genes and lifestyle factors, the most important of which is being overweight. (However, it's worth noting that not all people with type 2 diabetes are overweight.)

Eating sugar — even lots of it — is not responsible for diabetes. Indeed, you likely know people who are "sugarholics" who don't have (and never will develop) diabetes. If eating sugar is at all related to diabetes, it is indirect in that eating excess quantities of sugar often means you're consuming excess calories. It is these excess calories that may lead to overweight, and overweight, in turn, puts you at increased risk for developing type 2 diabetes. *How* you get overweight isn't relevant in terms of your diabetes risk; it is simply *being* overweight.

Changing the Way I Eat Is Pointless — If I'm Going to Get Diabetes, I Can't Do Anything to Prevent It

Many people with a family history of type 2 diabetes feel that they'll inevitably also get type 2 diabetes. Well, it's true that your risk of developing type 2 diabetes does go up if you have close relatives with the condition, but it's a myth that you're powerless to prevent it. The reality is that there's lots you can do to prevent it!

The most important thing you can do to lower your risk of developing type 2 diabetes is to follow a healthy lifestyle. Eating fewer calories, less fat, and more fibre and exercising regularly coupled with losing weight (if you're overweight) can reduce your risk of developing type 2 diabetes by up to 60 percent. Sixty percent. Wow, talk about exploding a myth!

Lifestyle change is always the best way of reducing your risk of developing type 2 diabetes, but it's worth noting that several medications are available, including acarbose, metformin, and thiazolidinediones, which have also been shown to reduce the risk of developing type 2 diabetes (or, at the very least, to delay its onset). We discuss these drugs in Chapter 1.

If I'm Sick I Have to Force Myself to Eat Normally

If you have diabetes and you get sick with a cold or other relatively minor illness that lays you up at home (but isn't so severe that you need to seek urgent medical attention or be hospitalized), you may feel that you have to force yourself to continue to eat as you would normally for fear that to do otherwise will cause your blood sugars to go out of whack. The problem is, however, that if you're like most people, when you're feeling really crummy the last thing in the world you want to do is eat three square meals.

If you have diabetes and you become ill with a cold or other flulike illness, you will be at risk of both *high* blood glucose (due to the physical stress on your body of the illness) and *low* blood glucose (from the action of your blood glucose–lowering medications). You will also be at risk of dehydration.

If you feel up to it, eating and drinking as you would normally is ideal. However, it's a myth that you need to force yourself to do this. You do, however, need to maintain your hydration and get nutrients into your body.

To maintain your hydration, drink plenty of fluids. Choices include water, soup (such as beef barley or that all-time sick-day friend, chicken soup), fruit juice, pop (regular, sugar-containing pop if you're not getting sufficient carbohydrates any other way that day), a Popsicle, milk, Gatorade, or commercial milkshakes (made specifically for those with diabetes).

For nutrition, eat small quantities of food frequently. Good choices include a slice of bread or toast, soda crackers, melba toast, oatmeal, fruit, Jell-O, yogurt, and sherbet.

Have a supply of foods and drinks, including some of these we just mentioned, set aside in your house in a designated container ("sick day box") in case you need them in a pinch. If you're feeling crummy, the last thing in the world you're going to want to do is go grocery shopping!

When you're ill — especially if you have type 1 diabetes or if you have insufficiently controlled type 2 diabetes — you must check your blood glucose levels frequently, in some cases as much as or more than a dozen times per day. Also, you need to know what to do with your diabetes medications, whether you need to check for ketones (a type of acid) in your blood or urine, when you should go to the hospital, and so forth. If you haven't had this discussion with your diabetes educators and your doctor, be sure to call them to arrange a meeting. Better to have a plan of action in place now than finding yourself suddenly in a quandary when you become ill. You can learn more about what to do with your medications when you are ill by having a look at an article on the subject on the CDA website (http://guidelines.diabetes.ca/Browse/Appendices/Appendix7).

Chapter 21

Ten Tips for Healthy Eating

In This Chapter
▶ Looking at how to keep time on your side
▶ Discovering how to eat what you want and what you need

*W*e have a hunch that if we asked you to list off reasons to eat healthfully you'd likely be able to do so pretty readily. You'd probably think of benefits like feeling better, helping with weight control, reducing your risk of heart disease, improving your cholesterol, lowering your blood pressure and your blood glucose levels, and so on.

Eating healthfully is often challenging, however, so in this chapter we provide ten tips to help you in your quest.

Eat Three Meals per Day

Eating three balanced meals per day is the foundation of an overall healthy nutrition strategy and will provide your body with the energy and nutrients needed throughout the day.

An additional, important reason to eat three meals per day if you have diabetes is so that your body can better handle the carbohydrates you eat. Carbohydrate is the nutrient that raises blood glucose. With diabetes, your body has, by definition, a tendency toward high blood glucose. By distributing your daily carbohydrates over three meals, you'll help your body deal with this nutrient better than if you consumed all your day's carbohydrates in one go. As a result of dividing up your carbohydrates over the course of the day, you may have better blood glucose control.

Limit the Time between Meals to Less Than Six Hours

The main reason for people living with diabetes to avoid going more than six hours between meals is that this can lead to problems with blood glucose control. In particular, delaying a meal often leads to overeating at the next meal, which will raise your blood glucose. Also, many diabetes medications have a fairly long action, and if you don't eat at regular intervals, the medicines can lead to hypoglycemia.

Although going longer than six hours between meals is less than ideal, we are strong believers that your diabetes management should, whenever possible, revolve around your life, not vice versa. Therefore, if your lifestyle dictates that you will be going more than six hours between meals, you can help smooth out your blood glucose control, avoid hypoglycemia, and avoid overeating come the next meal by having a snack about halfway between your meals. A snack could consist of a fruit, yogurt, two digestive biscuits, a slice of toast and 1 tbsp (15 ml) of peanut butter, or 1 ounce (30 g) of low-fat cheese with four to five high-fibre crackers.

If your lifestyle fits best with going more than six hours between meals, speak to your registered dietitian and your doctor to see how your treatment regimen can fit with this eating schedule.

Keep Your Sweets as Treasured Treats

If you have diabetes, there is no forbidden sweet. Indeed, you can eat anything your heart desires. You want chocolate cake? Go for it. Ice cream? Enjoy. Licorice? Yum. Having diabetes is not meant to be a punishment! All foods can fit, even sweet treats (though we admit that calling sweets "foods" is stretching it a bit).

There is, however, a *but*. The *but* is that although eating sugary snacks is okay, it must be done in very limited quantities. The Canadian Diabetes Association advises that no more than 10 percent of your daily calorie intake come in the form of sucrose (table sugar), as is used in baking and as is present in many sweet snack foods. For a person following a 2,000 calorie diet, this works out to 200 calories per day. Two hundred calories is found in many candy bars, about two-thirds of a cup (150 ml) of ice cream, or a small slice of cake or pie.

You should limit how many sweets you eat because they provide so-called empty calories (that is, calories without associated nutritional value) and raise blood glucose. Also, they replace more nutritious foods in your diet.

When reaching for a snack, you're better off foregoing junk food and instead opting for more nutritious foods like fruit or nuts. But having some sweet snacks — in limited quantities — is okay. Enjoy it. And don't feel guilty!

Choose Low-Fat Foods

Having diabetes considerably increases your risk of developing atherosclerosis (hardening of the arteries), which, in turn, increases the chances of your having a heart attack, a stroke, or a leg amputation. This risk, however (there's always a "however" or a "but" when it comes to diabetes risks!), is markedly reduced if you keep your cholesterol in check. In particular, and as we discuss in Chapter 2, most people with diabetes should have a blood LDL cholesterol (the "bad" cholesterol) level no higher than 2 mmol/L.

Choosing low-fat foods will help you get your LDL cholesterol into target range and keep it there. Bear in mind that not all fat is the same. As we review in Chapter 2, you should minimize your intake of saturated fat (as is found in meats) and your ingestion of trans fats. On the other hand, a diet rich in omega-3 fatty acids (as is found in certain types of fish) helps protect against atherosclerosis.

Low-fat foods often contain fewer calories than their non-low-fat counterparts. Therefore, choosing low-fat foods can help with weight management. Select low-fat cheese. Choose 1 percent or skim milk rather than whole milk (which contains 3.25 percent milk fat). Opt for low-fat yogurt, low-fat pudding, low-fat lean meats, chicken without the skin, and so forth. (However, when buying ultra-low-fat or fat-free foods be careful to read the labels because some of these products — especially certain types of peanut butter, salad dressings, and mayonnaise — may have sugar added.)

Nutrition therapy is very important in controlling your blood cholesterol levels, but medication therapy is also often required. We discuss this further in Chapter 4.

Choose Whole Grains and High-Fibre Foods

As we discuss in Chapter 2, whole grains and fibre are good food choices and provide many health benefits, including making controlling your weight and blood sugars easier, helping avoid constipation, reducing cholesterol, and, importantly, possibly reducing your risk of heart disease. Not too shabby.

Given this (and other) health benefits of consuming lots of whole grains and fibre, we encourage you to fill your grocery cart with foods that are rich in these nutrients. When making your food purchases, look for the term "whole grain" on the label. And, in this *buyer beware* world, it is important to know that foods labelled "multigrain" or "organic" may or may not be whole grain products, and that bread that has a brownish colour is not necessarily whole grain — rather, it may simply have been coloured brown by the addition of something like molasses.

A whole grain food is not necessarily high in fibre. Therefore, when buying your food, in addition to reviewing any health claims on the package, check the fibre content in the Nutrition Facts table. (We discuss health claims and Nutrition Facts tables in Chapter 6.)

If the health claim says the product is a

✔ *Source of fibre,* then it contains 2 grams or more of fibre per serving.

✔ *High source of fibre,* then it contains 4 grams or more of fibre per serving.

✔ *Very high source of fibre,* then it contains 6 grams or more of fibre per serving.

If the fibre content listed in the Nutrition Facts table is 15 percent or more of your "% Daily Value," then the food is a high source of fibre.

Eat Vegetables and Fruit at Most Meals

Consuming fruits and vegetables is integral to good diabetes health and should be a part of almost every meal. Canada's Food Guide recommends that teens and adults consume seven to ten servings of vegetables and fruits daily. Cynthia routinely finds that most people she counsels aren't getting enough vegetables and fruits.

Perhaps you love eating fruits and vegetables, in which case you'll need no convincing to make them a part of your daily eating plan. Or perhaps you don't love them but like them enough that you also don't need any arm twisting. But what if — heavens! — you really just don't like fruits or vegetables at all; what then? Well, all we can say is that sometimes you "gotta do what you gotta do," and if the taste of fruits and vegetables isn't of sufficient appeal for you to munch on them, then eat them for the most altruistic of reasons — your good health.

If you don't like cooked vegetables, you may like raw vegetables or salads. Try adding (or hiding) vegetables in soups or casseroles. Don't forget vegetable juices, but choose the unsalted variety. If you don't like fresh fruit, canned fruit packed in its own juice is fine. Also, be sure to try the Apple Crisp, Oatmeal Fruit Crepes, or the smoothies in this book.

Because fruit contains sugar, it sometimes gets a bad wrap. Perhaps you've eaten some fruit and found your blood glucose level rose afterward. However, this doesn't mean that fruit is unhealthy. What it does mean is that although you should eat fruit daily, you shouldn't eat it in unrestricted amounts. A medium-sized piece of fruit at each meal is generally sufficient. Also, if eating appropriate quantities of fruit still makes your blood glucose level go up unduly, you should get in touch with your dietitian, to ensure that you're eating the right amount of fruit, and your doctor, to see if your diabetes medications need adjusting.

Load Up with Calcium and Vitamin D

Having a diet rich in calcium and vitamin D is essential for good health, whether or not you have diabetes.

Calcium and you

Canada's Food Guide recommends two to four servings per day of Milk and Alternatives, based on age and gender. (As we discuss in Chapter 2, "alternatives" in this context refers to items such as cheese, yogurt, and soy-based products.) Calcium, which is plentiful in Milk and Alternatives, is important for strong bones and teeth and is needed for proper muscle and nerve function.

These are examples of good sources of calcium:

- 1 cup (250 ml) cow's milk or fortified rice or soy beverage has 300 mg.
- 1 cup (250 ml) fortified orange juice has 300 mg.
- ¾ cup (175 ml) plain yogurt has 290 mg.
- 1 oz. (30 g) cheddar, Edam, or Gouda cheese has 245 mg.
- ½ can salmon with the bones has 240 mg.
- ½ can sardines with the bones has 200 mg.

Osteoporosis Canada (www.osteoporosis.ca), an "organization serving people who have, or are at risk for, osteoporosis," recommends you ingest a total of 800 to 1,200 mg of calcium per day, based on age. This total includes both the calcium you get from food sources and any calcium supplements you may be taking.

Vitamin D and you

It seems like every day some new medical research comes out shedding ever more light on the importance of getting sufficient vitamin D in your diet. As we discuss in Chapter 2, lack of vitamin D can lead to osteoporosis (which in turn makes one susceptible to fractures) and has also been associated with an increased risk of developing many other diseases, including atherosclerosis and cancer. In order for vitamin D to do its job of maintaining strong bones, it needs to have sufficient amounts of calcium with which to work; bones are, after all, primarily made of calcium. Vitamin D enhances the intestine's ability to absorb calcium into the body.

It's hard to get sufficient vitamin D in your diet. For example, one cup (250 ml) of milk fortified with vitamin D has 100 units of vitamin D (which is far less than a person's daily needs), and other foods like margarine, eggs, salmon, sardines, herring, mackerel, swordfish, and cod liver oil contain only small amounts of vitamin D.

Another way of getting vitamin D is to make it yourself! In this case, we're not talking about creating your own home lab, but, rather, the process where your own sun-exposed skin makes vitamin D. Unfortunately, one drawback of living in this great country of ours is that short winter days and the need to bundle up when outdoors means that Canadians typically aren't getting enough vitamin D from October to April. Also, even when the weather turns warm and people are out in the sun, the commonplace use of sunscreen also limits the amount of vitamin D that the skin can make. These are some key reasons why many Canadians (whether or not living with diabetes) need to take vitamin D supplements.

Many Canadian adults require vitamin D supplements. The amount you need — which may vary from 400 units per day to 1,000 units per day or more — will depend on your age, gender, and other factors. Be sure to talk to your doctor and your dietitian to find out what the right amount is for you.

Considering Multivitamins — Do You Need Them?

Every year Canadians spend hundreds of millions of dollars on vitamin supplements. Is this money well spent? Should you be taking a multivitamin?

If you're eating a well-balanced diet following the nutrition principles outlined in Chapter 2 of this book and as taught by your registered dietitian, and, when necessary, taking a *specific* vitamin supplement (like Vitamin D), then you're getting all the vitamins you need and all that taking a multivitamin supplement does is give you very expensive, vitamin-laden urine (!) or similarly expensive fat cells (where many excess vitamins will end up residing).

Bottom line: Taking a multivitamin is seldom of benefit unless you're pregnant, in which case you should indeed be taking a daily multivitamin.

If you're wondering whether or not you should take a multivitamin (or, for that matter, any other vitamin supplement), we recommend you speak with your dietitian. He or she will be able to give you excellent advice tailored to your particular situation and needs.

Drink Water

The human body is an incredibly intricate, finely tuned, and wondrous machine. The human body is also 60 percent water. Ah, water truly is the sweet elixir of life!

As we discuss in detail in Chapter 2, consuming enough water to make up for your daily water losses from urine, stool, sweat, breathing, and so forth is essential. Drinking water will also help you feel full and thus can reduce your appetite and help you with weight control.

In general, make a point of drinking at least 1.5 litres (6 cups) of water per day. If, however, you are losing more than normal amounts of water from your body — as would be the case if you have a fever, are exercising, have high blood glucose, and so on — then you need to consume greater quantities of water.

Enjoy Variety — All Foods Can Fit!

We never use the term "diabetic diet." A so-called diabetic diet is simply a healthy eating program that includes appropriate proportions of carbohydrates, proteins, and fats; limited quantities of saturated fats and salt; sufficient fibre; and so on. A diabetes nutrition program doesn't exclude anything, not even sweets, as we discuss earlier in this chapter.

If you find your diet overly restrictive, get in touch with your dietitian. Your dietitian will sit down with you and review your diet in detail and find ways of modifying your nutrition program so that you find it, ahem, palatable and suited to your individual needs.

Part V
Appendixes

Small Meal Plan

The small meal plan provides approximately 1,400 calories and includes three meals and a night snack.

Breakfast	Lunch	Dinner	Snack
3 Carbohydrate Choices (45 g)	3 Carbohydrate Choices (45 g)	4 Carbohydrate Choices (60 g)	1 Carbohydrate Choice (15 g)
Free vegetables	Free vegetables	Free vegetables	Free vegetables
0–1 Protein Choices	1–2 Protein Choices	3 Protein Choices	0–1 Protein Choices
0–1 Fat Choices	1–2 Fat Choices	1–2 Fat Choices	0 Fat Choices

Large Meal Plan

The large meal plan provides approximately 2,000 calories and includes three meals and two snacks.

Breakfast	Lunch	Snack	Dinner	Snack
4 Carbohydrate Choices (60 g)	4 Carbohydrate Choices (60 g)	1 Carbohydrate Choice (15 g)	5 Carbohydrate Choices (75 g)	2 Carbohydrate Choices (30 g)
Free vegetables	Free vegetables	Free vegetables	Free vegetables	Free vegetables
0–2 Protein Choices	2–3 Protein Choices	0 Protein Choices	5 Protein Choices	1 Protein Choice
0–2 Fat Choices	1 Fat Choice	0 Fat Choices	1–2 Fat Choices	0–1 Fat Choices

In this part . . .

The Web is a wild and wonderful place, but getting accurate information about diabetes and nutrition online can sometimes be a challenge. In Appendix A we look at helpful and reliable places on the Web to learn about — and be kept up-to-date about — diabetes and nutrition. We also help you plan out a month of menus with, well, a month of menus.

Appendix A

Nutrition and Recipe Websites for People with Diabetes

. . . .

A number of excellent Websites provide helpful information about various aspects of living with diabetes. Some sites focus specifically on healthy eating, and some sites have a wide array of recipes. In this appendix, we list some of these sites. If you have a site you find particularly helpful we'd love to hear about it; please feel free to email us at diabetes@ianblumer.com.

General Diabetes Websites

Here are some helpful sites if you're looking for general information to help you manage your diabetes.

The Canadian Diabetes Association (CDA)

www.diabetes.ca

The CDA site is particularly helpful because it looks at diabetes issues from a Canadian perspective. Of special value is the listing of resources (including addresses and phone numbers) available in your province or territory and, in some cases, even within your community. A number of recipes can also be found on this site.

The American Diabetes Association

www.diabetes.org

This helpful site offers tons of information, but as you can imagine, it uses American units (for glucose, cholesterol, and so on), which can make it confusing for those of us north of the 49th parallel. A large collection of recipes is available on this site.

Ian Blumer's Practical Guide to Diabetes

www.ourdiabetes.com

This is, as you likely guessed, Ian's Website. Here you'll find a collection of practical tips to help you look after your diabetes and to stay healthy.

Online Diabetes Resources by Rick Mendosa

www.mendosa.com

On his site, Rick Mendosa, a medical writer who himself has diabetes, has catalogued a vast amount of information on the web concerning diabetes. Also available are some excellent articles that he's written on various topics related to diabetes.

Children with Diabetes

www.childrenwithdiabetes.com

This site is geared toward families with a child living with diabetes. It provides a huge collection of recipes, including many submitted by its readers (which is good in that they come personally recommended; however, it also means the recipes may not have been evaluated by a registered dietitian).

General Nutrition Websites

These Websites contain information on general principles of healthy eating.

Dietitians of Canada

www.dietitians.ca

This site is a "voice of the profession." Here you will find dietitians in your part of Canada as well as general nutrition information.

Health Canada

Heath Canada has terrific, not-to-be-missed information.

Health Canada's Main Website

www.hc-sc.gc.ca

This is a good place to start your tour of what Health Canada's site has to offer.

Health Canada information on food labelling

http://www.hc-sc.gc.ca/fn-an/label-etiquet/index-eng.php

This is the place to go to discover helpful facts about food labelling.

Health Canada's database on nutrients

www.healthcanada.gc.ca/cnf

This site contains Health Canada's exhaustive database of "up to 143 nutrients in over 5,500 foods."

Kraft Canada

www.kraftcanada.com

This commercial Website has lots of information on diabetes, including a number of diabetes-friendly recipes.

EatRight Ontario!

www.eatrightontario.ca

This Government of Ontario site was "designed to improve your health and quality of life through healthy, nutritious eating." Here you'll find information on nutrients, nutrition labelling, menu planning, and more.

CalorieKing Food Database

www.calorieking.com

The CalorieKing food database contains a nutrition breakdown of an exhaustive list of foods, including convenience foods and those served at popular restaurant chains.

Diabetes Nutrition-Focused Websites

Here are sites that focus specifically on diabetes nutrition. These sites also contain recipes geared toward people living with diabetes. (Many of the sites we list earlier in this appendix also contain diabetes-friendly recipes.)

Diabetic Gourmet Magazine

www.diabeticgourmet.com

Here you'll find a whole host of recipes.

The Diabetes Network

www.diabetesnet.com/diabetes_food_diet

The Diabetes Network has an abundance of helpful resources, including recipes and information on carbohydrate counting and the glycemic index.

Reality Bites

www.mymealplan.ca/recipes.php

Reality Bites has a whole raft of recipes geared toward people living with diabetes.

dLife

www.dlife.com

dLife ("for your diabetes life") has a large selection of recipes, including cooking videos you'll find on the "dLife kitchen."

Appendix B

A Month of Menus

• •

*P*lanning a menu is simple for some people living with diabetes, but for many others it's challenging or even downright daunting. Many people tell us they simply "don't know what to put on the plate" or what is suitable to eat. Some people want variety without knowing how to get it, and others tell us they deal with all these challenges by eating the same thing day after day after day.

If you face any of these hurdles, you've come to the right place. This book is designed to help you find a wide variety of healthy eating choices, and this appendix, in particular, is geared toward helping you plan out, as the title indicates, a month of menus.

This month of menus provides food choices for both small and larger caloric needs or appetites. We offer numerous ideas for snacks, too. Each row of the tables represents a day, and throughout the tables we offer chapter numbers indicating where you can locate the recipes we mention.

Small Meal Plan

The small meal plan provides approximately 1,400 calories and includes three meals and a night snack.

The table below represents the food group choices and grams of carbohydrate for a small meal plan. This plan provides approximately 50 percent of total calories from carbohydrate, 20 percent of total calories from protein, and 30 percent of total calories from fat. This percentage falls within the current goal for main nutrient balance according to the Canadian Diabetes Association.

This meal plan is just a sample. You can request a personalized meal plan to suit your lifestyle from your registered dietitian at your local diabetes education centre.

Think of the following table as a template — a "fill in the blanks" if you will. In this table the "blanks" are terms such as "carbohydrate choice" or "vegetables" and so forth. After this table we then look at many food choices you can substitute for the "blanks."

Breakfast	Lunch	Dinner	Snack
3 Carbohydrate Choices (45 g)	3 Carbohydrate Choices (45 g)	4 Carbohydrate Choices (60 g)	1 Carbohydrate Choice (15 g)
Free vegetables	Free vegetables	Free vegetables	Free vegetables
0–1 Protein Choices	1–2 Protein Choices	3 Protein Choices	0–1 Protein Choices
0–1 Fat Choices	1–2 Fat Choices	1–2 Fat Choices	0 Fat Choices

In the following month of menus, we build on those guidelines, plugging in different types and amounts of various foods that, taken together, provide approximately 1,400 calories per day and will do so in a balanced, healthy way.

Breakfast	Lunch	Dinner	Snack
Cranberry Walnut Muffin (Chapter 7) 1 oz (30 g) low-fat cheese 1 cup (250 ml) 1% milk	Salmon sandwich: 2 slices whole grain bread ¼–½ cup (50–125 ml) salmon 1 tbsp (15 ml) light mayonnaise Diced celery/lettuce Tossed salad with 1 tbsp (15 ml) light dressing 1 peach Water	1 cup (250 ml) Vegetarian Curry Tofu with Noodles (Chapter 16) ½ cup (125 ml) Marinated Mushrooms with Herbs (Chapter 9) ½ mango 1 cup (250 ml) 1% milk	1 rye toast 1–2 tbsp (15–30 ml) peanut butter
2 Oatmeal Pancakes (Chapter 7) with 2 tbsp (30 ml) light syrup 1 small banana Coffee	1 cup (250 ml) Classic Caesar Salad (Chapter 9) 4 rectangular melba toasts 1 oz (30 g) low-fat cheese 1 pear 1 cup (250 ml) 1% milk	¾ cup (175 ml) Hamburger Stroganoff (Chapter 15) with ½ cup (125 ml) noodles ½ cup (125 ml) squash ½ cup (125 ml) yellow beans ¾ cup (175 ml) yogurt with ¼ cup (50 ml) Baked Homemade Granola (Chapter 7) Tea	1 medium apple 1 oz (30 g) low-fat cheese

Eating Well with Canada's Food Guide

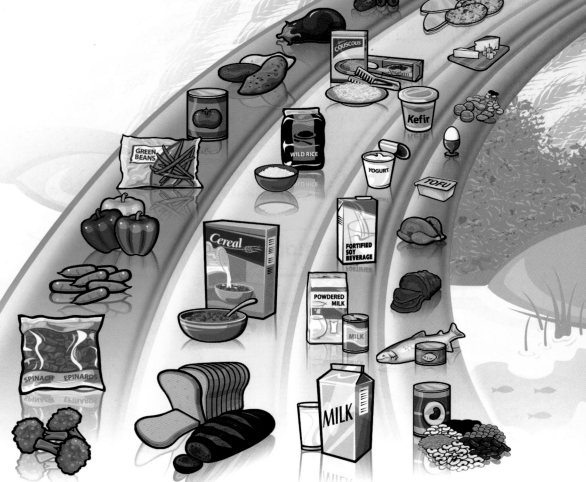

Canada

Eat well and be active today and every day!

The benefits of eating well and being active include:

- Better overall health.
- Lower risk of disease.
- A healthy body weight.
- Feeling and looking better.
- More energy.
- Stronger muscles and bones.

Be active

To be active every day is a step towards better health and a healthy body weight.

It is recommended that adults accumulate at least 2 ½ hours of moderate to vigorous physical activity each week and that children and youth accumulate at least 60 minutes per day. You don't have to do it all at once. Choose a variety of activities spread throughout the week.

Start slowly and build up.

Eat well

Another important step towards better health and a healthy body weight is to follow *Canada's Food Guide* by:

- Eating the recommended amount and type of food each day.
- Limiting foods and beverages high in calories, fat, sugar or salt (sodium) such as cakes and pastries, chocolate and candies, cookies and granola bars, doughnuts and muffins, ice cream and frozen desserts, french fries, potato chips, nachos and other salty snacks, alcohol, fruit flavoured drinks, soft drinks, sports and energy drinks, and sweetened hot or cold drinks.

Read the label

- Compare the Nutrition Facts table on food labels to choose products that contain less fat, saturated fat, trans fat, sugar and sodium.
- Keep in mind that the calories and nutrients listed are for the amount of food found at the top of the Nutrition Facts table.

Limit trans fat

When a Nutrition Facts table is not available, ask for nutrition information to choose foods lower in trans and saturated fats.

Nutrition Facts
Per 0 mL (0 g)

Amount	% Daily Value
Calories 0	
Fat 0 g	0 %
Saturates 0 g	0 %
+ Trans 0 g	
Cholesterol 0 mg	
Sodium 0 mg	0 %
Carbohydrate 0 g	0 %
Fibre 0 g	0 %
Sugars 0 g	
Protein 0 g	

Vitamin A	0 %	Vitamin C	0 %
Calcium	0 %	Iron	0 %

Take a step today...

- ✓ Have breakfast every day. It may help control your hunger later in the day.
- ✓ Walk wherever you can – get off the bus early, use the stairs.
- ✓ Benefit from eating vegetables and fruit at all meals and as snacks.
- ✓ Spend less time being inactive such as watching TV or playing computer games.
- ✓ Request nutrition information about menu items when eating out to help you make healthier choices.
- ✓ Enjoy eating with family and friends!
- ✓ Take time to eat and savour every bite!

For more information, interactive tools, or additional copies visit Canada's Food Guide on-line at:
www.healthcanada.gc.ca/foodguide

or contact:

Publications
Health Canada
Ottawa, Ontario K1A 0K9
E-Mail: publications@hc-sc.gc.ca
Tel.: 1-866-225-0709
Fax: (613) 941-5366
TTY: 1-800-267-1245

Également disponible en français sous le titre :
Bien manger avec le Guide alimentaire canadien

This publication can be made available on request on diskette, large print, audio-cassette and braille.

HC Pub.: 4651   Cat.: H164-38/1-2011E-PDF   ISBN: 978-1-100-19255-0

Advice for different ages and stages...

Children

Following *Canada's Food Guide* helps children grow and thrive.

Young children have small appetites and need calories for growth and development.

- Serve small nutritious meals and snacks each day.
- Do not restrict nutritious foods because of their fat content. Offer a variety of foods from the four food groups.
- Most of all... be a good role model.

Women of childbearing age

All women who could become pregnant and those who are pregnant or breastfeeding need a multivitamin containing **folic acid** every day. Pregnant women need to ensure that their multivitamin also contains **iron**. A health care professional can help you find the multivitamin that's right for you.

Pregnant and breastfeeding women need more calories. Include an extra 2 to 3 Food Guide Servings each day.

Here are two examples:
- Have fruit and yogurt for a snack, or
- Have an extra slice of toast at breakfast and an extra glass of milk at supper.

Men and women over 50

The need for **vitamin D** increases after the age of 50.

In addition to following *Canada's Food Guide*, everyone over the age of 50 should take a daily vitamin D supplement of 10 µg (400 IU).

How do I count Food Guide Servings in a meal?

Here is an example:

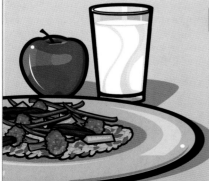

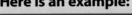

Vegetable and beef stir-fry with rice, a glass of milk and an apple for dessert		
250 mL (1 cup) mixed broccoli, carrot and sweet red pepper	=	2 **Vegetables and Fruit** Food Guide Servings
75 g (2 ½ oz.) lean beef	=	1 **Meat and Alternatives** Food Guide Serving
250 mL (1 cup) brown rice	=	2 **Grain Products** Food Guide Servings
5 mL (1 tsp) canola oil	=	part of your **Oils and Fats** intake for the day
250 mL (1 cup) 1% milk	=	1 **Milk and Alternatives** Food Guide Serving
1 apple	=	1 **Vegetables and Fruit** Food Guide Serving

Recommended Number of *Food Guide Servings* per Day

	Children			Teens		Adults			
Age in Years	2-3	4-8	9-13	14-18		19-50		51+	
Sex	Girls and Boys			Females	Males	Females	Males	Females	Males
Vegetables and Fruit	4	5	6	7	8	7-8	8-10	7	7
Grain Products	3	4	6	6	7	6-7	8	6	7
Milk and Alternatives	2	2	3-4	3-4	3-4	2	2	3	3
Meat and Alternatives	1	1	1-2	2	3	2	3	2	3

The chart above shows how many Food Guide Servings you need from each of the four food groups every day.

Having the amount and type of food recommended and following the tips in *Canada's Food Guide* will help:

• Meet your needs for vitamins, minerals and other nutrients.
• Reduce your risk of obesity, type 2 diabetes, heart disease, certain types of cancer and osteoporosis.
• Contribute to your overall health and vitality.

What is One Food Guide Serving?
Look at the examples below.

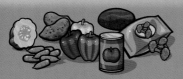 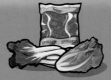 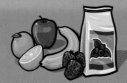

Fresh, frozen or canned vegetables
125 mL (½ cup)

Leafy vegetables
Cooked: 125 mL (½ cup)
Raw: 250 mL (1 cup)

Fresh, frozen or canned fruits
1 fruit or 125 mL (½ cup)

100% Juice
125 mL (½ cup)

Bread
1 slice (35g)

Bagel
½ bagel (45 g)

Flat breads
½ pita or ½ tortilla (35 g)

Cooked rice, bulgur or quinoa
125 mL (½ cup)

Cereal
Cold: 30 g
Hot: 175 mL (¾ cup)

Cooked pasta or couscous
125 mL (½ cup)

Milk or powdered milk (reconstituted)
250 mL (1 cup)

Canned milk (evaporated)
125 mL (½ cup)

Fortified soy beverage
250 mL (1 cup)

Yogurt
175 g
(¾ cup)

Kefir
175 g
(¾ cup)

Cheese
50 g (1 ½ oz.)

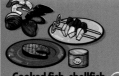

Cooked fish, shellfish, poultry, lean meat
75 g (2 ½ oz.)/125 mL (½ cup)

Cooked legumes
175 mL (¾ cup)

Tofu
150 g or
175 mL (¾ cup)

Eggs
2 eggs

Peanut or nut butters
30 mL (2 Tbsp)

Shelled nuts and seeds
60 mL (¼ cup)

Oils and Fats

- Include a small amount – 30 to 45 mL (2 to 3 Tbsp) – of unsaturated fat each day. This includes oil used for cooking, salad dressings, margarine and mayonnaise.
- Use vegetable oils such as canola, olive and soybean.
- Choose soft margarines that are low in saturated and trans fats.
- Limit butter, hard margarine, lard and shortening.

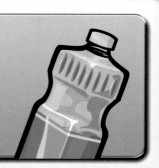

Make each Food Guide Serving count...
wherever you are – at home, at school, at work or when eating out!

▸ **Eat at least one dark green and one orange vegetable each day.**
- Go for dark green vegetables such as broccoli, romaine lettuce and spinach.
- Go for orange vegetables such as carrots, sweet potatoes and winter squash.

▸ **Choose vegetables and fruit prepared with little or no added fat, sugar or salt.**
- Enjoy vegetables steamed, baked or stir-fried instead of deep-fried.

▸ **Have vegetables and fruit more often than juice.**

▸ **Make at least half of your grain products whole grain each day.**
- Eat a variety of whole grains such as barley, brown rice, oats, quinoa and wild rice.
- Enjoy whole grain breads, oatmeal or whole wheat pasta.

▸ **Choose grain products that are lower in fat, sugar or salt.**
- Compare the Nutrition Facts table on labels to make wise choices.
- Enjoy the true taste of grain products. When adding sauces or spreads, use small amounts.

▸ **Drink skim, 1%, or 2% milk each day.**
- Have 500 mL (2 cups) of milk every day for adequate vitamin D.
- Drink fortified soy beverages if you do not drink milk.

▸ **Select lower fat milk alternatives.**
- Compare the Nutrition Facts table on yogurts or cheeses to make wise choices.

▸ **Have meat alternatives such as beans, lentils and tofu often.**

▸ **Eat at least two Food Guide Servings of fish each week.***
- Choose fish such as char, herring, mackerel, salmon, sardines and trout.

▸ **Select lean meat and alternatives prepared with little or no added fat or salt.**
- Trim the visible fat from meats. Remove the skin on poultry.
- Use cooking methods such as roasting, baking or poaching that require little or no added fat.
- If you eat luncheon meats, sausages or prepackaged meats, choose those lower in salt (sodium) and fat.

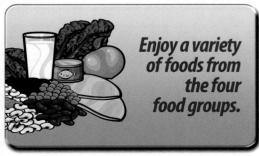

Enjoy a variety of foods from the four food groups.

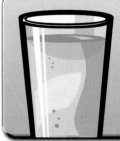

Satisfy your thirst with water!

Drink water regularly. It's a calorie-free way to quench your thirst. Drink more water in hot weather or when you are very active.

* Health Canada provides advice for limiting exposure to mercury from certain types of fish. Refer to www.healthcanada.gc.ca for the latest information.

Breakfast	Lunch	Dinner	Snack
2 slices rye toast 2 tbsp (30 ml) peanut butter ½ cup (125 ml) fruit cocktail Flavoured tea	1⅓ cups (325 ml) Vegetarian Three-Bean Chili (Chapter 16) Tossed salad with 1 tbsp (15 ml) light dressing Water	3 oz (90 g) Greek Fish (Chapter 13) ½ cup (125 ml) mashed potato ½ cup (125 ml) Tomato Cucumber Salad (Chapter 9) ½ cup (125 ml) Swiss Chard and Pine Nuts (Chapter 12) 1 cup (250 ml) grapes ½ cup (125 ml) 1% milk	½ cup (125 ml) mixed fruit ¼ cup (50 ml) low-fat cottage cheese
1 cup (250 ml) whole grain cereal 1 cup (250 ml) 1% milk ¼ cup (50 ml) sliced almonds Tea	1 Mexican Quesadilla (Chapter 16) Raw veggies and 1–2 tbsp (15–30 ml) light dip ½ cup (125 ml) applesauce Diet pop	3 oz (90 g) Roast Beef 2 tbsp (30 ml) low-fat gravy 1 medium roasted potato ½ cup (125 ml) corn ½ cup (125 ml) green beans 1 cup (250 ml) 1% milk	½ English Muffin with 1 tsp (5 ml) soft margarine 1 oz (30 g) fat-free ham
1⅛ cups (275 ml) Mango, Orange, Banana Smoothie (Chapter 7) 1 slice whole grain toast with 2 tbsp (30 ml) peanut butter	1 cup (250 ml) Veggie Soup (Chapter 8) 1 beef sandwich: 2 slices multigrain bread 1–2 oz (30–60 g) roast beef Mustard/lettuce 1 tsp (5 ml) soft margarine 3 arrowroot cookies Water	3 oz (90 g) Chicken in Dijon Sauce (Chapter 14) ⅔ cup (150 ml) brown rice ½ cup (125 ml) Stir Fried Snow Peas (Chapter 12) ½ cup (125 ml) carrots 1 cup (250 ml) strawberries 1 cup (250 ml) 1% milk	5 Triscuits 1 oz (30 g) low-fat cheese

Breakfast	*Lunch*	*Dinner*	*Snack*
1 slice multigrain toast with 1 tsp (5 ml) soft margarine and 2 tsp (10 ml) diet jam	1 English Muffin with 1 oz (30 g) low-fat cheese, 1 fried egg, and lettuce/ tomato	1 slice Salmon Loaf with ¼ cup (50 ml) Cucumber Sauce (Chapter 13)	¾ cup (175 ml) oatmeal
¾ cup (175 ml) yogurt	1 pear	½ cup (125 ml) Garlic Mashed Potatoes (Chapter 11)	¼ cup (50 ml) almonds
¼ cup (50 ml) Baked Homemade Granola (Chapter 7)	Water	Sliced tomato	
		½ cup (125 ml) broccoli	
Tea		1 cup (250 ml) honeydew melon	
		1 cup (250 ml) 1% milk	
1 slice Banana Bread (Chapter 7)	Corned beef sandwich: 2 slices rye bread 1–2 oz (30–60 g) corned beef Mustard 1 tsp (5 ml) soft margarine	1 cup (250 ml) Butter Chicken (Chapter 14)	½ cup (125 ml) Aboriginal Wild Rice Pudding with Splenda (Chapter 17)
1 oz (30 g) low-fat cheese		1 small naan bread	
½ cup (125 ml) 1% chocolate milk	½ cup (125 ml) Chunky Apple Coleslaw (Chapter 9)	Tossed salad and 1 tbsp (15 ml) light dressing	
	½ cup (125 ml) mixed fruit cup	¾ cup (175 ml) yogurt	
	Diet pop	Water	
1 whole grain English Muffin with 1 egg, 1 tsp (5 ml) soft margarine, and lettuce/tomato	1 cup (250 ml) French Onion Soup (Chapter 8)	1½ cups (375 ml) Stir-Fried Beef with Rice Noodles (Chapter 15)	½ slice Banana Bread (Chapter 7)
	1 slice garlic bread with 1 oz (30 g) low-fat cheese	1 cup (250 ml) Fruity Spinach Salad (Chapter 9)	¼ cup (50 ml) nuts
½ cup (125 ml) juice	2 kiwis	2 Jam Jewel Cookies (Chapter 17)	
	Water	Tea	

Breakfast	Lunch	Dinner	Snack
Raspberry Muffin (Chapter 7)	½ Curried Turkey in a Pita (Chapter 14)	3 oz (90 g) Parmesan Chicken (Chapter 14)	2 Flax Cookies (Chapter 17)
1 oz (30 g) low-fat cheese	Carrot sticks	¾ cup (175 ml) whole wheat pasta	10 almonds
1 orange	1 cup (250 ml) strawberries	½ cup (125 ml) Zesty Asparagus (Chapter 12)	
Coffee	1 cup (250 ml) 1% milk	⅔ cup (150 ml) Orange Glazed Carrots (Chapter 12)	
		¾ cup (175 ml) frozen yogurt	
		Water	
1 cup (250 ml) Shake Me Up Shake (Chapter 7)	1 cup (250 ml) Mediterranean-Style Tuna Casserole (Chapter 13)	1 cup (250 ml) Bulgur and Chickpea Salad with Lemon Dressing (Chapter 9)	¼ cup (50 ml) Toasted Walnut Hummus (Chapter 10)
1 slice flaxseed toast with 1–2 tbsp (15–30 ml) peanut butter	Tossed salad with 1–2 tbsp (15–30 ml) diet dressing	½ cup (125 ml) green beans	Raw veggies
2 tsp (10 ml) diet jam	Diet Jell-O	½ cup (125 ml) applesauce	
	Tea	1 cup (250 ml) 1% milk	
¾ cup (175 ml) yogurt	1 cup (250 ml) Chinese Jewelled Rice (Chapter 13)	1 cup (250 ml) Shepherd's Pie (Chapter 15)	1 Pizza Face (Chapter 18)
1 small banana	Celery sticks	1 small whole wheat roll with 1 tsp (5 ml) soft margarine	½ cup (125 ml) 1% milk
¼ cup (50 ml) Baked Homemade Granola (Chapter 7)	1 pear	Tossed salad and 1 tbsp (15 ml) light dressing	
Coffee	Water	Baked Apple with Raspberries (Chapter 18)	
		Tea	

Breakfast	Lunch	Dinner	Snack
2 slices whole grain toast with 1 slice pea meal bacon and 2 tsp (10 ml) soft margarine ½ cup (125 ml) juice	1 cup (250 ml) Asian Noodle Salad (Chapter 9) 1 cup (250 ml) 1% milk	1 cup (250 ml) Groundnut Stew (Chapter 15) 1 cup (250 ml) couscous ½ cup (125 ml) Ethiopian Cabbage (Chapter 12) Diet Jell-O ½ cup (125 ml) 1% milk	3 Shanghai Dumplings with ½ tsp (2 ml) sauce (Chapter 10)
1 piece Baked Scone (Chapter 7) with 1 tsp (5 ml) soft margarine 1 cup (250 ml) mixed fruit Herbal tea	Tuna sandwich: 2 slices whole grain bread ¼–½ cup (50–125 ml) tuna 1–2 tbsp (15–30 ml) light mayonnaise Celery/lettuce/onion 1 small banana Water	4 slices Barbequed Eggplant (Chapter 16) 1 cup (250 ml) Classic Caesar Salad (Chapter 9) ½ cup (125 ml) Balsamic Brussels Sprouts (Chapter 12) 1 small whole wheat roll with 2 tsp (10 ml) soft margarine 1 Little Jam Cupcake with Splenda (Chapter 18) Green tea	1 Banana Chocolate Chip Muffin with Splenda (Chapter 18) 1 tbsp (15 ml) peanut butter
1 cup (250 ml) Akoori Scrambled Eggs (Chapter 7) 2 slices rye toast with 2 tsp (10 ml) soft margarine 1 cup (250 ml) 1% milk	1 cup (250 ml) Kale Soup (Chapter 8) 5 Triscuits 1 oz (30 g) low-fat cheese ¾ cup (175 ml) yogurt Water	1 cup (250 ml) Saffron Fish (Chapter 13) ⅔ cup (150 ml) basmati rice ½ cup (125 ml) cooked spinach 1 tsp (5 ml) soft margarine 1 peach 1 cup (250 ml) 1% milk	1 slice Feta Bruschetta (Chapter 10)

Breakfast	Lunch	Dinner	Snack
½ large flax bagel with 2 tbsp (30 ml) light cream cheese 1 cup (250 ml) cantaloupe Tea	1 cup (250 ml) Mixed Bean Salad (Chapter 9) Veggies and 1–2 tbsp (15–30 ml) light dip 1 cup (250 ml) 1% milk	2 cups (500 ml) Walnut, Pear, and Chicken Salad (Chapter 9) 1 slice rye bread with 1 tsp (5 ml) soft margarine ¾ cup (175 ml) yogurt Water	1 piece Apple Crisp with Splenda (Chapter 18) 1 oz (30 g) low-fat cheese
1 cup (250 ml) canned fruit ¼ cup (50 ml) low-fat cottage cheese 1 slice multigrain toast with 1 tsp (5 ml) soft margarine Coffee	1 cup (250 ml) Veggie Soup (Chapter 8) ¾ cup (175 ml) Couscous Chickpea Salad (Chapter 9) 1 Chocolate Zucchini Muffin (Chapter 17) Diet pop	2 Chinese Tofu Mushroom Caps (Chapter 16) 1 cup (250 ml) Chinese Vegetable Fried Rice (Chapter 11) 10 lychees ½ cup (125 ml) 1% milk	1 piece Baked Scone (Chapter 7) 1 oz (30 g) low-fat cheese
2 chapatis (Chapter 16) ⅔ cup (150 ml) Dal (Chapter 11) Coffee	2 chapatis (Chapter 16) 1 boiled egg ½ cup (125 ml) mixed vegetables ¾ cup (175 ml) yogurt Tea	3 oz (90 g) Tandoori Chicken (Chapter 14) ⅔ cup (150 ml) basmati rice 1 cup (250 ml) Green Pea, Cauliflower, and Tomato Curry (Chapter 12) ½ cup (125 ml) 1% milk	¼ cup (50 ml) Mango Bean Mix (Chapter 11) 6 mini nachos

Breakfast	Lunch	Dinner	Snack
1 slice rye toast with 1 tsp (5 ml) soft margarine 1 oz (30 g) low-fat cheese 1 cup (250 ml) grapes Green tea	1 toasted tomato and cheese sandwich: 2 slices rye bread Sliced tomatoes 2 oz (60 g) low-fat cheese 2 tsp (10 ml) soft margarine Veggies and 1 tbsp (15 ml) light dip 1 slice Pumpkin Pie with Splenda (Chapter 17) Diet pop	¾ cup (175 ml) Nutty Rice and Mushroom Stir-Fry (Chapter 16) ½ cup (125 ml) Squash Apple Bake (Chapter 12) ¾ cup (175 ml) yogurt Water	3 cups (750 ml) light popcorn
2 Oatmeal Fruit Crepes (Chapter 7) with 2 tbsp (30 ml) light syrup 1 cup (250 ml) 1% milk	1 cup (250 ml) Best Beef Soup (Chapter 8) 1 slice whole wheat toast with 1 tsp (5 ml) soft margarine Tossed salad and 1 tbsp (15 ml) light dressing 2 Chocolate Chip Cookies (Chapter 17) Water	3 oz (90 g) Cinnamon Lime Chicken (Chapter 14) 24 Sweet Potato Fries (Chapter 11) ½ cup (125 ml) Beet and Feta Salad (Chapter 9) 1 slice Blueberry Pie with Splenda (Chapter 17) Tea	1 slice rye toast 1 boiled egg 1 tsp (5 ml) soft margarine

Breakfast	Lunch	Dinner	Snack
½ large whole grain bagel with 1 oz (30 g) melted low-fat cheese ½ grapefruit Coffee	Meatloaf sandwich: 2 slices multigrain bread 1 slice meatloaf (Chapter 15) 1 tsp (5 ml) soft margarine 1 tbsp (15 ml) light mayonnaise ½ cup (125 ml) Tomato Cucumber Salad (Chapter 9) 1 Mini Cheesecake (Chapter 17) Flavoured water	3 oz (90 g) Crispy Coated Sole (Chapter 13) Slice of lemon 2 Potato Latkes (Chapter 11) 2 tbsp (30 ml) light sour cream 1 cup (250 ml) mixed vegetables 1 piece Carrot Cake (Chapter 17) Tea	1 Baked Custard (Chapter 17) ½ cup (125 ml) 1% milk
1 whole grain English Muffin with 2 tbsp (30 ml) peanut butter 1 small banana Green tea	1⅓ cup (325 ml) Pork Chow Mein (Chapter 15) 1 dill pickle 15 cherries Coffee	3 oz (90 g) barbecued steak 1 medium baked potato with 1 tbsp (15 ml) light sour cream and chives 1 cup (250 ml) Broccoli with Feta and Roasted Peppers (Chapter 12) ⅔ cup (150 ml) Grilled Vegetables (Chapter 12) 1 piece Happy Birthday Cake with Splenda (Chapter 18) ½ cup (125 ml) 1% milk	30 pretzel sticks 1 tbsp (15 ml) almond butter

Breakfast	Lunch	Dinner	Snack
4 small Cottage Cheese Pancakes (Chapter 7) with 2 tbsp (30 ml) light syrup 1 cup (250 ml) mixed fruit Tea	Chicken salad sandwich: 2 slices whole wheat bread 1–2 oz (30–60 g) diced chicken 1–2 tbsp (30–60 ml) light mayonnaise Diced celery/lettuce Diet Jell-O 1 cup (250 ml) 1% milk	¾ cup (175 ml) Mac and Cheese (Chapter 18) Tossed salad with 1 tbsp (15 ml) light dressing 2 kiwis 1½ cups (375 ml) tomato juice	5 Triscuits 1 full Devilish Egg (Chapter 10)
¾ cup (175 ml) oatmeal 2 tbsp (30 ml) raisins 1 tbsp (15 ml) ground flaxseed 1 cup (250 ml) 1% milk	1 grilled cheese sandwich: 2 slices multigrain bread 1–2 oz (30–60 g) low-fat cheese 2 tsp (10 ml) soft margarine Red pepper and celery sticks 1 dill pickle 1 medium apple Water	1 Italian White Pizza (Chapter 16) 1 cup (250 ml) Classic Caesar Salad (Chapter 9) Diet Jell-O Tea	1 cup (250 ml) cantaloupe ¼ cup (50 ml) low-fat cottage cheese
2 Muffets *or* Shredded Wheat with 1 cup (250 ml) 1% milk 10 almonds Green tea	1 cup (250 ml) Fruity Spinach Salad (Chapter 9) 1 slice whole grain bread with 1 tsp (5 ml) soft margarine 1 boiled egg ¾ cup (175 ml) yogurt 3 ginger snap cookies Water	¼ lb (110 g) Seared Scallops (Chapter 13) 1 cup (250 ml) Greek Potatoes (Chapter 11) ½ cup (125 ml) Beet and Feta Salad (Chapter 9) ½ cup (125 ml) Orange Frost (Chapter 17) ½ cup (125 ml) 1% milk	½ cup (125 ml) grapes 1 oz (30 g) low-fat cheese

Breakfast	Lunch	Dinner	Snack
4 rectangular melba toasts 1 oz (30 g) low-fat cheese 1 large apple Coffee	1 slice Asparagus Cheddar Quiche (Chapter 12) Tossed salad with 1 tbsp (15 ml) light dressing 2 Flax Cookies (Chapter 17) 1 cup (250 ml) 1% milk	1 cup (375 ml) Pecan, Mango, and Brie Salad (Chapter 9) 3 Breaded Chicken Fingers (Chapter 18) ⅔ cup (150 ml) Pasta Primavera (Chapter 11) 1 piece Sour Cream Chocolate Chip Cake (Chapter 17) Water	7 whole wheat soda crackers 2 tbsp (30 ml) almond butter
1 strip bacon 1 egg 2 slices of whole grain toast with 2 tsp (10 ml) soft margarine ¾ cup (175 ml) pineapple Tea	1⅛ cups (275 ml) Broccoli Cheese Soup (Chapter 8) 2 Wasa crackers 1 oz (30 g) low-fat cheese ⅔ cup (150 ml) Strawberry Dream (Chapter 17) Diet pop	1 cup (250 ml) African Curry (Chapter 14) 1 cup (250 ml) Quinoa Risotto (Chapter 11) ⅔ cup (150 ml) Orange-Glazed Carrots (Chapter 12) Diet Jell-O Water	1 slice Asparagus Cheddar Quiche (Chapter 12) ½ cup (125 ml) tomato juice
1 cup (250 ml) whole grain cereal with 1 cup (250 ml) 1% milk ¼ cup (50 ml) almonds Coffee	1 cup (250 ml) Cheesy Turkey Bake (Chapter 14) Veggies and 1 tbsp (15 ml) light dip ½ cup (125 ml) low-fat pudding Water	1 slice Spinach Mushroom Lasagna (Chapter 11) Tossed salad and 1 tbsp (15 ml) light dressing Chocolate Mud Cake (Chapter 18) Diet pop	½ sandwich: 1 tbsp (15 ml) peanut butter and 1–2 tsp (5–10 ml) diet jam on 1 slice whole grain bread

Breakfast	Lunch	Dinner	Snack
2 chapatis (Chapter 16) ¾ cup (175 ml) yogurt 1 oz (30 g) low-fat cheese Coffee	Tossed salad with ½ cup (125 ml) chickpeas and 1 tbsp (15 ml) light dressing 1 chapati (Chapter 16) ½ cup (125 ml) canned fruit Tea	¾ cup (175 ml) Chickpea Curry (Chapter 11) 1 small naan bread ¾ cup (175 ml) yogurt Water	⅓ cup (75 ml) Black Bean Salsa (Chapter 10) 1 chapati (Chapter 16)
1 whole grain English Muffin with 2 tsp (10 ml) soft margarine and 1 tsp (5 ml) diet jam 1 cup (250 ml) strawberries ½ cup (125 ml) yogurt Tea	1 cup (250 ml) Carrot Parsnip Soup (Chapter 8) ½ sandwich: 1 slice rye bread 1 oz (30 g) pastrami Mustard/lettuce 1 tsp (5 ml) soft margarine ½ cup (125 ml) grapes Water	1½ cups (375 ml) Szechuan Noodles (Chapter 11) ½ cup (125 ml) cauliflower ½ cup (125 ml) mixed vegetables 1 piece Luscious Lemon Pudding Cake (Chapter 17) 1 cup (250 ml) 1% milk	3 Sushi slices (Chapter 10)
1 low-fat granola bar 1 large apple 1 oz (30 g) low-fat cheese Coffee	1 slice multigrain bread 1 slice pea meal bacon ½ cup (125 ml) Light Potato Salad (Chapter 9) 1 cup (250 ml) cantaloupe Flavoured water	½ cup (125 ml) Sloppy Joe (Chapter 18) on 1 medium whole grain bun Veggies and 1 tbsp (15 ml) light dip 1 cup (250 ml) blueberries 1 cup (250 ml) 1% milk	½ Raspberry Muffin (Chapter 7)

Large Meal Plan

The large meal plan provides approximately 2,000 calories and includes three meals and two snacks.

The following table represents the food group choices and grams of carbohydrate for a large meal plan. This plan provides approximately 50 percent of total calories from carbohydrate, 20 percent of total calories from protein, and 30 percent of total calories from fat. This percentage falls within the current goal for main nutrient balance according to the Canadian Diabetes Association.

This meal plan is just a sample. You can request a personalized meal plan to suit your lifestyle from your registered dietitian at your local diabetes education centre.

Breakfast	*Lunch*	*Snack*	*Dinner*	*Snack*
4 Carbohydrate Choices (60 g)	4 Carbohydrate Choices (60 g)	1 Carbohydrate Choice (15 g)	5 Carbohydrate Choices (75 g)	2 Carbohydrate Choices (30 g)
Free vegetables	Free vegetables	Free vegetables	Free vegetables	Free vegetables
0–2 Protein Choices	2–3 Protein Choices	0 Protein Choices	5 Protein Choices	1 Protein Choice
0–2 Fat Choices	1 Fat Choice	0 Fat Choices	1–2 Fat Choices	0–1 Fat Choices

In the following month of menus, we build on those guidelines, plugging in different types and amounts of various foods that, taken together, provide approximately 2,000 calories.

Breakfast	*Lunch*	*Snack*	*Dinner*	*Snack*
Cranberry Walnut Muffin (Chapter 7)	1 cup (250 ml) cream of mushroom soup	3 ginger snap cookies	1½ cups (375 ml) Vegetarian Curry Tofu with Noodles (Chapter 16)	2 slices rye toast
1 oz (30 g) low-fat cheese	Salmon sandwich: 2 slices whole grain bread ½–¾ cup (125–175 ml) salmon 1 tbsp (15 ml) light mayonnaise Diced celery/ lettuce		½ cup (125 ml) Marinated Mushrooms with Herbs (Chapter 9)	1–2 tbsp (15–30 ml) peanut butter
1 orange				
1 cup (250 ml) 1% milk			½ mango	
	Tossed salad		1 cup (250 ml) 1% milk	
	1 tbsp (15 ml) light dressing			
	1 peach			
	Water			
3 Oatmeal Pancakes (Chapter 7)	1 cup (250 ml) Classic Caesar Salad (Chapter 9)	1 Brownie (Chapter 18)	1⅓ cups (325 ml) Hamburger Stroganoff (Chapter 15) with ¾ cup (175 ml) noodles	1 large apple
2 tbsp (30 ml) light syrup	8 rectangular melba toasts			1 oz (30 g) low-fat cheese
1 small banana	2 oz (60 g) low-fat cheese		½ cup (125 ml) squash	
Coffee	1 pear		½ cup (125 ml) yellow beans	
	1 cup (250 ml) 1% milk		¾ cup (175 ml) yogurt with ¼ cup (50 ml) Baked Homemade Granola (Chapter 7)	
			Tea	

Breakfast	*Lunch*	*Snack*	*Dinner*	*Snack*
2 slices rye toast 2–3 tbsp (30–45 ml) peanut butter 1 cup (250 ml) fruit cocktail Flavoured tea	1⅓ cups (325 ml) Three-Bean Chili (Chapter 16) Tossed salad 1 tbsp (15 ml) light dressing ½ cup (125 ml) low-fat pudding Water	1 cup (250 ml) cantaloupe	5 oz (150 g) Greek Fish (Chapter 13) 1 cup (250 ml) mashed potato ½ cup (125 ml) Tomato Cucumber Salad (Chapter 9) ½ cup (125 ml) Swiss Chard and Pine Nuts (Chapter 12) 1 cup (250 ml) grapes ½ cup (125 ml) 1% milk	½ cup (125 ml) mixed fruit ¼ cup (50 ml) low-fat cottage cheese 2 digestive cookies
1½ cup (375 ml) whole grain cereal 1 cup (250 ml) 1% milk ¼ cup (50 ml) sliced almonds Tea	2 Mexican Quesadillas (Chapter 16) Raw veggies and 1–2 tbsp (15–30 ml) light dip Diet Jell-O Diet pop	2 Jam Jewel Cookies (Chapter 17)	5 oz (150 g) Roast Beef 2 tbsp (30 ml) low-fat gravy 1 large roasted potato ½ cup (125 ml) corn ½ cup (125 ml) green beans 1 cup (250 ml) 1% milk	1 English muffin 2 tsp (10 ml) soft margarine 1 oz (30 g) fat-free ham

Breakfast	Lunch	Snack	Dinner	Snack
1⅛ cups (275 ml) Mango, Orange, Banana Smoothie (Chapter 7) 2 slices whole grain toast 2–3 tbsp (30–45 ml) peanut butter	1 cup (250 ml) Veggie Soup (Chapter 8) 1½ beef sandwiches: 3 slices multi-grain bread 2–3 oz (30–60 g) roast beef Mustard/lettuce 3 tsp (15 ml) soft margarine 3 arrowroot cookies Water	1 pear	5 oz (150 g) Chicken in Dijon Sauce (Chapter 14) 1 cup (250 ml) brown rice ½ cup (125 ml) Stir-Fried Snow Peas (Chapter 12) ½ cup (125 ml) carrots 1 cup (250 ml) strawberries 1 cup (250 ml) 1% milk	5 Triscuits 1 oz (30g) low-fat cheese 1½ cups (375 ml) tomato juice
2 slices mul-tigrain toast with 2 tsp (10 ml) soft margarine 2–3 tsp (10–15 ml) diet jam ¾ cup (175 ml) yogurt ¼ cup (50 ml) Baked Homemade Granola (Chapter 7) Tea	1 English Muffin 1 oz (30 g) low-fat cheese 1 fried egg Lettuce/tomato 1 pear ½ cup (125 ml) frozen yogurt Water	½ cup (125 ml) applesauce	2 slices Salmon Loaf with ½ cup (125 ml) Cucumber Sauce (Chapter 13) ½ cup (125 ml) Garlic Mashed Potatoes (Chapter 11) Sliced tomato ½ cup (125 ml) broccoli 1 cup (250 ml) honeydew melon 1 cup (250 ml) 1% milk	¾ cup (175 ml) oatmeal ¼ cup (50 ml) almonds 1 small banana

Breakfast	Lunch	Snack	Dinner	Snack
1 slice Banana Bread (Chapter 7) 1 oz (30 g) low-fat cheese ½ cup (125 ml) grapes ½ cup (125 ml) 1% chocolate milk	Corned beef sandwich: 2 slices rye bread 1–2 oz (30–60 g) corned beef Mustard 1 tsp (5 ml) soft margarine ½ cup (125ml) Chunky Apple Coleslaw (Chapter 9) 1 cup (250 ml) mixed fruit cup Diet pop	1 piece Rhubarb Cake with Splenda (Chapter 17)	1½ cups (375 ml) Butter Chicken (Chapter 14) 1 medium naan bread Tossed salad and 1 tbsp (15 ml) light dressing ¾ cup (175 ml) yogurt Water	¾ cup (175 ml) Aboriginal Wild Rice Pudding with Splenda (Chapter 17) ½ cup (125 ml) 1% milk
1 whole grain English Muffin, with 1 egg, 1 tsp (5 ml) soft margarine, lettuce/tomato 1 medium apple ½ cup (125 ml) juice	1 cup (250 ml) French Onion Soup (Chapter 8) 2 slices garlic bread with 2 oz (60 g) low-fat cheese 2 kiwis Water	¾ cup (175 ml) yogurt	2 cups (500 ml) Stir-Fried Beef with Rice Noodles (Chapter 15) 1 cup (250 ml) Fruity Spinach Salad (Chapter 9) 2 Jam Jewel Cookies (Chapter 17) Tea	1 slice Banana Bread (Chapter 7) ¼ cup (50 ml) nuts

Breakfast	*Lunch*	*Snack*	*Dinner*	*Snack*
Raspberry Muffin (Chapter 7) 1 oz (30 g) low-fat cheese 1 orange ¾ cup (175 ml) yogurt Coffee	1 Curried Turkey in a Pita (Chapter 14) Carrot sticks 1 cup (250 ml) strawberries ½ cup (125 ml) 1% milk	One serving of Fruit Trifle (Chapter 17)	5 oz (150 g) Parmesan Chicken (Chapter 14) 1 cup (250 ml) whole wheat pasta ½ cup (125 ml) Zesty Asparagus (Chapter 12) ⅔ cup (150 ml) Orange-Glazed Carrots (Chapter 12) ¾ cup (175 ml) frozen yogurt Water	2 Flax Cookies (Chapter 17) 10 almonds ½ cup (125 ml) low-fat chocolate milk
1 cup (250 ml) Shake Me Up Shake (Chapter 7) 2 slices flaxseed toast 2–3 tbsp (30–45 ml) peanut butter 1 tbsp (15 ml) diet jam Coffee	1 cup (250 ml) cream of tomato soup 1 cup (250 ml) Mediterranean-Style Tuna Casserole (Chapter 13) Tossed salad with 1–2 tbsp (15–30 ml) diet dressing Diet Jell-O Tea	3 Rocky Road Balls (Chapter 17)	1½ cups (375 ml) Bulgur and Chickpea Salad with Lemon Dressing (Chapter 9) ½ cup (125 ml) green beans ½ cup (125 ml) applesauce 1 cup (250 ml) 1% milk	½ cup (125 ml) Toasted Walnut Hummus (Chapter 10) Raw veggies

Breakfast	Lunch	Snack	Dinner	Snack
1½ cup (375 ml) yogurt 1 small banana ¼ cup (50 ml) Baked Homemade Granola (Chapter 7) Coffee	1½ cup (375 ml) Chinese Jewelled Rice (Chapter 13) Celery sticks 1 pear Water	1 medium apple	1⅔ cups (400 ml) Shepherd's Pie (Chapter 15) 1 small whole wheat roll with 1 tsp (5 ml) soft margarine Tossed salad and 1 tbsp (15 ml) light dressing Baked Apple with Raspberries (Chapter 18) Tea	2 Pizza Faces (Chapter 18) 1 cup (250 ml) 1% milk
3 slices whole grain toast 1 egg 2 tsp (10 ml) soft margarine ½ cup (125 ml) juice	1 cup (250 ml) Asian Noodle Salad (Chapter 9) 1 cup (250 ml) honeydew melon 1 cup (250 ml) 1% milk	¾ cup (175 ml) yogurt	1 cup (250 ml) Groundnut Stew (Chapter 15) 1 cup (250 ml) couscous 1 cup (250 ml) Ethiopian Cabbage (Chapter 12) Diet Jell-O ½ cup (125 ml) 1% milk	6 Shanghai Dumplings with 1 tsp (5 ml) sauce (Chapter 10)

Breakfast	Lunch	Snack	Dinner	Snack
2 pieces Baked Scone (Chapter 7) with 2 tsp (10 ml) soft margarine 1 cup (250 ml) mixed fruit cup Herbal tea	Tuna sandwich: 2 slices whole grain bread ½–¾ cup (125–175 ml) tuna 2 tbsp (30 ml) light mayonnaise Celery/lettuce/ onion 1 small banana 1 cup (250 ml) 1% milk	30 pretzel sticks	4 slices Barbequed Eggplant (Chapter 16) 1 cup (250 ml) Classic Caesar Salad (Chapter 9) ½ cup (125 ml) Balsamic Brussels Sprouts (Chapter 12) 1 medium whole wheat roll with 2 tsp (10 ml) soft margarine 1 Little Jam Cupcake with Splenda (Chapter 18) Green tea	1 Banana Chocolate Chip Muffin with Splenda (Chapter 18) 1 tbsp (15 ml) peanut butter ½ cup (125 ml) 1% milk
1 cup (250 ml) Akoori Scrambled Eggs (Chapter 7) 2 slices rye toast with 2 tsp (10 ml) soft margarine ½ cup (125 ml) canned fruit 1 cup (250 ml) 1% milk	1 cup (250 ml) Kale Soup (Chapter 8) 10 Triscuits 2 oz (60 g) low-fat cheese ¾ cup (175 ml) yogurt Water	1 orange	1 cup (250 ml) Saffron Fish (Chapter 13) 1 cup (250 ml) basmati rice ½ cup (125 ml) cooked spinach 1 tsp (5 ml) soft margarine 1 peach 1 cup (250 ml) 1% milk	2 slices Feta Bruschetta (Chapter 10)

Breakfast	Lunch	Snack	Dinner	Snack
1 large flax bagel 4 tbsp (60 ml) light cream cheese Tea	1 cup (250 ml) Mixed Bean Salad (Chapter 9) Veggies and 1–2 tbsp (15–30 ml) light dip 1 medium apple 1 cup (250 ml) 1% milk	1 low-fat granola bar	3 cups (750 ml) Walnut, Pear, and Chicken Salad (Chapter 9) 1 slice rye bread 1 tsp (5 ml) soft margarine ¾ cup (175 ml) yogurt Water	1 piece Apple Crisp with Splenda (Chapter 18) 1 oz (30 g) low-fat cheese ½ cup (125 ml) low-fat chocolate milk
1 cup (250 ml) canned fruit ½ cup (125 ml) low-fat cottage cheese 2 slices multigrain toast with 2 tsp (10 ml) soft margarine Coffee	1 cup (250 ml) Veggie Soup (Chapter 8) 7 whole wheat soda crackers ¾ cup (175 ml) Couscous Chickpea Salad (Chapter 9) 1 Chocolate Zucchini Muffin (Chapter 17) Diet pop	¾ cup (175 ml) yogurt	4 Chinese Tofu Mushroom Caps (Chapter 16) 1 cup (250 ml) Chinese Vegetable Fried Rice (Chapter 11) 10 lychees 1 cup (250 ml) 1% milk	1 piece Baked Scone (Chapter 7) 1 oz (30 g) low-fat cheese 1 cup (250 ml) 1% milk
2 chapatis (Chapter 16) ⅔ cup (150 ml) Dal (Chapter 11) ¾ cup (175 ml) yogurt Coffee	3 chapatis (Chapter 16) 2 boiled eggs ½ cup (125 ml) mixed vegetables ¾ cup (175 ml) yogurt Tea	⅓ cup (75 ml) Toasted Walnut Hummus (Chapter 10) Raw veggies	5 oz (150 g) Tandoori Chicken (Chapter 14) 1 cup (250 ml) basmati rice 1 cup (250 ml) Green Pea, Cauliflower, and Tomato Curry (Chapter 12) ½ cup (125 ml) 1% milk	½ cup (125 ml) Mango Bean Mix (Chapter 11) 12 mini nachos

Breakfast	Lunch	Snack	Dinner	Snack
2 slices rye toast	1½ toasted tomato and cheese sandwiches: 3 slices rye bread Sliced tomatoes 2–3 oz (60–90 g) low-fat cheese 3 tsp (15 ml) soft margarine	1 piece Apple Crisp with Splenda (Chapter 18)	1⅓ cups (325 ml) Nutty Rice and Mushroom Stir-Fry (Chapter 16)	3 cups (750 ml) light popcorn
2 tsp (10 ml) soft margarine				½ cup (125 ml) low-fat chocolate milk
1 oz (30 g) low-fat cheese			½ cup (125 ml) Squash Apple Bake (Chapter 12)	
1 cup (250 ml) grapes			¾ cup (175 ml) yogurt	
Green tea	1 slice Pumpkin Pie with Splenda (Chapter 17)		Water	
	Diet pop			
3 Oatmeal Fruit Crepes (Chapter 7) with 2 tbsp (30 ml) light syrup	1½ cup (375 ml) Best Beef Soup (Chapter 8)	½ cup (125 ml) Orange Frost (Chapter 17)	5 oz (150 g) Cinnamon Lime Chicken (Chapter 14)	2 slices rye toast
	1 slice whole wheat toast with 1 tsp (5 ml) soft margarine		24 Sweet Potato Fries (Chapter 11)	1 boiled egg
1 cup (250 ml) 1% milk	Tossed salad and 1 tbsp (15 ml) light dressing		½ cup (125 ml) corn	1 tsp (5 ml) soft margarine
	3 Chocolate Chip Cookies (Chapter 17)		½ cup (125 ml) Beet and Feta Salad (Chapter 9)	
	Water		1 slice Blueberry Pie with Splenda (Chapter 17)	
			Tea	

Breakfast	Lunch	Snack	Dinner	Snack
1 large whole grain bagel with 2 oz (60 g) melted low-fat cheese Coffee	Meatloaf sandwich: 2 slices multi-grain bread 1 slice meatloaf (Chapter 15) 1 tsp (5 ml) soft margarine 1 tbsp (15 ml) light mayonnaise ½ cup (125 ml) Tomato Cucumber Salad (Chapter 9) 2 Mini Cheesecake (Chapter 17) Flavoured water	3 cups (750 ml) light popcorn	5 oz (150 g) Crispy Coated Sole (Chapter 13) Slice of lemon 3 Potato Latkes (Chapter 11) 2 tbsp (30 ml) light sour cream 1 cup (250 ml) mixed vegetables 1 piece Carrot Cake (Chapter 17) Tea	1 Baked Custard (Chapter 17) 1 small banana ½ cup (125 ml) 1% milk
1 whole grain English Muffin with 2 tbsp (30 ml) peanut butter 1 small banana ½ cup (125 ml) juice Green tea	1⅓ cups (325 ml) Pork Chow Mein (Chapter 15) 1 dill pickle 15 cherries 1 cup (250 ml) 1% milk Coffee	½ cup (125 ml) Aboriginal Wild Rice Pudding with Splenda (Chapter 17)	5 oz (150 g) BBQ steak 1 large baked potato with 2 tbsp (30 ml) light sour cream and chives 1 cup (250 ml) Broccoli with Feta and Roasted Peppers (Chapter 12) ⅔ cup (150 ml) Grilled Vegetables (Chapter 12) 1 piece Happy Birthday Cake with Splenda (Chapter 18) ½ cup (125 ml) 1% milk	45 pretzel sticks 1 tbsp (15 ml) almond butter ½ cup (125 ml) 1% milk

Breakfast	Lunch	Snack	Dinner	Snack
8 small Cottage Cheese Pancakes (Chapter 7) 4 tbsp (60 ml) light syrup 1 cup (250 ml) mixed fruit cup Tea	Chicken salad sandwich: 2 slices whole wheat bread 2–3 oz (60–90 g) diced chicken 1–2 tbsp (30–60 ml) light mayonnaise Diced celery/lettuce Diet Jell-O 2 plums 1 cup (250 ml) 1% milk	½ mango	1⅛ cups (275 ml) Mac and Cheese (Chapter 18) Tossed salad with 1 tbsp (15 ml) light dressing 2 kiwis 1½ cups (375 ml) tomato juice	10 Triscuits 1 full Devilish Egg (Chapter 10)
¾ cup (175 ml) oatmeal 2 tbsp (30 ml) raisins 1 tbsp (15 ml) ground flaxseed 1 slice rye toast with 1 tsp (5 ml) soft margarine 2 tsp (10 ml) diet jam 1 cup (250 ml) 1% milk	1½ grilled cheese sandwiches: 3 slices multigrain bread 2–3 oz (60–90 g) low-fat cheese 3 tsp (15 ml) soft margarine Red pepper and celery sticks 1 dill pickle 1 medium apple Water	2 Cocoa Oatmeal Cookies (Chapter 17)	1 Italian White Pizza (Chapter 16) 1 cup (250 ml) Classic Caesar Salad (Chapter 9) 1 pear Diet Jell-O Tea	1 cup (250 ml) cantaloupe ¼ cup (50 ml) low-fat cottage cheese ½ cup (125 ml) low-fat chocolate milk

Breakfast	Lunch	Snack	Dinner	Snack
2 Muffets *or* Shredded Wheat 10 almonds 1 cup (250 ml) 1% milk ½ English Muffin with 1 tsp (5 ml) soft margarine Green tea	1 cup (250 ml) Fruity Spinach Salad (Chapter 9) 2 slices whole grain bread with 1 tsp (5 ml) soft margarine 1–2 boiled eggs ¾ cup (175 ml) yogurt 3 ginger snap cookies Water	1 orange	½ lb (227 g) Seared Scallops (Chapter 13) 1 cup (250 ml) Greek Potatoes (Chapter 11) ½ cup (125 ml) Beet and Feta Salad (Chapter 9) ½ cup (125 ml) Orange Frost (Chapter 17) 1 cup (250 ml) 1% milk	1 cup (250 ml) grapes 1 oz (30 g) low-fat cheese
8 rectangular melba toasts 2 oz (60 g) low-fat cheese 1 large apple Coffee	1 slice Asparagus Cheddar Quiche (Chapter 12) Tossed salad with 1 tbsp (15 ml) light dressing 4 Flax Cookies (Chapter 17) 1 cup (250 ml) 1% milk	¾ cup (175 ml) pineapple	1½ cups (375 ml) Pecan, Mango, and Brie Salad (Chapter 9) 4 Breaded Chicken Fingers (Chapter 18) 1⅓ cups (325 ml) Pasta Primavera (Chapter 11) 1 piece Sour Cream Chocolate Chip Cake (Chapter 17) Water	7 whole wheat soda crackers 2 tbsp (30 ml) almond butter ½ cup (125 ml) 1% milk

Breakfast	*Lunch*	*Snack*	*Dinner*	*Snack*
2 slices strip bacon 1 egg 2 slices whole grain toast with 2 tsp (10 ml) soft margarine ¾ cup (175 ml) pineapple ¾ cup (175 ml) yogurt Tea	1⅛ cups (275 ml) Broccoli Cheese Soup (Chapter 8) 4 Wasa crackers 1–2 oz (30–60 g) low-fat cheese ⅔ cup (150 ml) Strawberry Dream (Chapter 17) Diet pop	1 banana	1½ cups (375 ml) African Curry (Chapter 14) 1 cup (250 ml) Quinoa Risotto (Chapter 11) 1 cup (250 ml) Orange-Glazed Carrots (Chapter 12) Diet Jell-O Water	1 slice Asparagus Cheddar Quiche (Chapter 12) 1½ cups (375 ml) tomato juice
1 cup (250 ml) whole grain cereal 1 cup (250 ml) 1% milk ¼ cup (50 ml) almonds 1 cup (250 ml) blueberries Coffee	1½ cups (375 ml) Cheesy Turkey Bake (Chapter 14) Veggies and 1 tbsp (15 ml) light dip ½ cup (125 ml) low-fat pudding Water	½ cup (125 ml) canned fruit	1½ slices Spinach Mushroom Lasagna (Chapter 11) Tossed salad and 1 tbsp (15 ml) light dressing Chocolate Mud Cake (Chapter 18) Diet pop	1 sandwich: 2 slices whole grain bread 1–2 tbsp (15–30 ml) peanut butter and 1 tbsp (15 ml) diet jam
3 chapatis (Chapter 16) ¾ cup (175 ml) yogurt 1–2 oz (30–60 g) low-fat cheese Coffee	Tossed salad and 1 tbsp (15 ml) light dressing ½ cup (125 ml) chickpeas 2 chapatis (Chapter 16) ½ cup (125 ml) canned fruit Tea	2 clementines	¾ cup (175 ml) Chickpea Curry (Chapter 11) 1 medium naan bread ¾ cup (175 ml) yogurt Water	⅔ cup (150 ml) Black Bean Salsa (Chapter 10) 1 chapati (Chapter 16)

Breakfast	Lunch	Snack	Dinner	Snack
1 whole grain English Muffin with 2 tsp (10 ml) soft margarine and 1 tbsp (15 ml) diet jam 2 cups (500 ml) strawberries ¾ cup (175 ml) yogurt Tea	1 cup (250 ml) Carrot Parsnip Soup (Chapter 8) 1 sandwich: 2 slices rye bread 2–3 oz (60–90 g) pastrami Mustard/lettuce 2 tsp (10 ml) soft margarine ½ cup (125 ml) grapes Water	2 Snickers Cookies (Chapter 17)	2¼ cups (550 ml) Szechuan Noodles (Chapter 11) ½ cup (125 ml) cauliflower ½ cup (125 ml) mixed vegetables 1 piece Luscious Lemon Pudding Cake (Chapter 17) 1 cup (250 ml) 1% milk	5 Sushi slices (Chapter 10)
2 low-fat granola bars 1 large apple 1 oz (30 g) low-fat cheese Coffee	2 slices multigrain bread 2 slices pea meal bacon ½ cup (125 ml) Light Potato Salad (Chapter 9) 1 cup (250 ml) cantaloupe Flavoured water	¾ cup (175 ml) yogurt	1 cup (250 ml) Sloppy Joe (Chapter 18) 1 large whole grain bun Veggies and 1 tbsp (15 ml) light dip 1 cup (250 ml) blueberries ½ cup (125 ml) 1% milk	1 Raspberry Muffin (Chapter 7)

Index

....

About the Author

Ian Blumer, MD, FRCPC, is a diabetes specialist in the Greater Toronto Area. He has a teaching appointment with the University of Toronto, is the medical advisor to the Charles H. Best Diabetes Centre in Whitby, Ontario, and is a member of the Board of Directors of the Canadian Diabetes Association (CDA).

Dr. Blumer is the author of *What Your Doctor* Really *Thinks*, and the co-author of *Diabetes For Canadians For Dummies* (now in its third edition), *Understanding Prescription Drugs For Canadians For Dummies* (co-written with Dr. Heather McDonald-Blumer), and *Celiac Disease For Dummies* (co-written with Dr. Sheila Crowe). Under the pen name of Sidney Gale he has also published the young adult novel *Unto the Breach*. He can be found on the Web at www.ourdiabetes.com. Dr. Blumer would love to get your comments about this book; please email him at diabetes@ianblumer.com.

Cynthia Payne RD, CDE, is a Registered Dietitian and Certified Diabetes Educator. She currently works at Northumberland Hills Hospital in Cobourg, Ontario. Additionally, Cynthia has a private nutrition counselling practice at Pharmacy 101 in Cobourg, and has worked at Alderville First Nations Health Centre providing nutrition counselling and workshops.

Cynthia is a well-known and sought-after public speaker to professional and lay audiences, and a former nutrition columnist. She is a member of Dietitians of Canada; the College of Dietitians of Ontario; the Diabetes Educator section of the Canadian Diabetes Association; the Kawartha Branch of Certified Diabetes Educators and the Consulting Dietitians of Ontario.

Cynthia has a wonderful husband, Keith and two amazing children, Kristen and Jeff, who keep her busy. When she is not at the hockey arena, Cynthia enjoys swimming, canoeing, kayaking, walking, skating and skiing.

Dedication

Ian: This book is dedicated to Dr. Steven Edelman who, with Sandra Bourdette, founded Taking Control of Your Diabetes (www.tcoyd.org), an organization "guided by the belief that every person with diabetes has the right to live a healthy, happy, and productive life." Steve's commitment, passion, energy, and selfless dedication, always mixed with humour and a spirit of fun, are inspirational. How great to be his friend; how wonderful to be a part of his organization.

Cynthia: This book is dedicated to people living with diabetes. My hope is that this book can make a difference in their lives by making meal time easier to plan and so much more enjoyable than they ever imagined. This is more than a cookbook; my hope is for people to gain some ingredients for success in their management towards a healthy life with diabetes.

Authors' Acknowledgments

Ian: I would like to thank Hannah Draper and Lisa Berland for their editorial expertise, Pauline Ricablanca for her overseeing the book's development, and, as always, I am ever so grateful to have been able to once again work with the unflappable Robert Hickey.

I cannot possibly express my level of gratitude and appreciation for the boundless efforts and expertise that my co-author Cynthia Payne has brought to this book. Working with Cynthia to create this book has been a truepleasure. Cynthia; thank you so much!

Cynthia: I would like to thank my family and friends for being at my side and encouraging me through the process of this book's conception, development, and birth.

I need to thank my mother, Bonnie Payne, for helping me out with some of the cooking and recipe testing and for calming me down near deadline time. Thanks for always being there for me, Mom.

I would like to thank my husband Keith and children, Kristen and Jeffrey, for putting up with me as I worked weekends and evenings on this book as well as their willingness to eat what was put in front of them.

Thank you to the many taste testers: my co-workers: Pam Bates, RN CDE; Doris Brunton, Jennifer Case, Melissa Geleynse, RD; Stephanie Ross, RN CDE NP; Angel Targon, RN; Debbie Bontje, RN CDE; Christine McCleary, RD CDE, and the other staff who just happened to be in the cafeteria or who were in their departments and were willing to sample a morsel when I passed through.

Other friends were honest taste testers: Debbie, Doug, Ryan and Alexis Smith; Betty Adams; Gill Kassela; Jolien Todd; Linda Redner-Hunter; Diane Dudnick; Joanne Cherry-Lauzon; Yvon Lauzon; Dave Hammond; Janet Harris, RD CDE; Marcey Wilson, RD; Don and Annette Ashfield; Pete Marrocco; Cathy McGinn; Elaine and Dave Trahair; and Jackie and Jim Hudson.

Many special thanks to my parents, my brothers and their families for letting me cook for them and being honest with the outcome: Bonnie and Ron Payne; Stephen, Cindy, Corrina, Kyle and Bradley Payne; and Greg, Roberta, Nicole and Stephanie Payne.

I appreciate the help of Christine McCleary, RD CDE; Pam Bates, RN CDE; Melissa Geleynse, RD; Janet Harris, RD CDE; Janice Stringham, RD CDE; and Grace Pineau, RD CDE, for their assistance in the information in some of the chapters — smart women!

I can not go any further without thanking Dr. Ian Blumer for giving me the opportunity to write this book with him and to learn from his patience, encouragement, brilliance and wisdom. Thanks to Marian Barltrop, RN CDE, for thinking of me when this opportunity arose. I met an amazing editor, Robert Hickey, who was so understanding, knowledgeable and patient and who made this adventure very pleasant.

I have much appreciation and thanks for my father, Ron, and my many patients who let me live diabetes through them, teaching me so much.

Publisher's Acknowledgments

Acquisitions Editor: Tracy Boggier

Production Editor: Pauline Ricablanca

Reprint Editor: Paige Newman

Project Coordinator: Patrick Redmond

Cover Photos: iStock.com/ratmaner, Courtesy of Abbott Diabetes Care Ltd.